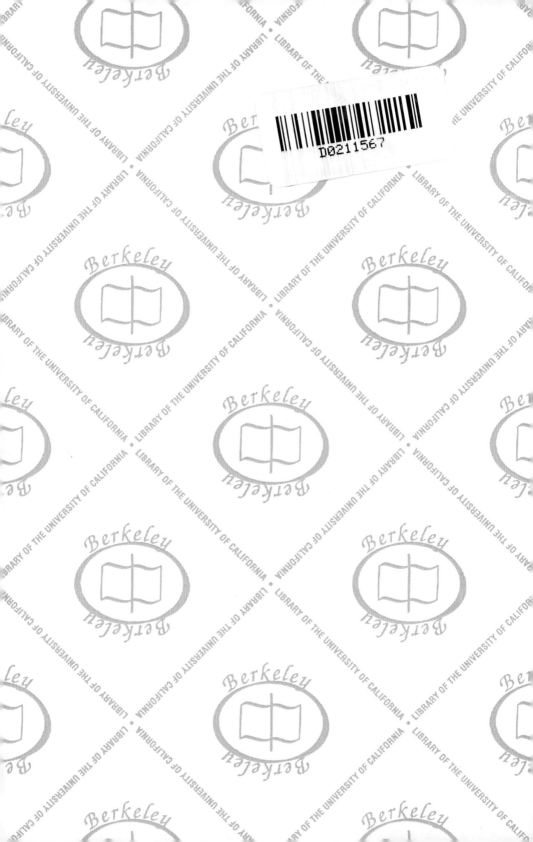

Wills Eye Hospital
OFFICE AND EMERGENCY ROOM DIAGNOSIS AND TREATMENT OF EYE DISEASE

Contributors

Melissa M. Brown, M.D.

Catharine J. Crockett, M.D.

Bret L. Fisher, M.D.

Patrick M. Flaharty, M.D.

Mark A. Friedberg, M.D.

James T. Handa, M.D.

Victor A. Holmes, M.D.

Bruce J. Keyser, M.D.

Marlon Maus, M.D.—Medical Illustrator

Ronald L. McKey, M.D.

Christopher J. Rapuano, M.D.

Paul A. Raskauskas, M.D.

Eric P. Suan, M.D.

Wills Eye Hospital
OFFICE AND EMERGENCY ROOM DIAGNOSIS AND TREATMENT OF EYE DISEASE

Mark A. Friedberg, M.D.

Christopher J. Rapuano, M.D.

J. B. LIPPINCOTT COMPANY   Philadelphia
Grand Rapids   New York   St. Louis   San Francisco
London   Sydney   Tokyo

Acquisitions Editor: Darlene Barela Cooke
Editorial Assistant: Catherine Hoffman
Production Manager: Janet Greenwood
Compositor: Harper Graphics
Printer/Binder: R.R. Donnelley & Sons

1   3   5   6   4   2

Library of Congress Cataloging-in-Publication Data

Wills Eye Hospital office and emergency room diagnosis and treatment
  of eye disease / [edited by] Mark A. Friedberg. Christopher J.
  Rapuano : contributors. Melissa M. Brown . . . [et al.].
      p.   cm.
    Includes bibliographical references.
    ISBN 0-397-51046-2
    1. Eye—Diseases and effects—Diagnosis. 2. Ophthalmology.
  I. Friedberg, Mark A.   II. Rapuano, Christopher J.   III. Brown,
  Melissa M.   IV. Wills Eye Hospital (Philadelphia, Pa.)   V. Title:
  Office and emergency room diagnosis and treatment of eye disease.
    [DNLM: 1. Emergencies—outlines.   2. Eye Diseases—diagnosis
  -outlines.   3. Eye Diseases—therapy—outlines.   WW 18 W741]
  RE46.W78 1990
  617.7—dc20
  DNLM/DLC
  for Library of Congress   89-13498
                                                                  CIP

The authors and publisher have exerted every effort to ensure that drug selection
and dosage set forth in this text are in accord with current recommendations and
practice at the time of publication. However, in view of ongoing research, changes
in government regulations, and the constant flow of information relating to drug
therapy and drug reactions, the reader is urged to check the package insert for each
drug for any change in indications and dosage and for added warnings and
precautions. This is particularly important when the recommended agent is a new
or infrequently employed drug.

Consultants

Cornea

Major Consultant
Elisabeth J. Cohen, M.D.

Consultants
Juan J. Arentsen, M.D.
Peter R. Laibson, M.D.
Michael A. Naidoff, M.D.
Irving M. Raber, M.D.

Glaucoma

Consultants
L. Jay Katz, M.D.
Marlene R. Moster, M.D.
George L. Spaeth, M.D.
Richard P. Wilson, M.D.

Neuro-ophthalmology

Major Consultants
Peter J. Savino, M.D.
Robert C. Sergott, M.D.

Oculo-plastics

Consultants
Edward H. Bedrossian, Jr., M.D.
Joseph C. Flanagan, M.D.
Ignatius S. Hneleski, Jr., M.D.
Thaddeus S. Nowinski, M.D.
Mary A. Stefanyszyn, M.D.

Oncology

Consultants
James J. Augsburger, M.D.
Jerry A. Shields, M.D.

Pediatrics

Consultants
Joseph H. Calhoun, M.D.
Leonard B. Nelson, M.D.
Robert D. Reinecke, M.D.

Retina

Major Consultant
William Tasman, M.D.

Consultants
William H. Annesley, Jr., M.D.
Jonathan B. Belmont, M.D.
William E. Benson, M.D.
Gary C. Brown, M.D.
Jay L. Federman, M.D.
David H. Fischer, M.D.
Alfred C. Lucier, M.D.
J. Arch McNamara, M.D.
Hermann D. Schubert, M.D.
Lov K. Sarin, M.D.

General

Consultants
Edward A. Jaeger, M.D.
John B. Jeffers, M.D.
Stephen B. Lichtenstein, M.D.

Foreword

It gives me a great deal of pleasure to write the foreword to this book, which was created as a group effort by the second-year resident class at the Wills Eye Hospital. This is an enterprise that is unique in more than one way. First, and perhaps most important, the project represents recognition by residents in training of the need for a legacy to those who will follow in their footsteps. In a time of entrepreneurism, frequent breaches of ethical behavior, and uncertainties about the course of medicine in general and ophthalmology in particular, this is refreshing indeed.

To achieve their goal the authors have prepared a concise volume in outline form that contains differential diagnostic clues and therapeutic regimens to be kept in mind when a patient is examined. Because of the large and diversified number of patients that Wills residents have the opportunity to see, they have been able to base their thoughts and ideas on their personal experience as ophthalmologists in training—a second unique feature of the book.

Basically, whether residents, fellows, or Board Certified practitioners of many years' standing, we are all, by virtue of the rapid medical and technological advances taking place daily, ophthamologists in training. Recognizing that fact, the present second-year class of Wills' residents has arranged with the publisher for future second-year classes to update their volume so that it can be kept as current as possible.

WILLIAM TASMAN, M.D.

Preface

Our goal has been to produce a concise book, providing essential diagnostic tips and specific therapeutic information pertaining to eye disease. We realized the need for this book while managing emergency room patients at one of the largest and busiest eye hospitals in the country. Until now, reliable information could only be obtained in unwieldy textbooks or inaccessible journals.

As residents at Wills Eye Hospital we have benefited from the input of some of the world-renowned ophthalmic experts in writing this book. More importantly, we are aware of the questions that the ophthalmology resident, the attending ophthalmologist, and the emergency room physician (not trained in ophthalmology) want answered immediately.

The book is written for the eye care provider who, in the midst of evaluating an eye problem, needs quick access to additional information. We try to be as specific as possible, describing the therapeutic modalities used at our institution. Many of these recommendations are, therefore, not the only manner in which to treat a particular disorder, but indicate personal preference. They are guidelines, not rules.

Because of the forever changing wealth of ophthalmic knowledge, omissions and errors are possible, particularly with regard to management. Drug dosages have been checked carefully, but the physician is urged to check the *Physicians Desk Reference* or *Facts and Comparisons* when prescribing unfamiliar medications. Not all contraindications and side effects are described.

We feel this book will make a welcome companion to the many physicians involved with treating eye problems. It is everything you wanted to know and nothing more.

CHRISTOPHER J. RAPUANO, M.D.
MARK A. FRIEDBERG, M.D.

Acknowledgments

We are indebted to a great number of people who helped make this book possible.

We would like to thank the attendings at Wills Eye Hospital, without whose guidance we would not have been able to write this book. In particular we would like to thank Dr. Elisabeth Cohen and Dr. Edward Jaeger, who were enthusiastic and supportive from the beginning of this project. We are grateful to Ms. Fleur Weinberg and Ms. Gloria Parker for their help in library research.

Finally, special thanks go to our wives, Ronda Friedberg and Sara Rapuano, for all their love and support.

Contents

11 Neuro-ophthalmology   233

12 Retina   277

13 Uveitis   331

14 Systemic Disorders   367

15 General Ophthalmic Problems   399

16 Appendixes   419

1

Differential Diagnosis of Ocular Symptoms

Burning

More common   Blepharitis, dry eye syndrome, conjunctivitis (discharge or eyelid sticking additionally).

Less common   Corneal problem (fluorescein staining of the cornea usually), inflamed pterygium/pingueculum, episcleritis, superior limbic keratoconjunctivitis.

Crossed Eyes in Children

See "Esodeviations in Children" (eyes turned in), Section 9.3, or "Exodeviations in Children" (eyes turned out), Section 9.4.

Decreased Vision

I. Transient visual loss   (Vision returns to normal within 24 hours, usually within 1 hour.)

More common   Few seconds (usually bilateral): Papilledema.

Few minutes: Amaurosis fugax (TIA) (unilateral), vertebrobasilar artery insufficiency (bilateral).

10-60 minutes: Migraine (with or without a subsequent headache).

Less common   Impending central retinal vein occlusion, ischemic optic neuropathy, ocular ischemic syndrome (carotid occlusive disease), glaucoma, a sudden change in blood pressure, central nervous system (CNS) lesion, optic disc drusen.

1

II. Visual loss lasting >24 hours
   A. Sudden, painless loss
      More common Retinal artery or vein occlusion, ischemic optic neuropathy, vitreous hemorrhage, retinal detachment, optic neuritis (usually pain with eye movements).
      Less common Other retinal or CNS disease.
   B. Gradual, painless loss (over weeks, months, or years)
      More common Cataract, refractive error, open-angle glaucoma, chronic retinal disease (e.g., age-related macular degeneration [ARMD], diabetic retinopathy).
      Less common Chronic corneal disease (e.g., corneal dystrophy), optic neuropathy/atrophy (e.g., CNS tumor).
   C. Painful visual loss: Acute-angle closure glaucoma, optic neuritis (pain with eye movements), uveitis, corneal hydrops (keratoconus).

NOTE Always remember nonphysiologic visual loss.

Discharge See "Red Eye" in this chapter.

Distortion (of Vision)

More common Refractive error, macular disease (e.g., central serous chorioretinopathy or ARMD), corneal irregularity.
Less common Cataract, topical eye drops (miotics), retinal detachment, migraine (transient), CNS abnormality.

Double Vision

I. Monocular (The double vision remains when the uninvolved eye is occluded.)
   More common Refractive error, corneal opacity or irregularity, cataract.
   Less common Dislocated natural lens or lens implant, extra pupillary openings, macular disease, retinal detachment, nonphysiologic.
II. Binocular (The double vision is eliminated when either eye is occluded.)
   A. Typically intermittent: Myasthenia gravis, intermittent decompensation of an existing phoria.
   B. Constant: Isolated sixth-, third-, or fourth-nerve palsy; orbital disease (e.g., thyroid eye disease, orbital inflammatory pseudotumor, tumor); cavernous sinus/superior orbital fissure syndrome; status post ocular surgery (e.g., residual anesthesia, displaced muscle); status post trauma (e.g., orbital wall fracture with extraocular muscle entrapment, orbital edema); internuclear ophthalmoplegia, vertebrobasilar artery insufficiency, other CNS lesions, spectacle problem.

Dry Eyes   See Section 4.2.

Eyelid Crusting

> *More common*   Blepharitis, conjunctivitis.
> *Less common*   Canaliculitis, nasolacrimal duct obstruction, dacryocystitis.

Eyelid Droop   See "Ptosis" and "Pseudoptosis" in Chapter 2.

Eyelid Swelling

A. Associated with inflammation (usually erythematous)
  More common   Hordeolum, blepharitis, conjunctivitis, preseptal or orbital cellulitis, trauma, contact dermatitis.
  Less common   Ectropion, corneal abnormality, urticaria/angioedema, insect bite, dacryoadenitis, erysipelas, eyelid or lacrimal gland mass.
B. Noninflammatory: Chalazion; prolapse of orbital fat (retropulsion of the globe increases the prolapse); laxity of the eyelid skin; cardiac, renal, or thyroid disease; lacrimal gland or eyelid mass.

Eyelid Twitch

Fatigue, lack of sleep, habit, corneal or conjunctival irritation (especially from an eyelash or cyst), dry eye, blepharospasm (bilateral), hemifacial spasm, albinism (photosensitive), rarely a serum electrolyte abnormality or anemia.

Flashes of Light

> *More common*   Retinal break or detachment, posterior vitreous detachment, migraine, rapid eye movements (particularly in darkness).
> *Less common*   CNS (particularly occipital lobe) disorders, retinitis.

Floaters   See "Spots in Front of the Eyes" in this chapter.

Foreign-Body Sensation

Dry eye syndrome, blepharitis, conjunctivitis, trichiasis, corneal abnormality (e.g., corneal abrasion or foreign body, recurrent erosion, superficial punctate keratitis), contact-lens-related problem, episcleritis.

Halos Around Lights

Cataract, acute-angle closure glaucoma or corneal edema from another cause (e.g., corneal endothelial dystrophy, aphakic/pseudophakic bullous keratopathy), corneal haziness or mucus, drugs (e.g., digitalis, chloroquine).

Headache   See Section 15.3.

Itchy Eye

Conjunctivitis (especially viral, vernal, and allergic), blepharitis, dry eye syndrome, topical drug allergy or contact dermatitis, giant papillary conjunctivitis or another contact-lens-related problem.

Light Sensitivity   See "Photophobia" in this chapter.

Night Blindness

More common   Refractive error (especially undercorrected myopia), advanced glaucoma, small pupil (especially from miotic drops), retinitis pigmentosa, congenital stationary night blindness, drugs (e.g., phenothiazines, chloroquine, quinine).
Less common   Vitamin A deficiency, gyrate atrophy, choroideremia.

Pain (Ocular)

A. Typically mild to moderate: Dry eye syndrome, blepharitis, conjunctivitis, episcleritis, inflamed pingueculum or pterygium, foreign body (corneal or conjunctival), corneal disorder (e.g., superficial punctate keratitis), others.
B. Typically moderate to severe: Corneal disorder (abrasion, erosion, infiltrate/ulcer), anterior uveitis, scleritis, acute-angle closure glaucoma.

Photophobia

More common   Corneal abnormality (e.g., abrasion) or anterior uveitis.
Less common   Conjunctivitis (mild photophobia), posterior uveitis, albinism, total color blindness, aniridia.
With normal eye examination   Migraine, meningitis, retrobulbar optic neuritis, subarachnoid hemorrhage, trigeminal neuralgia, or a lightly pigmented eye.

Proptosis   See "Orbital Disease," Section 7.1.

Ptosis   See "Ptosis" and "Pseudoptosis" in Chapter 2.

Red Eye

 I. Discharge present
   More common   Conjunctivitis, ophthalmia neonatorum in infants, blepharitis.
   Less common   Acute allergic reaction, dacryocystitis, canaliculitis.
 II. No discharge present
   A. Pain present: See "Pain" above.
   B. Minimal or no pain present
     More common   Subconjunctival hemorrhage, injected pterygium/pingueculum, blepharitis, dry eye syndrome.
     Less common   Conjunctival tumor.

Spots in Front of the Eyes

 A. Transient: Migraine.
 B. Permanent or longstanding
   More common   Posterior vitreous detachment, posterior uveitis, vitreous hemorrhage.
   Less common   Retinal detachment, corneal opacity.

NOTE   Some patients are referring to a blind spot in their visual field due to a retinal, optic nerve, or CNS disorder.

Tearing

 I. Adults
   A. Pain present: Corneal abnormality (e.g., abrasion, foreign body/rust ring, recurrent erosion), anterior uveitis, eyelash (trichiasis, entropion), cyst or foreign body rubbing against the cornea, conjunctival abnormality (e.g., foreign body, laceration).
   B. Minimal or no pain present: Dry eye syndrome, nasolacrimal duct obstruction, punctal occlusion or other tear drainage abnormality, ectropion, conjunctivitis (especially allergic and toxic), lacrimal gland mass or inflammation.
 II. Children: Nasolacrimal duct obstruction, congenital glaucoma, corneal or conjunctival foreign body or other irritative disorder.

Watery Eyes   See "Tearing" in this chapter.

White Pupil   See "Leukocoria," Section 9.1.

2

Differential Diagnosis of Ocular Signs

Anterior Chamber/Anterior Chamber Angle

Blood in Schlemm's canal on gonioscopy Compression of episcleral vessels by a gonioprism (iatrogenic), Sturge-Weber syndrome, arteriovenous fistula (e.g., carotid-cavernous sinus fistula), superior vena cava obstruction, hypotony.

Hyphema Following trauma or intraocular surgery, bleeding from iris or corneal wound neovascularization, herpes simplex or zoster iritis, blood dyscrasia or clotting disorder (e.g., hemophilia), or intraocular tumor (e.g., juvenile xanthogranuloma, retinoblastoma, leukemia, others).

Hypopyon Infectious corneal ulcer, endophthalmitis, severe iritis, reaction to an intraocular lens or retained lens protein following cataract surgery, intraocular tumor necrosis (e.g., retinoblastoma [a pseudohypopyon]), or a tight contact lens.

Cornea/Conjunctival Findings

Band Keratopathy See Section 4.11.

Corneal Crystals Schnyder's crystalline dystrophy, multiple myeloma, cystinosis, gout, uremia, hypergammaglobulinemia, drugs (e.g., indomethacin or chloroquine).

7

Corneal Edema

A. Congenital: Congenital glaucoma, congenital hereditary endothelial dystrophy, birth trauma (forceps injury).
B. Acquired: Early postoperative, aphakic or pseudophakic bullous keratopathy, Fuchs' endothelial dystrophy, contact-lens overwear, trauma, acute-angle closure glaucoma and other causes of acute elevation in intraocular pressure, corneal hydrops (acute keratoconus), herpes simplex keratitis, iritis, failed corneal graft, iridocorneal endothelial (ICE) syndrome.

Corneal Filaments See "Filamentary Keratopathy," Section 4.3.

Dilated Episcleral Vessels (in the absence of ocular irritation or pain) Underlying uveal melanoma, arteriovenous fistula (e.g., carotid-cavernous fistula), polycythemia vera, leukemia, ophthalmic vein or cavernous sinus thrombosis.

Enlarged Corneal Nerves

Most important Multiple endocrine neoplasia type IIb or Sipple syndrome (medullary carcinoma of the thyroid gland, pheochromocytoma, mucosal neuromas; may have marfanoid habitus).
Others Keratoconus, keratitis, neurofibromatosis, Fuchs' endothelial dystrophy, Refsum's syndrome, trauma, congenital glaucoma, failed corneal graft, leprosy.

Membranous Conjunctivitis (Removal of the membrane is difficult and causes bleeding). Streptococcus, pneumococcus, chemical burn, ligneous conjunctivitis, corynebacterium diptheria. Rarely adenovirus or herpes simplex virus. See also "Pseudomembranous conjunctivitis" in this chapter.

Opacification of the Cornea in Infancy Congenital glaucoma, birth trauma (forceps injury), congenital hereditary endothelial or stromal dystrophy (bilateral), developmental abnormality of the anterior segment (especially Peter's anomaly), metabolic abnormalities (bilateral) (e.g., mucopolysaccharidoses, mucolipidoses), interstitial keratitis, herpes simplex virus, corneal ulcer, corneal dermoid, sclerocornea.

Pannus (superficial vascular invasion of the cornea) Rosacea, tight contact lens or contact-lens overwear, phlyctenule, chlamydia (trachoma and inclusion conjunctivitis), superior limbic keratoconjunctivitis (micropannus only), staphylococcal hypersensitivity, vernal keratoconjunctivitis, herpes simplex virus, chemical burn.

Large Papillae on the Superior Tarsus Vernal conjunctivitis, giant papillary conjunctivitis, exposed suture, prosthesis-induced, superior limbic keratoconjunctivitis, trachoma.

Pigmentation of the Conjunctiva Racial pigmentation (perilimbal), nevus, primary acquired melanosis, melanoma, ocular and oculodermal melanocytosis (congenital, blue in color, not conjunctival, but episcleral), Addison's disease, mascara, pregnancy, radiation, drug or metal (e.g., argyrosis from silver).

Pseudomembranous Conjunctivitis (Removal of the membrane is easy, and no bleeding results). All of the causes of membranous conjunctivitis, as well as ocular pemphigoid, Stevens-Johnson syndrome, superior limbic keratoconjunctivitis, gonococcus, staphylococcus, and others.

Symblepharon (fusion of the eyelid [palpebral] conjunctiva with the conjunctiva covering the globe [bulbar conjunctiva]) Ocular pemphigoid, Stevens-Johnson syndrome, chemical burn, trauma, drugs, longstanding inflammation.

Whorl-like Opacity in the Corneal Epithelium Amiodarone, chloroquine, Fabry's disease, phenothiazines, indomethacin, vortex dystrophy.

Eyelid Abnormalities

Eyelid Edema or Swelling

More common Orbital fat herniation from aging, conjunctivitis, allergy, chalazion, orbital disease.

Less common Cardiac disease, renal disease, urticaria/angioneurotic edema, dacryoadenitis, hypothyroidism, superior vena cava syndrome.

Eyelid Lesion See "Malignant Tumors of the Eyelid," Section 6.11.

Pseudoptosis Dermatochalasis (laxity of the eyelid skin from old age), enophthalmos (e.g., from a traumatic blow-out fracture), phthisis bulbi, microphthalmia (small eye), chalazion or other eyelid tumor, eyelid edema.

Ptosis

More common Aging (e.g., levator dehiscence), following intraocular surgery or trauma, congenital.

Less common Myasthenia gravis, Horner's syndrome, third-nerve palsy, chronic progressive external ophthalmoplegia, corneal or anterior segment disease (e.g., corneal abrasion), prolonged use of topical steroids, botulinum toxin injection.

Fundus Findings

Bone Spicules (Widespread Pigment Clumping)

More common   Retinitis pigmentosa and its associated syndromes, disseminated chorioretinitis (especially old syphilis), trauma senile pigmentary changes.

Less common   Following spontaneous reattachment of a retinal detachment (e.g., toxemia of pregnancy, Harada's disease), Kearns-Sayre syndrome, abetalipoproteinemia, vitamin A deficiency, viral infections (e.g., rubella), drugs (e.g., thioridazine and other phenothiazines), retinopathy of prematurity (when seen years later as an adult), cystinosis, old vascular occlusions.

Bull's Eye Macular Lesion   Age-related macular degeneration (ARMD), Stargardt's disease, cone dystrophy, chloroquine retinopathy, Spielmeyer-Vogt syndrome.

Cotton Wool Spots, without other abnormalities (white fluffy lesions with feathered edges, often obscuring retinal vessels)

More common   AIDS retinopathy, hypertension, diabetes, collagen vascular disease (e.g., systemic lupus erythematosus), retinal artery/arteriole occlusion.

Less common   Retinal vein occlusion, cardiac valvular disease, carotid artery obstruction, chest trauma (Purtscher's retinopathy), anemia, leukemia, lymphoma.

Choroidal Folds   Orbital or choroidal tumor, thyroid orbitopathy, orbital inflammatory pseudotumor, posterior scleritis, hypotony, retinal detachment, marked hyperopia, scleral laceration, papilledema.

Choroidal Neovascularization (gray-green membrane or blood seen deep to the retina)

More common   ARMD, ocular histoplasmosis syndrome, high myopia, angioid streaks, choroidal rupture from trauma.

Less common   Drusen of the optic nerve head, tumors, following retinal laser photocoagulation, idiopathic.

Embolus   (See "Amaurosis Fugax" [Section 12.6], "Branch Retinal Artery Occlusion" [Section 12.2], or "Central Retinal Artery Occlusion" [Section 12.1]).

- Platelet-fibrin   (Dull gray and elongated [as opposed to round]: Carotid disease. NOTE   Similar-appearing fibrin emboli may also arise from the heart.)

- Cholesterol   (Sparkling yellow, usually at an arterial bifurcation: Carotid disease.)
- Calcium   (Dull white, typically around or on the disc: Cardiac disease.)
- Cardiac myxoma   (Common in young patients, particularly in the left eye. Often occludes the ophthalmic or central retinal artery behind the globe and is not visualized.)
- Talc and cornstarch   (Small yellow-white glistening particles in macular arterioles. May produce peripheral retinal neovascularization: IV drug abuse.)
- Lipid or air   (Cotton wool spots, not emboli, are often seen. Results from chest trauma [Purtscher's retinopathy] and fracture of long bones.)
- Others (Tumors, parasites, other foreign bodies.)

Macular exudates

More common   Diabetes, choroidal (subretinal) neovascular membrane, hypertension.

Less common   Macroaneurysm, Coats' disease (children), peripheral retinal capillary hemangioma, retinal vein occlusion, papilledema, radiation.

Normal Fundus in the Presence of Decreased Vision   Retrobulbar optic neuritis, cone degenerations, Stargardt's disease/fundus flavimaculatus, other optic neuropathy (e.g., tumor, alcohol/tobacco), rod monochromatism, nonphysiologic visual loss.

Optociliary Shunt Vessels on the Disc   Orbital or intracranial tumor (especially meningioma), status post central retinal vein occlusion, chronic papilledema (e.g., pseudotumor cerebri), chronic open-angle glaucoma, optic nerve glioma.

Retinal Neovascularization

A. Posterior pole: Diabetes, following a central retinal vein occlusion.
B. Peripheral: Sickle cell retinopathy, following branch retinal vein occlusion, diabetes, sarcoidosis, retinopathy of prematurity, embolization from IV drug abuse, others (leukemia, anemia, Eales' disease, etc.).

Roth Spots (hemorrhages with white centers)

More common   Leukemia, septic chorioretinitis (e.g., secondary to subacute bacterial endocarditis), diabetes.

Less common   Pernicious anemia (and rarely other forms of anemia), sickle cell disease, scurvy, systemic lupus erythematosus, other collagen vascular diseases.

Sheathing of Retinal Veins (Periphlebitis)

More common   Syphilis, sarcoidosis, pars planitis, sickle cell disease.

Less common   Tuberculosis, multiple sclerosis, Eales' disease, viral retinitis (HIV, herpes, etc.), Behçet's disease, fungal retinitis, septicemia (or bacteremia).

Tumor   See "Malignant Melanoma of the Choroid," Section 8.3.

Glaucoma

Acute Rise in Intraocular Pressure   Acute-angle closure glaucoma, glaucomatocyclitic crisis (Posner-Schlossman syndrome), inflammatory open-angle glaucoma, malignant glaucoma, postoperative glaucoma, suprachoroidal hemorrhage, retrobulbar hemorrhage.

Iris

Iris Heterochromia (irides of different colors)

A. Involved iris is lighter than normal: Congenital Horner's syndrome, Fuchs' heterochromic iridocyclitis, chronic uveitis, juvenile xanthogranuloma, metastatic carcinoma, Waardenburg's syndrome (white forelock, decreased hearing, telecanthus).
B. Involved iris is darker than normal: Ocular melanocytosis (or oculodermal melanocytosis), hemosiderosis, siderosis, retained intraocular foreign body, ocular malignant melanoma, diffuse iris nevus, retinoblastoma, leukemia, lymphoma, iridocorneal endothelial (ICE) syndrome.

Iris Lesion

A. Melanotic (brown): Nevus, melanoma, adenoma or adenocarcinoma of the iris pigment epithelium (NOTE in heavily pigmented irides, cysts, foreign bodies, neurofibromas, and other lesions may appear pigmented.)
B. Amelanotic (white, yellow, or orange): Amelanotic melanoma, inflammatory nodule or granuloma (sarcoidosis, tuberculosis, leprosy, other granulomatous disease), neurofibroma, patchy hyperemia of syphilis, juvenile xanthogranuloma, foreign body, cyst, leiomyoma, seeding from a posterior segment tumor.

Neovascularization of the Iris   Diabetic retinopathy, central retinal vein or artery occlusion, branch retinal vein occlusion, ocular ischemic syndrome (carotid occlusive disease), chronic uveitis, chronic retinal detachment, intraocular tumor (e.g., retinoblastoma), other retinal vascular disease.

Lens

Iridescent Lens Particles   Drugs, hypocalcemia, myotonic dystrophy, familial, idiopathic.

Lenticonus

A. Anterior (marked convexity of the anterior lens): Rule out Alport's syndrome (hereditary nephritis).
B. Posterior (marked concavity of the posterior lens surface): Usually idiopathic—may be associated with persistent hyperplastic primary vitreous.

Neuro-ophthalmic Abnormalities

Afferent Pupillary Defect

A. Severe (2-3 +): Optic nerve disease (e.g., ischemic optic neuropathy, optic neuritis, tumor, glaucoma), central retinal artery or vein occlusion, less commonly a lesion of the optic chiasm/tract.
B. Mild (1 +): Any of the above, amblyopia, vitreous hemorrhage, macular degeneration, branch retinal vein or artery occlusion, retinal detachment, or other retinal disease.

Anisocoria (Pupils of Different Sizes)   See Section 11.1.

Limitation of Ocular Motility

A. With exophthalmos and resistance to retropulsion: See "Orbital Disease," Section 7.1.
B. Without exophthalmos and resistance to retropulsion: Isolated third-, fourth-, or sixth-nerve palsy; multiple ocular motor nerve palsies (see "Cavernous Sinus/Superior Orbital Fissure Syndrome," Section 11.8); myasthenia gravis; chronic progressive external ophthalmoplegia; orbital blow-out fracture with muscle entrapment; ophthalmoplegic migraine; Duane's syndrome; other CNS disorders.

Optic Disc Atrophy

More common   Glaucoma, status post central retinal vein or artery occlusion, ischemic optic neuropathy, chronic optic neuritis, chronic papilledema, compression of the optic nerve or chiasm or tract by a tumor or aneurysm, traumatic optic neuropathy.
Less common   Syphilis, retinal degeneration (e.g., retinitis pigmentosa), toxic/metabolic optic neuropathy, Leber's optic atrophy, Leber's congenital

amaurosis, retinal storage disease (e.g., Tay-Sachs), radiation neuropathy, other forms of congenital or hereditary optic atrophy (nystagmus almost always present in the congenital forms).

Optic Disc Swelling (Edema) See "Papilledema," Section 11.12.

Optociliary Shunt Vessels See "Fundus Findings" in this chapter.

Paradoxical Pupillary Reaction (pupil dilates in light and constricts in darkness) Congenital stationary night blindness, cone dystrophy, optic neuritis, dominant optic atrophy. Rarely amblyopia and strabismus.

Orbit

Extraocular Muscle Thickening on CT Scan

More common Thyroid orbitopathy, orbital inflammatory pseudotumor.
Less common Tumor (especially lymphoma, metastasis, or spread of a lacrimal gland tumor to muscle), carotid-cavernous fistula, cavernous hemangioma (usually appears in the muscle cone without muscle thickening), rhabdomyosarcoma (child).

Lacrimal Gland Lesions See "Lacrimal Gland Mass," Section 7.7.

Optic Nerve Lesion (Isolated)

More common Optic nerve glioma (especially children), optic nerve meningioma (especially adults).
Less common Metastasis, leukemia, orbital inflammatory pseudotumor, sarcoidosis, increased intracranial pressure with secondary optic nerve swelling.

Orbital Lesions/Proptosis See "Orbital Disease," Section 7.1.

Pediatrics

Leukocoria (White Pupillary Reflex) See Section 9.1.

Nystagmus in Infancy Congenital nystagmus, albinism, Leber's congenital amaurosis, thalamic injury, spasmus nutans, optic nerve or chiasmal glioma, optic nerve hypoplasia, congenital cataract, aniridia.

Postoperative Problems

Shallow Anterior Chamber

A. Accompanied by increased intraocular pressure: Pupillary block glaucoma, suprachoroidal hemorrhage, malignant glaucoma.
B. Accompanied by decreased intraocular pressure: Wound leak, choroidal detachment.

Refractive Problem

Progressive Hyperopia   Orbital tumor pressing on the posterior surface of the eye, serous elevation of the retina (e.g., central serous chorioretinopathy), posterior scleritis, presbyopia, hypoglycemia, cataract.

Progressive Myopia   High (pathologic) myopia, diabetes, cataract, use of miotic drops, staphyloma and elongation of the globe, childhood (physiologic).

Visual Field Abnormalities

Altitudinal Field Defect

More common   Ischemic optic neuropathy, hemibranch artery or vein occlusion.
Less common   Glaucoma, optic nerve or chiasmal lesion, optic nerve coloboma.

Arcuate Scotoma

More common   Glaucoma.
Less common   Ischemic optic neuropathy (especially nonarteritic), optic disc drusen, high myopia.

Binasal Field Defect

More common   Glaucoma, bitemporal retinal disease (e.g., retinitis pigmentosa).
Rare   Bilateral occipital disease, tumor or aneurysm compressing both optic nerves or chiasm.

Bitemporal Hemianopsia

More common   Chiasmal lesion (e.g., pituitary adenoma, meningioma, craniopharyngioma, aneurysm, glioma).

Less common   Tilted optic discs.

Rare   Nasal retinitis pigmentosa.

Blind Spot Enlargement   Papilledema, glaucoma, optic nerve drusen, optic nerve coloboma, medullated nerve fibers off the disc, drugs, myopic disc with a crescent, others.

Central Scotoma   Macular disease, optic neuritis, ischemic optic neuropathy (more typically produces an altitudinal field defect), optic atrophy (e.g., from tumor compressing the nerve or toxic/metabolic disease), rarely an occipital cortex lesion.

Homonymous Hemianopsia   Optic tract or lateral geniculate body lesion; temporal, parietal, or occipital lobe lesion of the brain (stroke and tumor more common; aneurysm and trauma less common). Migraine may cause a transient homonymous hemianopsia.

Constriction of the Peripheral Fields Leaving Only a Small Residual Central Field   Glaucoma, retinitis pigmentosa (or some other peripheral retinal disorder), chronic papilledema, status post panretinal photocoagulation, central retinal artery occlusion with cilioretinal artery sparing, bilateral occipital lobe infarction with macular sparing, nonphysiologic visual loss, rarely drugs.

Vitreous

Vitreous Opacities   Asteroid hyalosis, synchysis scintillans, vitreous hemorrhage, inflammatory cells in vitritis or posterior uveitis, "snow ball" opacities of pars planitis or sarcoidosis, normal vitreous strands from age-related vitreous degeneration, tumor cells. Rarely, amyloidosis or Whipple's disease.

3

Trauma

3.1 Chemical Burn

Treatment should be instituted IMMEDIATELY, even before taking the vision.

Emergent Treatment

1. Copious irrigation of the eyes, preferably with saline or Ringer's lactated solution, for at least 30 minutes. However, if nonsterile water is the only liquid available, it should be used. Do *not* use acidic solutions to neutralize alkalies or vice versa. It is helpful to place an eyelid speculum and topical anesthetic (e.g., proparacaine) in the eye prior to irrigation. Pull down the lower eyelid and evert the upper eyelid if possible to irrigate the fornices. Manual use of IV tubing connected to an irrigation solution facilitates the irrigation process.
2. Five minutes after ceasing irrigation (to allow for equilibration), litmus paper should be touched to the inferior cul-de-sac. If the pH is not neutral (i.e., 7), irrigation should be continued until it is.

A. Mild-to-Moderate Burns

Critical Signs   Corneal epithelial defects ranging from scattered superficial punctate keratitis (SPK) to focal epithelial loss to sloughing of the entire epithelium.

No significant areas of perilimbal ischemia are seen (no sign of interrupted blood flow through the conjunctival or episcleral vessels).

Other Signs   Focal areas of conjunctival chemosis, hyperemia, and/or hemorrhages, mild eyelid edema, mild anterior-chamber reaction, first- and second-degree burns of the periocular skin.

Work-up

1. History: Time of injury? Chemical to which the patient was exposed? Duration of the exposure until irrigation was started? Duration of the irrigation?
2. Slit-lamp examination with fluorescein staining. Evert the eyelids to search for foreign bodies. Check the intraocular pressure (IOP).

NOTE   In the presence of a distorted cornea, IOP may be most accurately measured with a McKay-Marg tonometer.

Treatment—After Irrigation

1. Thoroughly search the fornices and remove any sequestered particles of caustic material and necrotic conjunctiva which may contain residual chemicals. Calcium hydroxide particles may be more easily removed with a cotton-tipped applicator soaked in sodium EDTA.
2. Cycloplegic (e.g., scopolamine ¼%). Avoid phenylephrine because of its vasoconstrictive properties.
3. Topical antibiotic ointment (e.g., erythromycin).
4. Pressure patch for 24 hours.
5. Oral pain medication (e.g., acetaminophen $+/-$ codeine) as needed.

- If the IOP is elevated, acetazolamide (e.g., Diamox) 250 mg po qid or 500 mg sequel po bid or methazolamide (e.g., Neptazane) 25-50 mg po 2-3 × / day may be given. Add a topical beta-blocker (e.g., timolol ½% bid or levobunolol ½% bid) if additional IOP control is required.

Follow-up   Recheck and repatch with antibiotic ointment plus a cycloplegic drop every day until the corneal defect is healed. Watch for corneal ulceration and infection.

B. Moderate-to-Severe Burns

Critical Signs   Pronounced chemosis and perilimbal blanching; corneal edema and opacification, sometimes with little-to-no view of the anterior chamber, iris, or lens; a moderate-to-severe anterior-chamber reaction (may not be appreciated if the cornea is opaque).

Other Signs Increased IOP, second- and third-degree burns of the surrounding skin, and a local necrotic retinopathy due to direct penetration of alkali through the sclera.

NOTE If you suspect an epithelial defect, but do not see one on fluorescein staining, repeat the fluorescein application to the eye. Sometimes the defect is slow to take up the dye. Occasionally the whole epithelium has sloughed off and all that is left is Bowman's membrane, which takes up fluorescein poorly.

Work-up Same as for mild-to-moderate burns (A).

Treatment—After Irrigation

1. Admission to the hospital may be necessary for close monitoring of IOP and corneal healing.
2. Debride necrotic tissue containing foreign matter.
3. Topical antibiotic (e.g., gentamicin drops 4 × /day or erythromycin ointment 2-4 × /day).
4. Cycloplegic (e.g., scopolamine ¼% or atropine 1% qid).
5. Topical steroid (e.g., prednisolone acetate 1% or dexamethasone 0.1% 4-9 × /day) if significant inflammation of the anterior chamber or cornea is present.
6. Pressure patch between drops/ointment.
7. Antiglaucoma medications if the IOP is elevated or cannot be determined. See the antiglaucoma recommendations above.
8. Lysis of conjunctival adhesions using a glass rod covered by an antibiotic ointment, sweeping the fornices bid. If symblepharon begin to form despite attempted lysis, consider using a scleral shell or ring to maintain the fornices.

• Consider a therapeutic soft contact lens or a collagen shield. (Usually used if healing is delayed beyond two weeks. Leave it in place for 6-8 weeks after resolution of the epithelial defect.)
• If any melting of the cornea occurs, collagenase inhibitors may be used (e.g., acetylcysteine 10-20% [e.g., Mucomyst] q 4 hours.)
• If the melting progresses (or the cornea perforates) consider cyanoacrylate adhesive. An emergent corneal transplant may be necessary; however, the prognosis is better if it is performed 12-18 months after the injury.

Follow-up These patients need to be followed closely either in the hospital or daily as outpatients. Topical steroids need to be tapered after 7 days because they can promote corneal melting. Long-term use of artificial tears and lubricating ointment (e.g., Refresh drops q 1-6 hours and Refresh PM ointment 1-4×/day) may be required. A severe dry eye may require a tarsorrhaphy, conjunctival flap, or mucous membrane graft. A conjunctival transplant may be performed in unilateral injuries which fail to heal within several weeks to several months.

3.2 Corneal Abrasion

Symptoms Pain, photophobia, foreign-body sensation, tearing, history of scratching the eye.

Critical Sign Epithelial staining defect with fluorescein.

Other Signs Conjunctival injection, swollen eyelid, mild anterior-chamber reaction.

Work-up

1. Slit-lamp examination: Use fluorescein and measure the size of the abrasion, diagram its location, and evaluate for an anterior-chamber reaction.
2. Evert the eyelids to make certain no foreign body is present.

Treatment

A. Non-contact-lens wearer
   1. Cycloplegic (e.g., cyclopentolate 2%).
   2. Antibiotic ointment (e.g., erythromycin).
   3. Pressure patch for 24 hours.

NOTE A pressure patch is generally not applied when the abrasion is at significant risk for infection (e.g., scratches from a tree branch or a false fingernail).

B. Contact-lens wearer
   1. Cycloplegic (e.g., cyclopentolate 2%).
   2. Tobramycin drops 4-6×/day. Can add tobramycin ointment qhs if the patient is significantly uncomfortable.
   3. No eye patch.

Follow-up

A. Non-contact-lens wearer with a small, noncentral abrasion
   1. Patient removes the patch after 24 hours.
   2. Topical antibiotic for 4 days (e.g., erythromycin ointment 2-3 × /day or sulfacetamide drops 4 × /day), after the patch is removed.
   3. Return if the symptoms persist or worsen.
B. Non-contact-lens wearer with a central or large corneal abrasion
   1. Return the next day to determine if the epithelial defect is improving.
   2. If the abrasion has resolved or only a superficial punctate keratitis remains, then treat with topical antibiotics for 4 more days (e.g., erythromycin ointment 2-3 × /day or sulfacetamide drops 4 × /day).
   3. If it is healing and the remaining abrasion is small and noncentral, then treat with topical antibiotics for 4 days as above.
   4. If the abrasion remains large or a central area of staining persists, then repeat the cycloplegic, antibiotic ointment, and pressure patch as above, and have the patient return the following day.
C. Contact-lens wearer
   Return every day until the epithelial defect resolves, then treat with topical tobramycin drops for 1-2 additional days. The patient may resume contact-lens wear after the eye feels perfectly normal for 3-4 days (after having had the lens examined for tears, scratches, protein build-up, etc., by their contact-lens specialist).

NOTE   If at any time a corneal infiltrate is observed, appropriate smears and cultures should be obtained and more aggressive therapy instituted (see Section 4.12).

3.3   Corneal Foreign Body / Rust Ring

Symptoms   Foreign-body sensation, tearing, blurred vision, photophobia, and commonly a history of a foreign body to the eye.

Critical Sign   Corneal foreign body, rust ring, or both.

Other Signs   Conjunctival injection, eyelid edema, mild anterior-chamber reaction and superficial punctate keratitis (SPK). A small infiltrate may surround the foreign body, especially if the foreign body has been present in the eye for more than 24 hours. This infiltrate is usually sterile.

Work-up

1. History: Was the patient wearing safety goggles? Did the foreign body arise from metal striking metal (which might suggest an intraocular foreign body)?
2. Slit-lamp examination: Locate the foreign body. Evert the eyelids and inspect the fornices for additional foreign bodies, especially in the presence of linear SPK. Measure the dimensions of the infiltrate, if present, and the degree of any anterior-chamber reaction.
3. Dilate the eye and examine the vitreous and retina when a history of hammering or forcibly striking metal is provided (or a possible intraocular foreign body from another cause is considered).

Treatment

1. Remove the corneal foreign body: Apply a topical anesthetic (e.g., proparacaine)—2 drops. Remove the foreign body with a foreign body spud or a 25-gauge needle under magnification, usually at a slit lamp.

   NOTE   Multiple superficial foreign bodies may be more easily removed by irrigation.

2. Remove the rust ring: Occasionally it can be shelled out in one piece with a foreign-body spud, but usually it is most easily removed with an ophthalmoscopic rust ring drill after topical anesthesia as above.

   NOTE   It is sometimes safer to leave a rust ring centered in the visual axis (especially when it is deep) to allow time for the rust to migrate to the corneal surface, at which point it can be more easily extracted.

3. Measure the size of the resultant corneal epithelial defect.
4. Cycloplegic (e.g., cyclopentolate 2%).
5. Antibiotic ointment (e.g., erythromycin).
6. Pressure patch for 24 hours.

Follow-up

A. Small (<1-2 mm diameter in size), clean, noncentral epithelial defect present after foreign-body removal: The patient may remove the patch after 24 hours and begin topical antibiotics for 3-4 days (e.g., sulfacetamide drops qid or erythromycin ointment 2-3 ×/day) and follow-up as needed.
B. Central or large epithelial defect, mucopurulent discharge, infiltrate, residual rust in cornea, or moderate anterior-chamber reaction: Follow-up in 24 hours to reevaluate.

NOTE An infiltrate accompanied by a significant anterior chamber re-action, purulent discharge, or extreme redness and pain, should be cultured to rule out an infection and treated with antibiotics more aggressively (see Section 4.12).

3.4 Conjunctival / Subconjunctival Foreign Body

Symptoms Ocular irritation or pain, foreign-body sensation, tearing, red eye. A history of trauma or a foreign body to the eye is often elicited.

Signs Linear, vertically oriented corneal scratches may be observed when a foreign body is under the upper eyelid. A conjunctival laceration is observed when a subconjunctival foreign body is present. A conjunctival or subcon-junctival hemorrhage may also be present.

Differential Diagnosis See "Foreign-Body Sensation" in Chapter 1.

Work-up

1. History: Determine whether an intraocular or intraorbital foreign body may be present and whether the globe may be ruptured. Be especially suspicious when a history of hammering or grinding metal is provided.
2. Ocular examination including an intraocular pressure measurement and a thorough slit-lamp evaluation. To evaluate the superior fornix double evert the eyelid over an instrument such as a Desmarres eyelid retractor. Careful inspection in the area of a conjunctival laceration is always required to definitively rule out a scleral laceration and an intraocular foreign body.
3. A dilated retinal examination is needed if a subconjunctival foreign body exists or the eye has had significant trauma. Carefully examine the area under the conjunctival lesion looking for retinal damage and possibly an intraocular foreign body.
4. Consider a B-scan ultrasound to rule out an intraocular foreign body.
5. Consider a CT scan of the orbit (axial and coronal views) to rule out an intraocular or intraorbital foreign body and a ruptured globe.

Treatment

1. Remove the foreign body under topical anesthesia (e.g., proparacaine):
   a. Multiple loose foreign bodies: These can often be removed with saline irrigation.

b. A foreign body on the conjunctival surface: Remove it with a cotton-tipped applicator soaked in topical anesthetic or a foreign-body spud.
c. A foreign body embedded in the conjunctiva or beneath the conjunctiva: Remove it with fine forceps.

NOTE   In the presence of multiple small foreign bodies, remove as many as possible. Small, relatively inaccessible subconjunctival foreign bodies may sometimes be left in the eye without harm. Occasionally they will surface with time, at which point they can be removed more easily.

2. Sweep the fornices of the eye with a glass rod (or sterile cotton-tipped applicator soaked with a topical anesthetic) to catch small loose material that may have been missed on examination.

See Section 3.5 if there is conjunctival laceration. If no laceration is noted:

3. A topical antibiotic (e.g., erythromycin ointment bid or sulfacetamide drops qid) may be used if superficial punctate keratitis or a corneal or conjunctival abrasion is present.
4. Artificial tears (e.g., Refresh qid × 2 days) may be given to a mildly irritated eye.

Follow-up   As needed, unless residual foreign bodies were left in or under the conjunctiva. A patient with residual foreign material is reexamined within 1 week.

3.5   Conjunctival Laceration

Symptoms   Mild pain, red eye, foreign-body sensation, usually a history of ocular trauma.

Signs   Fluorescein staining of the conjunctiva, noted after instillation of fluorescein dye and examination of the eye with the blue light of the slit lamp. With the white light, the conjunctiva can be seen to be torn and rolled up upon itself; the exposed white sclera may be noted. Conjunctival and subconjunctival hemorrhage are often present.

Work-up

1. History: Determine the nature of the trauma and whether a ruptured globe or intraocular or intraorbital foreign body may be present.
2. Complete ocular examination, including a careful exploration of the sclera (after topical anesthesia [e.g., proparacaine]) in the region of the conjunc-

tival laceration to rule out a scleral laceration or a subconjunctival foreign body. The entire area of sclera under the conjunctival laceration must be inspected. The fundus, especially the area underlying the conjunctival injury, needs careful evaluation by indirect ophthalmoscopy.
3. Consider a CT scan of the orbit (axial and coronal views) to rule out an intraocular or intraorbital foreign body or a ruptured globe (a B-scan ultrasound may additionally be helpful).
4. Exploration of the site in the operating room under general anesthesia may be necessary when a ruptured globe is suspected.

Treatment (In case of ruptured globe or penetrating ocular injury see Section 3.15.)

1. Antibiotic ointment (e.g., erythromycin) tid for 4-7 days. A pressure patch can be used for the first 24 hours.
2. Large lacerations (e.g., >1-1.5 cm) may be sutured (e.g., with 7-0 Vicryl), but most lacerations heal without surgical repair. When suturing, it is important not to bury folds of conjunctiva (e.g., by not correctly suturing the edges of the conjunctiva) nor to incorporate tenons capsule in the wound. Additionally, avoid suturing the plica semilunaris or caruncle (both near the medial canthus) to the conjunctiva.

Follow-up   If there is no concomitant ocular damage, patients with large conjunctival lacerations are reexamined within one week; patients with small injuries are seen only as needed.

3.6 Eyelid Laceration

All patients receive a complete ocular examination, including a dilated retinal examination, prior to laceration repair. A CT scan (axial and coronal views) of the orbit and brain needs to be obtained prior to repair in cases of significant orbital trauma or when suspicious of an orbital foreign body or a ruptured globe.

Treatment   All patients should be considered for tetanus prophylaxis (see Appendix 11 for indications).

A. Eyelid lacerations repaired in the operating room or requiring complicated surgical repair:

• Those associated with ocular trauma requiring surgery (e.g., ruptured globe.)

- Those involving the lacrimal drainage apparatus (i.e., punctum, canaliculus, common duct, or lacrimal sac.)
- Those involving the levator aponeurosis of the upper eyelid (producing ptosis) or the superior rectus muscle; orbital fat is often exposed.
- Those in which the medial canthal tendon is avulsed (exhibits a displaced medial canthus or abnormal laxity of the medial canthus.)
- Those associated with an intraorbital foreign body which may be removed.
- Those which cause extensive tissue loss (especially >⅓ of the eyelid) or severe distortion of anatomy.

The treatment of these lacerations is beyond the scope of this book.

B. Delayed repair is beneficial in some eyelid lacerations:

- Those wounds at significant risk for contamination.
- Those wounds from human bites (controversial).

These lacerations are treated as follows:
1. Clean the area of injury and surrounding skin (e.g., Betadine).
2. Irrigate the wound thoroughly with saline in a syringe.
3. Search the wound for foreign bodies, and remove them if present. Debride any severely infected or necrotic tissue. In general, minimal debridement of the eyelid is usually performed due to its vascular nature.
4. Leave the wound open and treat with a topical antibiotic (e.g., bacitracin tid).
5. Apply a sterile dressing to keep the wound clean.
6. 3-4 days later the patient needs surgical debridement and repair.
7. Systemic antibiotics as described below.

C. Eyelid lacerations repaired in the office or emergency room:
1. Clean the area of injury and surrounding skin (e.g., Betadine).
2. Local subcutaneous anesthetic (e.g., 2% lidocaine with epinephrine).
3. Irrigate the wound thoroughly with saline in a syringe.
4. Search the wound carefully for foreign bodies (and remove them if present).
5. Isolate the surgical field with a sterile eye drape.
6. Place a drop of topical anesthetic (e.g., proparacaine) into the eye and a protective eye shell over the eye before suturing.
7. Repair the laceration—one of many methods (Fig. 3.1):
   a. *Lacerations involving the eyelid margin:* The eyelid margin is closed with three sutures prior to closing the part of the laceration extending into the eyelid.

   Suture #1 (5-0 silk): Placed through the gray line (just anterior to the meibomian orifices) of one wound edge (approximately 2 mm

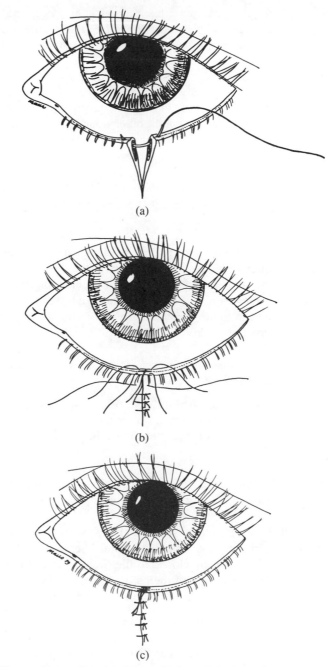

(a)

(b)

(c)

Figure 3.1 Eyelid margin repair. (a) Suture #1 (see text). (b) and (c) At the conclusion of the repair, the eyelid margin sutures are tied under the knot of the skin suture closest to the eyelid margin.

from the laceration margin and 2 mm deep) and then through the gray line of the other wound edge (to arise just anterior to the meibomian orifices of the opposite wound edge). Cut the suture long and do not tie it yet.

Suture #2 (6-0 silk): Passed posterior and parallel to suture #1 in the same manner, through the tarsus of one wound edge and then through the tarsus of the other wound edge. Avoid passing the suture through the palpebral conjunctiva. Cut the suture long and do not tie it yet.

Suture #3 (6-0 silk): Passed anterior and parallel to suture #1 again in the same manner, just posterior to the eyelash line through both wound edges.

Tie all three sutures, leaving the suture ends long.
Stretch the eyelid by pulling on the three suture arms and clamp the sutures with a hemostat to maintain the eyelid on stretch. The suture arms will be incorporated into the knot of the skin suture closest to the eyelid margin at the end of the repair.
Proceed to (b).

b. *Lacerations of the eyelid:* If the laceration is deep, a two-layer closure is required.

Interrupted 6-0 absorbable (e.g., Vicryl) sutures are used to close the tarsus (the deep layer) without passing through the conjunctiva (the posterior aspect of the eyelid). These sutures are cut close to the knot.

The skin and orbicularis (the superficial layer) are closed with interrupted 6-0 or 7-0 nonabsorbable sutures (e.g., nylon).

If the eyelid margin was repaired, the long ends of the three eyelid margin sutures are released from the hemostat and tied under the knot of the skin suture closest to the eyelid margin (to prevent these arms from rubbing against the cornea). The portions of the three arms extending beyond this skin suture are then cut.

The protective eye shell is removed.

8. Antibiotic ointment is applied to the wound bid (e.g., bacitracin).
9. A systemic antibiotic is given if contamination is suspected (e.g., dicloxacillin 250-500 mg po qid [adults]; 25-50 mg/kg/day divided into 4 doses [children] × 2 days. Alternative treatment is cephalexin in the

same dose as dicloxacillin. For human or animal bites, consider adding penicillin V [same dose as dicloxacillin]).

NOTES

1. Do not shave the eyebrow when it has been lacerated; in some cases the hair will not regrow or will do so irregularly.
2. Absorbable suture (e.g., Vicryl) may be used to close the skin when the patient is a child or cannot be counted upon to return.
3. In animal bites (especially dog bites), rabies needs to be considered.

Follow-up Eyelid margin sutures are left in place for 10-14 days. All other superficial sutures are removed in 4-6 days.

3.7 Traumatic Iritis

Symptoms Pain, photophobia, tearing, and a history of ocular trauma within the preceding few days.

Critical Signs White blood cells and flare in the anterior chamber (seen under high power magnification by focusing into the anterior chamber with a small bright beam from the slit lamp).

Other Signs Pain in the traumatized eye when a light is shined in either the nontraumatized or traumatized eye, lower (although sometimes higher) intraocular pressure (IOP) and a smaller pupil (which dilates poorly) in the traumatized eye, perilimbal conjunctival injection, and sometimes decreased vision.

Differential Diagnosis

- Traumatic corneal abrasion   (Corneal epithelial defect which stains with fluorescein. May have an accompanying anterior-chamber reaction.)
- Traumatic microhyphema   (*Red* blood cells suspended in the anterior chamber. Often accompanied by iritis.)
- Traumatic retinal detachment   (May produce an anterior-chamber reaction. May also see pigment in the anterior vitreous. A detachment is seen on dilated fundus examination.)

Work-up Complete ophthalmic examination, including an IOP measurement and a dilated fundus examination.

Treatment Cycloplegic agent (e.g., cyclopentolate 2% qid or scopolamine ¼% tid).

NOTE Some physicians additionally give a steroid drop (e.g., prednisolone acetate ⅛%-1% qid); we do not initially.

Follow-up

• Recheck in a few days to one week (usually one week unless the iritis is severe.)
• If there is no improvement after 5-7 days, a steroid drop (e.g., prednisolone acetate 1% qid) may be given in addition to the cycloplegic agent.
• If resolved, the cycloplegic agent is discontinued.
• Examination of the anterior chamber angle in both eyes by gonioscopy and the ora serrata by indirect ophthalmoscopy with scleral depression are performed one month after the trauma, looking for angle recession (which predisposes the eye to glaucoma) and retinal breaks or a retinal detachment.

3.8 Hyphema and Microhyphema

Symptoms Pain, blurred vision, history of trauma.

Critical Sign Blood in the anterior chamber:

• Hyphema = layering and/or clot.
• Microhyphema = suspended red blood cells only.

Work-up

1. History: Type of injury, exact time of injury, exact time of visual loss, if any.
2. Complete ocular examination, first ruling out a ruptured globe (see Section 3.15). Quantitate (percent) and/or draw the extent of layering of RBCs (mm) and the presence of any clot, measure the intraocular pressure (IOP), and perform a dilated retinal evaluation, if possible. Do not perform gonioscopy or scleral depression.
3. External and periocular examinations, evaluating for other traumatic injuries (e.g., an orbital fracture).
4. Black patients should have a sickle-cell prep (e.g., Sickle Dex) and, when admitted to the hospital, a hemoglobin electrophoresis in addition.
5. Consider a B-scan ultrasound if a retinal detachment cannot be ruled out due to a poor view of the fundus.
6. CT scan (axial and coronal views) of the orbits and brain when indicated.

Treatment

A. *Hyphema and unreliable microhyphema patients*
   1. Hospitalize the patient at bedrest with the head of the bed elevated 30 degrees; bathroom privileges only.
   2. Shield the involved eye at all times (no eye patch unless corneal pathology is present).
   3. Atropine 1% drops 3-4×/day.
   4. Aminocaproic acid (e.g., Amicar) 50 mg/kg po q 4 hours (maximum: 30 grams per day) as a liquid (inform the patient of potential postural hypotension).
   5. No aspirin-containing products.
   6. Mild analgesics only (e.g., acetaminophen +/− codeine).
   7. Antiemetic (e.g., prochlorperazine (e.g., Compazine) 10 mg im q 8 hours or 25 mg pr q 12 hours) prn.
   8. If the IOP is elevated (e.g., >20 mm Hg is a sickle cell or sickle trait positive patient or >30 mm Hg in other patients), treat with a topical beta-blocker (e.g., levobunolol ½% bid or timolol ½% bid). If the IOP is still elevated, consider adding methazolamide (e.g., Neptazane) 50 mg po 2-3×/day (acetazolamide may be used if the patient is sickle trait negative). For further control of IOP add IV mannitol once in a 24-hour period (1-2 g/kg iv over 45 minutes. NOTE: A 500-cc bag of mannitol 20% contains 100 grams of mannitol).

B. *Compliant microhyphema patients*
   1. To be seen on a daily basis as an outpatient for 5 additional days.
   2. Bedrest with the head of the bed elevated as much as possible. No strenuous activities.
   3. No aspirin-containing products.
   4. Mild analgesics only (e.g., acetaminophen).
   5. Atropine 1% drops 3-4×/day.
   6. Shield the involved eye at all times (no patch).
   7. The patient should be instructed to return immediately for reevaluation if he notes a sudden increase in pain or decrease in vision.

Follow-up

A. *Hyphema and unreliable microhyphema patients:* Check the visual acuity, IOP, and slit-lamp examination bid. Look for new bleeding, increased IOP, and corneal blood staining.

   • If the IOP rises (e.g., to a level >20 mm Hg in a sickle cell or sickle-trait-positive patient or >30 mm Hg in other patients), treat as described above.
   • If a heavy fibrinous anterior-chamber reaction develops or if the eye becomes more photophobic or irritated during hospitalization, consider adding topical steroids (e.g., prednisolone acetate 1% q 2-6 hours depending on the severity.)

- If a rebleed does not occur, the Amicar may be halved on post-trauma (or post-rebleed) day 3, and stopped on post-trauma (or post-rebleed) day 4. Observe the patient for one additional day before discharge.
- If there is a rebleed, continue the above treatment for an additional 5 days, observing closely for elevated IOP and corneal blood staining. Recalculate the Amicar dosage (to make certain it is correct) and check clotting studies (e.g., PT, PTT, bleeding time, platelet count). (Patients rarely rebleed on the appropriate dosage of Amicar.)
- If the patient's vision deteriorates significantly, the entire anterior chamber becomes filled with blood, a substantial clot persists in the anterior chamber for 7 days, corneal blood staining occurs, or the IOP cannot be lowered to a safe level despite maximal medical therapy, surgical evacuation of the hyphema may be indicated.

If no complications arise, the patient may be discharged the sixth day post-trauma.

Discharge instructions:
1. Atropine 1% drops 1-3 × /day (dosage depends on the amount of anterior-chamber reaction).
2. Topical steroid (e.g., prednisolone acetate 1%) 3-4 × /day if an inflammatory element results in patient discomfort.
3. Antiglaucoma medication if required to control increased IOP.
4. Glasses or eye shield during the day and the eye shield at night for 2 weeks post-trauma, after which the patient should be advised to wear protective eyewear (polycarbonate lenses) any time there exists the potential of an eye injury.
5. Refrain from strenuous physical activities for 2 weeks from the date of the initial injury and then *gradually* resume activities. Not until 4 weeks from the date of the original injury can one resume all normal activities.

Outpatient examinations following discharge:
1. 2-3 days later.
2. 3-4 weeks later for gonioscopy and dilated fundus examination with scleral depression (scleral depression and gonioscopy should not be performed until this time if it can be avoided).
3. Yearly (due to the potential of developing angle-recession glaucoma).

If any complications arise, more frequent follow-up examinations are required.

B. *Compliant microhyphema patients*   The vision, IOP, and anterior segment are evaluated daily until the fifth day post-trauma and then one week later. Gonioscopy and a dilated fundus examination with scleral depression are performed 3-4 weeks after the trauma as described above.

• If a rebleed or an intractable IOP rise occurs, the patient should be hospitalized and treated as above.

NOTES

1. A spontaneous hyphema in a child should make one suspect juvenile xanthogranuloma, child abuse, leukemia, or possibly retinoblastoma.
2. Postoperative hyphemas generally resolve spontaneously, usually requiring simple observation. The IOP must be monitored closely.
3. Gonioscopy should be performed in nontraumatic cases to rule out a bleeding blood vessel from a corneal wound.

3.9 Commotio Retinae

Symptoms   Decreased vision or asymptomatic; a history of recent ocular trauma can be elicited.

Critical Sign   A confluent area of retinal whitening.

Other Signs   The retinal blood vessels are seen more clearly in the area of retinal whitening. Other signs of ocular trauma may be noted.

Differential Diagnosis

• Retinal detachment   (Retinal vessels can be seen to rise upward with the detached retina. May see a retinal break or dialysis. Anterior vitreous pigment and an anterior-chamber reaction are common.)
• Branch retinal artery occlusion   (Rarely follows trauma. Whitening of the retina with edema occurs along the distribution of an artery; may see cotton wool spots, narrowed arterioles, and dilated veins with sludging of blood in the affected vessels.)
• White without pressure   (A common retinal anomaly unrelated to trauma. A prominent vitreous base is seen in the peripheral retina, often in several locations, including the other eye.)

Work-up   Complete ophthalmic examination, including a dilated fundus examination with scleral depression.

NOTE   Scleral depression is not performed when a hyphema, microhyphema, or iritis is present.

Treatment   No treatment is required, as this condition usually clears without therapy.

Follow-up   A dilated fundus examination is repeated in 1-2 weeks. Patients are instructed to return sooner if symptoms of decreased vision or floaters or flashing lights are experienced, or if a curtain appears to drop over part of the visual field.

3.10   Traumatic Choroidal Rupture

Symptoms   Decreased vision or asymptomatic. History of ocular trauma.

Critical Signs   A yellow or white crescent-shaped subretinal streak usually concentric to the optic disc. It may be single or multiple. Often the rupture cannot be seen until several days or weeks following the trauma, as it may be obscured by overlying blood.

Other Signs   Rarely the rupture may be radially oriented. A choroidal neovascular membrane (CNVM) may later develop.

Differential Diagnosis

• Lacquer cracks of high myopia   (Often bilateral. May additionally see a tilted disc, a scleral crescent adjacent to the disc, or a posterior staphyloma. A CNVM may also develop in this condition.)
• Angioid streaks   (Bilateral reddish-brown or gray subretinal streaks which radiate out from the optic disc, sometimes associated with a CNVM.)

Work-up

1. Complete ocular examination, including a dilated fundus evaluation to detect a traumatic choroidal rupture or an area of blood obscuring the fundus. A CNVM is best seen with a slit lamp and a fundus contact or 60 or 90 diopter lens.
2. Consider fluorescein angiography to confirm the presence of a choroidal rupture or to delineate a CNVM.

Treatment   Laser therapy is instituted when a CNVM more than 200 microns from the center of the fovea is discovered within the macula and there is no foveolar hemorrhage or exudate. Treatment should be applied within 72 hours of obtaining the fluorescein angiogram.

Follow-up   Following ocular trauma, patients with hemorrhage obscuring the underlying choroid are reevaluated every 1-2 weeks until the choroid can be well visualized. If a choroidal rupture is present, patients are instructed on the use of an Amsler grid and asked to test themselves daily, returning immediately if a change in the appearance of the grid is noted (see Appendix 3). Fundus examinations are performed every 3-6 months. Patients treated for a CNVM need to be followed closely after treatment, watching for a persistent or new CNVM (see Section 12.10 for further follow-up guidelines).

3.11   Orbital Blow-out Fracture

Symptoms   Pain (especially on attempted vertical eye movement), local tenderness, binocular double vision (the double vision disappears when one eye is covered), eyelid swelling after nose blowing, recent history of trauma.

Critical Signs   Restricted eye movement (especially in upward and/or lateral gaze), orbital subcutaneous emphysema, hypesthesia in the distribution of the infraorbital nerve (ipsilateral cheek and upper lip), enophthalmos (may initially be masked by orbital edema).

Other Signs   Nosebleed, eyelid edema and ecchymosis, ptosis.

Differential Diagnosis

- Orbital edema and hemorrhage without a blow-out fracture   (May have limitation of ocular movement, periorbital swelling, and ecchymosis, but these resolve over 7-10 days.)
- Cranial-nerve palsy   (Limitation of eye movement, but no restriction on forced duction testing.)

Work-up

1. Complete ophthalmologic examination, including a measurement of extraocular movements and globe displacement. Compare the sensation of the ipsilateral cheek with that on the contralateral side; palpate the eyelids for crepitus (subcutaneous emphysema); and evaluate the globe carefully for a rupture, hyphema/microhyphema, traumatic iritis, and retinal/choroidal damage. The intraocular pressure (IOP) should be measured.
2. Forced duction testing is performed if restriction of eye movement persists beyond one week (see Appendix 6).
3. CT scan of the orbits and brain (axial and coronal views) is obtained if the diagnosis is uncertain or if surgical repair is being considered.

Treatment

1. Nasal decongestants (e.g., Afrin nasal spray bid) for 10-14 days.
2. Broad-spectrum oral antibiotics (e.g., cephalexin [e.g., Keflex] 250-500 mg po qid or erythromycin 250-500 mg po qid) for 10-14 days.
3. Instruct the patient not to blow his nose.
4. Ice packs to the orbit for the first 24-48 hours.
5. Surgical repair at 10-14 days following trauma is undertaken if the patient has persistent diplopia when looking straight or attempting to read, if he has cosmetically unacceptable enophthalmos, or if a large fracture is present.

NOTE   Some physicians use oral steroids initially to decrease the inflammatory reaction (we generally do not).

Follow-up   Patients should be seen at 1 and 2 weeks post-trauma and evaluated for persistent diplopia or enophthalmos after the acute orbital edema has subsided. The presence of these findings may indicate entrapment of the orbital contents and the need for surgical repair. Patients should also be monitored for the development of associated ocular injuries (e.g., orbital cellulitis, angle recession glaucoma, and retinal detachment).Gonioscopy of the anterior chamber angle and a dilated retinal examination with scleral depression is performed 3-4 weeks after the trauma. Warning symptoms of retinal detachment and orbital cellulitis are explained to the patient.

3.12   Traumatic Retrobulbar Hemorrhage

Symptoms   Pain, decreased vision, recent history of trauma to the eye or orbit.

Critical Signs   Proptosis with resistance to retropulsion, diffuse subconjunctival hemorrhage without any visible sclera posterior to the hemorrhage.

Other Signs   Eyelid ecchymosis, chemosis, and elevated intraocular pressure (IOP). May have limited extraocular motility in any or all fields of gaze, crepitus, or infraorbital hypesthesia.

Differential Diagnosis

• Orbital cellulitis   (Fever, proptosis, chemosis, limitation of eye movements with pain on motion; also may follow trauma, but generally not as acute.)

- Orbital fracture (blow-out, medial wall, or tripod fracture) (Limited extraocular motility, infraorbital hypesthesia, and subcutaneous emphysema. Enophthalmos, not proptosis, may be present.)
- Ruptured globe (Subconjunctival edema and hemorrhage may mask a ruptured globe. A deep anterior chamber, a hyphema, and limitation of ocular motility are often present. IOP is commonly low, and there is usually no proptosis.)

Work-up

1. Complete ophthalmic examination, checking specifically for an afferent pupillary defect, loss of color vision (color plates), elevated or decreased IOP, pulsations of the central retinal artery, and choroidal folds (signs that vision is threatened). (Pulsations of the central retinal artery often precede a central retinal artery occlusion.)
2. CT scan of the orbit (axial and coronal views). The CT scan should be delayed until treatment has been instituted in cases in which vision is threatened.

Treatment   If the IOP is elevated (e.g., >30 mm Hg in a patient with a normal optic nerve or >20 mm Hg in a patient whose optic cup is very large and who normally has a lower IOP), any or all of the following methods are employed to lower the IOP. When vision is threatened all of them are instituted immediately.

1. Carbonic anhydrase inhibitor (e.g., acetazolamide 250 mg po × 2 simultaneously).
2. Topical beta-blocker (e.g., timolol ½% q 30 minutes × 2).
3. Hyperosmotic agent (e.g., mannitol 20% 1-2 g/kg iv over 45 minutes. NOTE   A 500-cc bag of mannitol 20% contains 100 grams of mannitol.)
4. Lateral canthotomy and cantholysis (See Fig. 3.2) (A hemostat is placed horizontally over the lateral canthus and clamped for one minute to compress the tissues and reduce bleeding. (a) It is released and sterile scissors are used to make a horizontal incision approximately 1 cm into the tissue compressed by the hemostat. (b) The skin and conjunctiva in the area of the incision are separated and the scissors are placed between them to cut the inferior arm of the lateral canthal tendon. (c) Hemostasis is generally achieved with pressure. A sterile dressing is placed over the wound.)

If the IOP is not lowered or if vision is still threatened after the above treatment, hospitalization is indicated. Emergent orbital decompression surgery may be required if the optic nerve becomes compromised, visual acuity decreases, or color vision is lost.

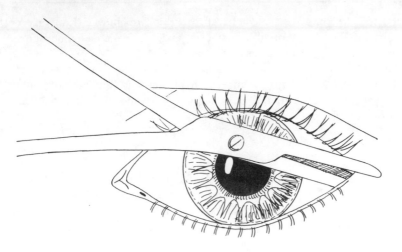

(a)

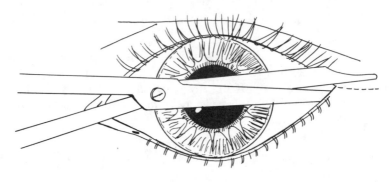

(b)

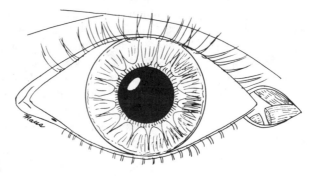

(c)

Figure 3.2 See text, page 37.

Follow-up   In vision-threatening cases, follow daily until stable. After the acute episode has resolved, reexamination should be performed every few weeks at first, watching for infection and abscess formation. Fibrosis may develop later, limiting extraocular motility.

3.13   Intraorbital Foreign Body

Symptoms   May be asymptomatic or may have decreased vision, pain, eyelid swelling, or double vision. The patient usually has a history of trauma (days to years prior).

Critical Signs   Orbital foreign body identified by x-ray, CT scan, and/or orbital ultrasound.

Other Signs   A palpable orbital mass, limitation of ocular motility, proptosis, swollen, erythematous eyelids and/or a conjunctival or eyelid laceration or scar. An inert orbital foreign body may not produce any signs. The presence of an afferent pupillary defect may be due to a traumatic optic neuropathy.

Types of Foreign Bodies
  A. *Poorly tolerated* (often lead to inflammation)   Organic (e.g., wood and vegetable matter) and sometimes copper foreign bodies.
  B. *Fairly well tolerated* (typically produce a chronic low grade inflammatory reaction)   Copper alloys (<85% copper, e.g., brass, bronze).
  C. *Well tolerated* (inert)   Stone, glass, plastic, iron, lead, steal, aluminum, and most other metals.

NOTE   BBs and shotgun pellets are typically made of 80-90% lead and 10-20% iron.

Work-up
  1. History: Determine the composition of the foreign body, the time period since the original injury, and the degree of symptoms.
  2. Complete ocular and periorbital examination, with special attention to the pupillary reaction, intraocular pressure (IOP), and retinal evaluation (determining whether an afferent pupillary defect and decreased vision can be accounted for by the retinal findings.) Examine carefully for an entry site.
  3. CT scan of the orbit and brain (axial and coronal views). Rule out a ruptured globe, determine the location of the intraorbital foreign body, and rule out

optic-nerve or CNS involvement. An MRI is contraindicated if a metal foreign body is suspected or cannot be ruled out.
4. B-scan orbital ultrasound if a foreign body is suspected but not detected by CT scan.
5. If possible, culture the object from which the foreign body arose. Culture any drainage sites.

Surgical Treatment Indications   The following may be indications for surgical exploration and attempted extraction of the foreign body.

1. Signs of infection (e.g., fever, proptosis, restricted motility, severe chemosis, a palpable orbital mass, or an abscess on CT scan).
2. Fistula formation.
3. Signs of optic-nerve compression (seen on CT scan in a patient with an afferent pupillary defect and poor vision).
4. The presence of a "poorly tolerated" intraorbital foreign body (see above) when it can be well localized.
5. A large or sharp-edged foreign body (independent of composition) that can be easily extracted.

Treatment

1. Hospitalization.
2. Systemic antibiotics (e.g., gentamicin 1.75 mg/kg load iv followed by 1 mg/kg q 8 hours, plus cefazolin 1 g iv q 8 hours or clindamycin 600 mg iv q 8 hours).[1]
3. Tetanus toxoid prn (see Appendix 11 for indications).
4. Surgical exploration and removal of the foreign body when indicated. No food or drink prior to surgery (NPO).

Follow-up   Daily, checking vision, assessing the degree (if any) of an afferent pupillary defect, measuring IOP, and evaluating motility, proptosis, and eye discomfort. If no complications develop and a decision to leave the foreign body within the orbit is made, the patient is discharged from the hospital after 4-10 days. Oral antibiotics (e.g., amoxicillin/clavulanate (e.g., Augmentin) 250-500 mg po q 8 hours) are given to complete a 10-14 day course of antibiotic therapy. The patient is told to return in one week for a checkup, sooner if the condition worsens.

---

[1]The dosages may need to be adjusted in the presence of renal dysfunction. Peak and trough levels of gentamicin are obtained ½ hour before and after the fifth dose, and BUN and creatinine levels are evaluated every other day.

See "Ruptured Globe and Penetrating Ocular Injury" (Section 3.15), "Traumatic Optic Neuropathy" (Section 3.17), "Orbital Cellulitis" (Section 7.4), "Hyphema and Microhyphema" (Section 3.8), and "Inflammatory Open-Angle Glaucoma" (Section 10.4) for the management of these entities.

3.14 Corneal Laceration

A. **Partial-thickness laceration**   (The anterior chamber is not entered and, therefore, the globe is not penetrated.)

Work-up

1. Complete ocular examination, carefully ruling out ocular penetration with a slit lamp. Carefully inspect the cornea, conjunctiva, and sclera. Make sure the anterior chamber is deep and without blood. Measure the intraocular pressure (IOP) by applanation tonometry only if the laceration site can be avoided (otherwise gently assess the IOP with your fingers).
2. Seidel test (see Appendix 4). If the Seidel test is positive and a full thickness laceration is present, then see (B) below.

Treatment

1. A cycloplegic (e.g., scopolamine ¼%), an antibiotic (e.g., erythromycin ointment or gentamicin drop), plus a pressure patch.
2. Occasionally a soft contact lens is used with an antibiotic drop (e.g., gentamicin qid) after cycloplegia as above.

NOTE   When a moderate-to-deep corneal laceration is accompanied by a wound gape, it is often best to suture the wound closed in the operating room.

Follow-up   Reevaluate daily as above until the epithelium heals.

B. **Full-thickness laceration**   See Section 3.15.

3.15 Ruptured Globe and Penetrating Ocular Injury

Symptoms   Pain, decreased vision, history of trauma.

Critical Signs

A. *Ruptured globe:* Severe subconjunctival edema and hemorrhage, abnormally deep anterior chamber, hyphema (often with clotted blood), limitation of extraocular motility (most restriction when moving toward the direction of the rupture), intraocular contents may be outside of the globe.
B. *Penetrating injury:* Full thickness scleral or corneal laceration accompanying signs of a ruptured globe. History of a sharp object entering the globe.

Other Signs   Low intraocular pressure (IOP) (although it may be normal or elevated), irregular pupil, iridodialysis, cyclodialysis, periorbital ecchymosis, subluxed lens, commotio retinae, choroidal rupture, retinal breaks, traumatic optic neuropathy.

Work-up/Treatment   Once the diagnosis of a ruptured globe or penetrating ocular injury is made by penlight (or slit-lamp examination if necessary), further examination should be deferred until the time of surgical repair in the operating room (to avoid placing any pressure on the globe and risking extrusion of the intraocular contents). The following measures should be taken:

1. Protect the eye with a shield.
2. No food or drink (NPO).
3. Systemic antibiotics (e.g., Adults: cefazolin 1 g iv q 8 hours + gentamicin 1.75 mg/kg iv load, then gentamicin 1 mg/kg iv q 8 hours. Children: cefazolin 25-50 mg/kg/day iv in three divided doses + gentamicin 2 mg/kg iv q 8 hours).[2]
4. Tetanus toxoid prn (see Appendix 11).
5. Antiemetic (e.g., prochlorperazine (e.g., Compazine) 10 mg im q 8 hour) prn.
6. Sedative (e.g., temazepam 15 mg po) prn.
7. Bed rest with bathroom privileges.
8. Determine when the patient had his last meal. The timing of surgical repair may be influenced by this information.
9. CT scan (axial and coronal views) of the orbits and brain +/− B-scan ultrasound are needed to localize the rupture site(s) and to rule out an intraocular or intraorbital foreign body.
10. Arrange for surgical repair to be done as soon as possible.

---

[2]Antibiotic doses may need to be reduced if renal function is impaired. Gentamicin peak and trough levels are obtained ½ hour before and after the fifth dose and BUN and creatinine levels are evaluated every other day.

NOTE   In any severely traumatized eye in which there is no chance of restoring vision, enucleation should be considered initially or within the first 7-14 days after the trauma.

3.16   Intraocular Foreign Body

Symptoms   Eye pain, decreased vision, or may be asymptomatic. A suggestive history is often provided (e.g., ocular foreign body after hammering metal).

Critical Signs   May or may not have a clinically detectable corneal or scleral perforation site or an intraocular foreign body. Intraocular foreign bodies are usually seen on CT scan and/or B-scan ultrasound.

Other Signs   Microcystic (epithelial) edema of the peripheral cornea (a clue that a foreign body may be hidden in the anterior chamber angle in the same sector of the eye), an iris transillumination defect (see below), an irregular pupil, anterior and/or posterior segment inflammation, vitreous hemorrhage, decreased intraocular pressure (IOP).

Types of Foreign Bodies

A. Frequently produce severe inflammatory reactions when left in the eye:
   1. Magnetic: Iron and steel.
   2. Nonmagnetic: Copper.
B. Typically produce mild inflammatory reactions when left in the eye:
   1. Magnetic: Nickel.
   2. Nonmagnetic: Aluminum, lead, mercury, and zinc.
C. Inert foreign bodies: Carbon, coal, glass, lead, plaster, platinum, porcelain, rubber, silver, and stone.

NOTES

1. Even inert foreign bodies can be toxic to the eye due to a coating or chemical additive.
2. Most BBs and gunshot pellets are made of 80-90% lead and 10-20% iron.

Work-up

1. History: Composition of foreign body, time of last meal, tetanus immunization status.

2. Ocular examination, including a visual-acuity assessment and a careful evaluation of whether the globe is intact. If there is an obvious perforation site, the remainder of the examination may be deferred until surgery. If there does not appear to be a risk of extrusion of the intraocular contents, the globe is inspected gently to localize the site of perforation and detect the foreign body.

   a. Slit-lamp examination, searching the anterior chamber and iris for a foreign body and looking for an iris transillumination defect (direct a small beam of light directly through the pupil and look at the iris for a red reflex penetrating through it.) Check the IOP.

   b. Consider gonioscopy of the anterior chamber angle if no wound leak can be detected and the globe appears intact. (This may produce an aqueous leak if the cornea has been perforated.)

   c. Dilated retinal examination using indirect ophthalmoscopy.

3. Obtain a CT scan of the orbit and brain (coronal and axial views). (An MRI is contraindicated in the presence of an intraocular foreign body that may be metallic).

4. B-scan ultrasound of the globe and orbit. (Note that intraocular air can mimic a foreign body).

5. Culture the object from which the foreign body arose (if possible). Culture any wound site if present.

6. Determine whether the foreign body is magnetic (e.g., examine the hammer, nail, or piece of metal off of which the foreign body broke).

Treatment

1. Hospitalization.
2. No food or drink (NPO).
3. Place a protective shield over the involved eye.
4. Tetanus prophylaxis as needed (see Appendix 11).
5. IV antibiotics (e.g., gentamicin 1.75 mg/kg iv load, then 1 mg/kg q 8 hours plus cefazolin 1 g iv q 8 hours or clindamycin 600 mg iv q 8 hours).[3]
6. Cycloplegic (e.g., atropine 1% tid).
7. Surgical removal of the intraocular foreign body may be advisable in the following situations:

---

[3]Dosages may need to be adjusted in the presence of renal dysfunction. Peak and trough levels of gentamicin are obtained ½ hour before and after the fifth dose, and BUN and creatinine levels are evaluated every other day.

a. When the foreign body is composed of iron, steel, or copper.
b. A large foreign body (even if inert) in the visual axis.
c. Any foreign body associated with severe recurrent inflammation.
d. A foreign body which may be extracted without much difficulty during the surgical repair of an ocular structure.

Follow-up Observe closely in the hospital for signs of inflammation. Periodic follow-up for years is required, watching for a delayed inflammatory reaction. When an intraocular foreign body is left in place, an electroretinogram (ERG) should be obtained as soon as it can be done safely and the patient should have serial ERGs performed looking for toxic retinal metallosis. If found, this retinal toxicity often reverses after the foreign body is removed.

3.17 Traumatic Optic Neuropathy

Symptoms Decreased vision after a traumatic injury, other symptoms from trauma (e.g., pain).

Critical Signs A new afferent pupillary defect in a traumatized eye that cannot be accounted for by retinal pathology (which would have to be severe) or chiasmal damage.

Other Signs Relatively poor color vision in the affected eye, a visual field defect, and other signs of trauma.

NOTE Optic disc pallor may not appear for weeks following a traumatic optic-nerve injury.

Etiology Shearing injury from blunt trauma; compression of the nerve by bone, hemorrhage, or perineural edema; laceration of the nerve by bone or an intraorbital foreign body (which may or may not still be present in the orbit).

Differential Diagnosis (Other causes of a traumatic afferent pupillary defect)

• Severe retinal trauma   (Retinal pathology evident on examination.)
• Traumatic vitreous hemorrhage   (Obscured retinal view on dilated-fundus examination. The relative afferent pupillary defect is mild.)
• Intracranial trauma with damage to the optic chiasm.

Work-up

1. Complete ocular examination (if a penetrating injury/ruptured globe is ruled out and it is determined to be safe to fully examine the globe without risking extrusion of the intraocular contents). A pupillary evaluation is essential in order to diagnose a traumatic optic neuropathy.
2. Color vision testing in each eye (color plates).
3. Visual fields by confrontation. (Formal visual-field testing may be deferred.)
4. CT scan of the head and orbit with coronal and axial views to rule out an intraorbital foreign body and to possibly determine the cause of the optic neuropathy.
5. B-scan orbital ultrasound when a foreign body is suspected, but not discovered by CT scan.

Treatment

1. Consider hospitalization in acute cases.
2. Systemic antibiotics in the presence of a sinus wall fracture or penetrating orbital injury (e.g., gentamicin 1.75 mg/kg iv load, then 1 mg/kg iv q 8 hours, plus cefazolin 1 g iv q 8 hours or clindamycin 600 mg iv q 8 hours).[4]

- Consider IV steroids (e.g., methylprednisolone 250 mg iv q 6 hours × 12 doses) plus an H_2-blocker (e.g., ranitidine 150 mg po bid) (controversial). See Appendix 5 when considering systemic steroids.
- Surgical intervention is indicated when vision is decreasing.

Follow-up   Daily. Evaluate vision, pupillary reactions, and color vision. If the vision deteriorates after the termination of steroids, they should be reinstituted as previously. If visual deterioration occurs despite steroids, surgery is indicated.

---

[4]Dosages may need to be adjusted in the presence of renal dysfunction. Peak and trough levels of gentamicin are obtained ½ hour before and after the fifth dose. BUN and creatinine levels are evaluated every other day.

4

Cornea

4.1 Superficial Punctate Keratitis (SPK)

Symptoms   Pain, photophobia, red eye, foreign-body sensation.

Critical Signs   Small pinpoint corneal epithelial defects (stain with fluorescein).

Other Signs   Conjunctival injection.

Etiology   SPK are nonspecific, but are most commonly seen with the following disorders:

- Dry eye syndrome   (Poor tear lake or a decreased tear break-up time.)
- Blepharitis   (Erythema, telangiectasias, and crusting of the eyelid margins.)
- Trauma   (Can occur from relatively mild trauma, such as chronic eye rubbing.)
- Exposure keratopathy   (Poor eyelid closure with failure to cover the entire globe.)
- Topical drug toxicity (e.g., neomycin, tobramycin, or any drops with preservatives including artificial tears)
- Ultraviolet burn/photokeratopathy   (Often in welders or from sun lamps.)
- Mild chemical injury
- Contact-lens-related disorder (e.g., chemical toxicity, tight-lens syndrome, contact-lens overwear syndrome, giant papillary conjunctivitis, etc.)

- Thygeson's superficial punctate keratopathy (Bilateral, recurrent SPK without conjunctival injection.)
- Foreign body under the upper eyelid (Typically linear SPK, fine scratches arranged vertically.)
- Conjunctivitis (Discharge, eyelids stuck together upon awakening.)
- Trichiasis/distiachiasis (Eyelash[es] rubbing on the cornea.)

Work-up

1. History: Trauma? Contact-lens wear? Eyedrops? Discharge or eyelid matting?
2. Slit-lamp examination using fluorescein stain: Evaluate the tear film, test eyelid closure, and evert the upper eyelids.
3. Inspect contact lenses for fit (if still in the eye) and for the presence of deposits, sharp edges, cracks, etc.

NOTE A soft contact lens should be removed prior to placing fluorescein in the eye.

Treatment See the appropriate section in order to treat the underlying disorder. SPK are often treated nonspecifically as follows:

A. Non-contact-lens wearer with a small amount of SPK
  1. Artificial tears, preferably nonpreserved (e.g., Refresh) qid.
  2. Can add a lubricating ointment qhs (e.g., Refresh PM).
B. Non-contact-lens wearer with a large amount of SPK
  1. Antibiotic ointment (e.g., erythromycin ointment), cycloplegics (e.g., tropicamide 1% plus cyclopentolate 2%), and a pressure patch for 24 hours.
  2. Antibiotic (e.g., erythromycin ointment 2-3×/day or sulfacetamide drops qid) × 4 days after the patch is removed.
C. Contact-lens wearer with a small amount of SPK
  1. Artificial tears, preferably nonpreserved (e.g., Refresh) qid.
  2. Lenses may or may not be worn, depending on the symptoms and the degree of SPK.
D. Contact-lens wearer with a large amount of SPK
  1. Discontinue contact-lens wear.
  2. Tobramycin drops 4-6×/day and tobramycin ointment qhs.
  3. Consider a cycloplegic drop (e.g., scopolamine 1/4%) for pain.

Follow-up

A. Non-contact-lens wearers with SPK (especially traumatic SPK) are not seen again solely for the SPK unless the patient is a child or is unreliable. Reliable patients are told to return if their symptoms worsen or do not improve. When underlying ocular pathology is responsible for the SPK, follow-up is in accordance with the guidelines for the underlying problem (see the specific section).

B. Contact-lens wearers with a large amount of SPK are seen every day until significant improvement is demonstrated. Contact lenses are not to be worn until the condition clears. The tobramycin may be stopped when the SPK resolves. The patient's contact-lens habits (e.g., wearing time and cleaning routine) are corrected and/or the contact lenses are changed if cither is thought to be responsible (see Section 4.17). Contact-lens wearers with a small amount of SPK are rechecked within several days to a week, depending on their symptoms and degree of SPK.

NOTE   In general, contact-lens wearers should not wear their lenses whenever their eyes feel irritated.

4.2   Dry Eye Syndrome

Symptoms   Burning or foreign-body sensation, may have *excess* tearing, often exacerbated by smoke, wind, heat, low humidity, or prolonged use of the eye. Usually bilateral and chronic (although patients sometimes present with recent onset in one eye). Often causes more discomfort than the clinical signs would suggest.

Critical Signs   (Either or both may be present.)

- Scanty tear meniscus seen at the inferior eyelid margin. The meniscus should be at least 1 mm in height with a convex shape.
- Decreased tear break-up time. The time measured from a blink to the appearance of a tear film defect (using fluorescein stain) should be greater than 10 seconds.

Other Signs   Punctate corneal and/or conjunctival fluorescein or rose bengal staining, usually in the interpalpebral area. Excess mucus or debris in the tear film and filaments on the cornea may be found.

Differential Diagnosis

- Blepharitis   (Eyelid margin crusting, thickening, erythema, and telangiectasias, often seen in combination with dry eyes.)

- Eyelid abnormality leading to exposure (exposure keratopathy) (Often secondary to a seventh-nerve palsy, trauma, a chemical or thermal burn, a congenital anomaly, senile ectropion, etc.)
- Nocturnal lagophthalmos (Eyelids remain partially open while asleep.)

Etiology

- Idiopathic
- Collagen vascular diseases (e.g., Sjögren's syndrome, rheumatoid arthritis, Wegener's granulomatosis, systemic lupus erythematosis)
- Conjunctival scarring (e.g., ocular pemphigoid, Stevens-Johnson syndrome, trachoma, chemical burn)
- Drugs (e.g., oral contraceptives, antihistamines, phenothiazines, atropine)
- Infiltration of the lacrimal glands (e.g., sarcoidosis, tumor, etc.)
- Postradiation therapy fibrosis of the lacrimal glands
- Vitamin A deficiency (Usually from malnutrition or intestinal malabsorption.)

Work-up

1. History and external examination to detect an underlying etiology.
2. Slit-lamp examination: Using fluorescein stain, examine the tear meniscus and tear break-up time.
3. Schirmer test
   Technique: Schirmer filter paper is placed at the junction of the middle and lateral third of the lower eyelid in each eye for 5 minutes after drying the eye of excess tears.
   a. Unanesthetized—Measures basal and reflex tearing.
      Normal = wetting of greater than or equal to 15 mm in 5 minutes
   b. Anesthetized—Topical anesthetic (e.g., proparacaine) applied before drying with cotton swab and placing filter paper—Measures basal tearing only.
      Normal = wetting of greater than or equal to 10 mm in 5 minutes
   We prefer the anesthetized method.

Treatment

MILD

Artificial tears qid (e.g., Refresh, Tears Plus, Hypo tears, etc.)

MODERATE

1. Increase frequency of artificial tear application to up to every 1-2 hours— use preservative free tears (e.g., Refresh).

2. Can add a lubricating ointment at bedtime (e.g., Refresh PM, Lacrilube, Duolube, etc.).

SEVERE

1. Lubricating ointment (e.g., Refresh PM) 2-3 × /day during the daytime with preservative-free artificial tears q 1-2 hours.
2. Patching with lubrication at night (may need to patch during the day).
3. Consider 10-20% acetylcysteine (e.g., Mucomyst) qid if mucus strands or filaments are present.
4. Consider an artificial-tear insert (e.g., Lacrisert) with tears and ointment.
5. If the above measures are unsuccessful consider punctal occlusion with collagen or silicone plugs or occlusion by electric cautery.
6. Consider a lateral tarsorrhaphy if all of the above fail. A temporary adhesive tape tarsorrhaphy (tape the lateral one-third of the eyelid closed) can also be used before a surgical tarsorrhaphy.

NOTES

1. In addition to treating the dry eye, treatment for contributing disorders (e.g., blepharitis and exposure keratopathy) needs to be instituted if present.
2. Always use preservative-free artificial tears if using them more frequently than every 3 hours.
3. If the history suggests the presence of a previously undiagnosed collagen vascular disease (e.g., history of arthritic pain), referral should be made to an internist or rheumatologist for further evaluation.

Follow-up   In days to weeks, depending upon the severity of the drying changes and the symptoms. Anyone with severe dry eyes caused by an underlying chronic systemic disease such as rheumatoid arthritis, sarcoidosis, or ocular pemphigoid may need to be monitored more closely.

NOTE   Patients with severe dry eyes should be discouraged from contact-lens wear.

4.3   Filamentary Keratopathy

Symptoms   Moderate-to-severe pain, red eye, foreign-body sensation, photophobia.

Critical Signs   Short strands of epithelial cells and mucus attached to the anterior surface of the cornea at one end of the strand. The strands stain with fluorescein.

Other Signs   Conjunctival injection, poor tear film, superficial punctate keratitis.

Etiology

- Dry eye syndrome   (Most common cause. Can be associated with an autoimmune collagen vascular disease such as Sjögren's syndrome [dryness of the mouth and other mucous membranes].)
- Superior limbic keratoconjunctivitis   (Superior conjunctival injection and fluorescein staining, superior corneal pannus.)
- Recurrent corneal erosions   (Recurrent spontaneous corneal abrasions often occurring upon awakening.)
- Patching (e.g., postoperative, following corneal abrasions)

Work-up

1. History, especially for the above conditions.
2. Slit-lamp examination with fluorescein staining.

Treatment

1. Treat the underlying condition (see the specific sections).
2. Consider debridement of the filaments: After applying topical anesthesia (e.g., proparacaine) remove filaments at their base with fine forceps or a cotton-tipped applicator.
3. Lubrication with one of the following regimens:
   a. Artificial tears (e.g., Refresh) 4-8×/day and artificial-tear ointment (e.g., Refresh PM) qhs.
   b. Sodium chloride 5% drops qid and ointment qhs.
   c. Acetylcysteine 10-20% (e.g., Mucomyst) qid.
4. If the symptoms are severe or the above treatment fails then consider a bandage soft contact lens, unless the patient has severe dry eyes. Extended wear bandage soft contact lenses may need to be worn for months.

Follow-up   In 1-4 weeks. If the condition is not improved, then consider or repeat the debridement and/or bandage soft contact lens if not yet tried. Lubrication must be maintained chronically if the underlying condition cannot be eliminated.

4.4   Exposure Keratopathy

Symptoms   Ocular irritation, burning, foreign-body sensation, and redness of one or both eyes. Usually worst in the morning.

Critical Signs Inadequate blinking or closure of the eyelids leading to corneal drying. Superficial punctate keratitis is found on the lower one-third of the cornea or as a horizontal band in the region of the palpebral fissure.

Other Signs Conjunctival injection, corneal infiltrate or ulcer, eyelid deformity, or abnormal eyelid closure.

Etiology

- Seventh-nerve palsy (orbicularis oculi weakness—e.g., Bell's palsy.)
- Eyelid deformity (e.g., ectropion or eyelid scarring from trauma, chemical burn, or herpes zoster ophthalmicus.)
- Nocturnal lagophthalmos (Failure to close the eyes during sleep.)
- Proptosis (e.g., due to an orbital process, such as thyroid eye disease.)
- Postptosis repair or postblepharoplasty procedures.

Differential Diagnosis See Section 4.1.

Work-up

1. History: Previous Bell's palsy or eyelid surgery? Thyroid disease?
2. Evaluate eyelid closure and corneal exposure. Ask the patient to close his eyes gently (as if he were sleeping).
3. Slit-lamp examination, evaluating the tear film and corneal integrity (with fluorescein dye). Look for signs of secondary infection (corneal infiltrate, anterior-chamber reaction, severe conjunctival injection).
4. Investigate why the patient has an underlying disorder (e.g., why a seventh-nerve problem exists).

Treatment (In the presence of secondary infection, see Section 4.12)

1. Correct the underlying disorder.
2. Artificial tears (e.g., Refresh tears q 1-6 hours).
3. Lubricating ointment (e.g., Refresh PM qhs or up to qid).
4. Consider eyelid taping or patching at bedtime to maintain the eyelids in the closed position. If severe, consider taping the lateral third of the eyelids closed (allowing the patient to see) during the day. (Taping is rarely a definitive therapy, but may be tried when the underlying disorder is thought to be temporary.)
5. When maximal medical therapy fails to prevent progressive corneal deterioration, one of the following surgical procedures may be beneficial:
   a. Eyelid reconstruction (e.g., for ectropion).
   b. Tarsorrhaphy.
   c. Orbital decompression (e.g., for proptosis).

    d. Conjunctival flap.

Follow-up Reevaluate every 1-2 days in the presence of corneal ulceration. Less frequent examinations (e.g., weeks to months) are required for less severe corneal pathology.

4.5 Neurotrophic Keratopathy

Symptoms Red eye, foreign-body sensation, swollen eyelid.

Critical Signs Loss of corneal sensation, epithelial defects with fluorescein staining.

Other Signs

    Early Perilimbal injection progressing to corneal superficial punctate keratitis.
    Late Corneal ulcer with associated iritis. The ulcer often has a gray, heaped-up border, tends to be in the lower half of the cornea, and is oval in shape.

Etiology

- Status post infection by varicella-zoster or herpes simplex virus
- Stroke
- Complication of trigeminal nerve surgery
- Complication of irradiation to the eye or an adnexal structure
- Tumor (especially an acoustic neuroma)

Work-up

1. History: Previous episodes of a red and painful eye (herpes)? Previous eye surgery, irradiation, stroke, or hearing problem?
2. Test corneal sensation with a sterile cotton wisp (before topical anesthesia).
3. Slit-lamp examination with fluorescein staining.
4. Check the skin for herpetic lesions or scars from a previous herpes zoster infection.
5. Look for signs of a corneal exposure problem (e.g., inability to close an eyelid, seventh-nerve palsy, absent Bell's phenomena).
6. If suspicious of a CNS lesion, obtain a CT scan (axial and coronal views) of the brain.

Treatment

Mild punctate epithelial staining   Artificial tears (e.g., Refresh drops) q 2 hours and artificial tear ointment (e.g., Refresh PM) qhs.

Small corneal epithelial defect   Erythromycin ointment and pressure patch for 24 hours. Then erythromycin ointment qid × 4 days or until resolved. Usually requires chronic artificial tear treatment as above.

Corneal ulcer   See "Infectious Corneal Infiltrate/Ulcer," Section 4.12, for the work-up and treatment of an infected ulcer. If the ulcer is sterile, then use erythromycin ointment and patching for several days. A tarsorrhaphy, bandage soft contact lens, or conjunctival flap may be required.

NOTE   Patients with neurotrophic keratopathy and a corneal exposure problem often will not respond to treatment unless a tarsorrhaphy is performed (eyelids partly sewn together). A temporary adhesive tape tarsorrhaphy (the lateral one-third of the eyelid is taped closed) may be beneficial.

Follow-up

Mild epithelial staining   In 3-7 days.

Corneal epithelial defect   Every 1-2 days until improvement demonstrated, then every 3-5 days until resolved.

Corneal ulcer   Hospitalization is required for severe ulcers as per Section 4.12. Follow daily until significant improvement is demonstrated.

4.6   Recurrent Corneal Erosion

Symptoms   Recurrent attacks of acute ocular pain, photophobia, and tearing often at the time of awakening or during sleep when the eyelids are rubbed or opened. A history of a prior corneal abrasion in the involved eye can often be elicited.

Critical Signs   Vary from localized roughening of the corneal epithelium (fluorescein dye may lightly outline the area) to a corneal abrasion. Epithelial changes may resolve within hours of the onset of symptoms so that no abnormality is present when the patient is examined.

Other Signs   Corneal epithelial dots or small cysts (microcysts), a fingerprint pattern, or maplike lines may be seen in both eyes if map-dot-fingerprint (MDF) dystrophy is the underlying problem.

Etiology Damage to the corneal epithelium or epithelial basement membrane from the following:

- Anterior corneal dystrophy (e.g., MDF, Meesmann's, and Reis-Bückler's dystrophies)
- Stromal corneal dystrophy (e.g., lattice, macular, and granular dystrophies)
- A previous traumatic corneal abrasion
- Radial keratotomy or cataract surgery

Work-up

1. History: Recent trauma? Previous corneal abrasion?
2. Slit-lamp examination with fluorescein staining.

Treatment

1. Acute episodes: A cycloplegic (e.g., cyclopentolate 2% or homatropine 2%), an antibiotic ointment (e.g., erythromycin), and a pressure patch are applied. The patch is left over the eye for 24-48 hours. This treatment may need to be repeated in large or persistent epithelial defects.
2. After epithelial healing is complete: Artificial tears (e.g., Refresh) 4-8 ×/day and artificial-tear ointment (e.g., Refresh PM) qhs for at least 3 months,

   or

   5% sodium chloride drops 4-8×/day and 5% sodium chloride ointment at bedtime for at least 3 months.
3. If the corneal epithelium is loose and heaped and is not healing, consider debridement of the abnormal epithelium. Apply a topical anesthetic (e.g., proparacaine) and use a sterile cotton-tipped applicator to gently remove the loose epithelium.
4. Erosions not responsive to the above treatment:
   a. Consider an extended wear bandage soft contact lens for several months.
   b. Consider anterior stromal puncture (Fig. 4.1). Generally used in extremely symptomatic, refractory cases, with erosions outside the visual axis. It can be performed with or without an intact epithelium. The patient must be very cooperative. This treatment causes small permanent corneal scars.

   Technique: Anesthetize the eye with a topical anesthetic (e.g., proparacaine). At the slit lamp use a 25-gauge needle to perform multiple punctures into the superficial cornea through Bowman's membrane, just into the anterior stroma. Depending on the size of the erosion, between twenty and fifty punctures are placed close together until the entire area of the erosion has been punctured. A cycloplegic drop, antibiotic ointment, and pressure patch as above are placed onto the eye following the procedure, and the patient is reexamined in 24 hours.

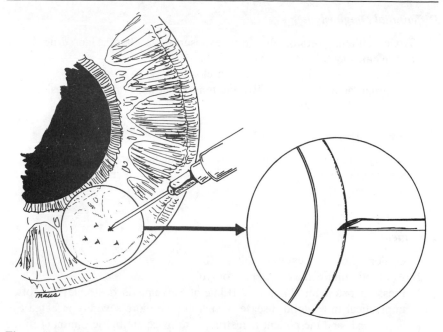

Figure 4.1 Anterior stromal puncture. In the area of the erosion, multiple superficial corneal punctures are made to the depth illustrated.

Follow-up Every 1-2 days until the epithelium has healed. Then every 1-6 months, depending on the severity and frequency of the episodes.

4.7 Thermal / Ultraviolet Keratopathy

Symptoms Moderate-to-severe ocular pain, foreign-body sensation, red eye, tearing, photophobia, blurred vision. Often a history of welding or using a sunlamp without protective eyewear can be elicited. The symptoms are typically worse 6-12 hours after the exposure.

Critical Sign Confluent superficial punctate keratopathy (SPK) in an interpalpebral distribution seen with fluorescein staining.

Other Signs Conjunctival injection, mild-to-moderate eyelid edema, mild-to-no corneal edema, and relatively miotic pupils which react sluggishly.

Differential Diagnosis

- Toxic epithelial keratopathy from exposure to a chemical or drug (e.g., neomycin, tobramycin, antiviral agents, etc.)
- Exposure keratopathy   (Poor eyelid closure.)
- Nocturnal lagophthalmos   (Eyelids remain partially open while asleep.)

Work-up

1. History: Welding? Sunlamp use? Topical medications?
2. Slit-lamp examination: Use fluorescein stain. Evert the eyelids to search for a foreign body.

Treatment

1. Cycloplegic (e.g., cyclopentolate 2%).
2. Antibiotic ointment (e.g., erythromycin).
3. Pressure patch for 24 hours. Bilateral patching is desirable, but often impractical in bilateral disease. Generally the more severely affected eye is patched, and the patient is instructed to place antibiotic ointment in the fellow eye upon arriving home. Sometimes patients are asked to patch their second eye upon going to sleep.
4. Oral pain medicine (e.g., acetaminophen $+/-$ codeine) prn.

Follow-up   Patients are instructed to remove the patch after 24 hours.

- If the eye feels much improved they are to begin topical antibiotics (e.g., erythromycin ointment 2-3 ×/day or sulfacetamide drops qid for 3-4 days.)
- If the eye is still significantly symptomatic they should return for reevaluation. If significant SPK are still present patients are retreated with a cycloplegic, antibiotic, and pressure patch as above.

4.8   Thygeson's Superficial Punctate Keratopathy

Symptoms   Foreign-body sensation, photophobia, and tearing. There is no history of recent conjunctivitis. The disease is usually bilateral and has a chronic course with exacerbations and remissions.

Critical Sign Coarse punctate gray-white corneal epithelial opacities, often central, slightly elevated with minimal-to-no staining with fluorescein.

Other Signs No conjunctival injection, no corneal edema, no anterior-chamber reaction.

Differential Diagnosis See Section 4.1.

Treatment

MILD

1. Artificial tears (e.g., Refresh) 4-8 × /day.
2. Artificial-tear ointment (e.g., Refresh PM) qhs.

MODERATE-TO-SEVERE

1. Mild topical steroid (e.g., fluorometholone qid) for 1 week. Then taper very slowly. May need chronic low-dose topical steroid therapy.
2. If no improvement with topical steroids, a therapeutic soft contact lens can be tried.

Follow-up Every week during an exacerbation, then every 3-12 months. Patients receiving topical steroids require periodic intraocular pressure checks.

4.9 Phlyctenulosis

Symptoms Tearing, irritation or pain, mild-to-severe photophobia. History of similar episodes. Corneal phlyctenules cause more severe symptoms than conjunctival phlyctenules.

Critical Signs

Conjunctival phlyctenule A small white nodule on the bulbar conjunctiva in the center of a hyperemic area. Often occurs at the limbus.
Corneal phlyctenule A small white nodule, initially at the limbus with dilated conjunctival blood vessels bordering it, that may migrate toward the center of the cornea, producing corneal neovascularization and ulceration behind the leading edge of the lesion. Often bilateral.

___

Other Signs   Conjunctival injection, blepharitis, corneal scarring.

___

Etiology   Delayed hypersensitivity reaction usually to one of the following:

- Staphylococcus   (Often related to blepharitis.)
- Tuberculosis (TB)
- Another infectious agent elsewhere in the body   (Rare.)

Differential Diagnosis

- Inflamed pingueculum   (Located within the palpebral fissure. Connective tissue is often seen to extend from the lesion to the limbus. Usually bilateral.)
- Infectious corneal ulcer   (Corneal phlyctenules which migrate from the limbus toward the center of the cornea may produce a sterile ulcer surrounded by a white infiltrate. When an infectious ulcer is suspected [e.g., increased pain, anterior-chamber reaction] appropriate diagnostic smears and cultures are necessary. See Section 4.12.)
- Ocular rosacea   (Corneal neovascularization with thinning and subepithelial infiltration may develop in an eye with rosacea. Telangiectasias, erythema, and/or pustules are found on the cheeks, nose, forehead, and eyelid margins.)
- Herpes simplex keratitis   (May produce corneal neovascularization running into a stromal infiltrate. A history of recurrent herpes is often elicited. Usually unilateral.)

Work-up

1. History: TB or recent infection?
2. Slit-lamp examination: Inspect the eyelid margin for signs of blepharitis and rosacea.
3. PPD with anergy panel (tuberculin skin test) in patients who have not had a known positive PPD in the past.

   NOTE   The PPD should be read between 48 and 72 hours after placement. A positive reaction is defined as skin induration (not just erythema) of 10 mm or more.

4. Chest x-ray if the PPD is positive or TB is suspected.

Treatment   Indicated for symptomatic patients.

1. Topical steroid (e.g., prednisolone acetate 1% 4-8 × /day, depending on the severity).

2. Eyelid hygiene 2-3 × /day (see Section 5.10).
3. Artificial tears (e.g., Refresh drops) 4-6 × /day.
4. Antibiotic ointment at bedtime (e.g., bacitracin or erythromycin ointment).
5. In severe cases of blepharitis use tetracycline or erythromycin 250 mg po qid (see Section 5.10).
6. If the PPD or chest x-ray is positive for TB, then refer the patient to a medical internist to consider antituberculous therapy.
7. Penetrating keratoplasty may benefit patients with central corneal scarring from previous phlyctenules.

Follow-up Recheck in several days. When the symptoms have significantly improved, start tapering the steroid rapidly. Maintain the antibiotic ointment as long as steroids are being used and for at least 2-3 weeks. Continue eyelid hygiene indefinitely and artificial tears prn.

4.10 Pterygium / Pingueculum

Symptoms May be asymptomatic or cause irritation, redness, or decreased vision.

Critical Sign

Pterygium Wing-shaped fold of fibrovascular tissue arising from the interpalpebral conjunctiva and extending onto the cornea.
Pingueculum Yellow-white flat or slightly raised conjunctival lesion, usually in the interpalpebral fissure adjacent to the limbus, but not involving the cornea.

Other Signs Either lesion may be highly vascularized and injected or may be associated with superficial punctate keratitis or a dellen (thinning of the cornea secondary to drying). An iron line (Stocker's line) may be seen in the cornea adjacent to a pterygium.

Differential Diagnosis

• Conjunctival intraepithelial neoplasia (Unilateral jellylike, velvety, or leukoplakic mass, often elevated, vascularized, and not in a wing-shaped configuration.)

- Dermoid (Congenital white lesion, usually at the inferotemporal limbus. Occasionally associated with a deformity of the ear—often preauricular skin tags—and/or vertebral skeletal defects [Goldenhar's syndrome].)
- Pannus (Blood vessels growing into the cornea, often secondary to contact lens wear, trachoma, phylectenular keratitis, atopic disease, blepharitis, ocular rosacea, herpes keratitis, and others. It is usually at the level of Bowman's membrane with minimal to no elevation.)
- See Section 8.1 for others.

Work-up Slit-lamp examination to identify the lesion and evaluate the adjacent corneal integrity and thickness.

Treatment

1. Protect the eyes from sun, dust, and wind (e.g., sunglasses or goggles if appropriate) as sunlight and chronic irritation are thought to be factors in pterygium/pingueculum growth.
2. Reduce ocular irritation if present:
   a. Mild: Artificial tears (e.g., Refresh 4-8 × /day) or a mild topical vasoconstrictor (e.g., naphazoline 3-4 × /day).
   b. Moderate-to-severe: Mild topical steroid (e.g., fluorometholone 3-4 × /day).
3. If a dellen is present then apply artificial-tear ointment (e.g., Refresh PM) and patch the eye for 24 hours.
4. Surgical removal may be considered when:
   a. The lesion is interfering with contact-lens wear.
   b. The patient is experiencing extreme irritation unrelieved by the above treatment.
   c. The pterygium involves the visual axis.

NOTE   A more aggressive pterygium may recur after surgical excision.

Follow-up Asymptomatic patients may be followed every 1-2 years.

- If treating with a topical vasoconstrictor, then the patient should be followed in 2 weeks. The drop may be stopped when the inflammation has subsided.
- If treating with a topical steroid, then follow every 1-2 weeks to monitor inflammation and intraocular pressure. Taper and discontinue the steroid drop over several days once the inflammation has abated.

4.11 Band Keratopathy

Symptoms   May be asymptomatic or complain of decreased vision, a foreign-body sensation, or a white spot on the cornea.

Critical Sign   Anterior corneal plaque of calcium in the palpebral fissure area, separated from the limbus by clear cornea. Holes are often present in the plaque, giving it a "Swiss cheese" appearance. It usually begins at the 3 and 9 o'clock positions, adjacent to the limbus, and can extend across the cornea.

Other Signs   May have other signs of chronic eye disease.

Etiology

   More common   Chronic uveitis (e.g., juvenile rheumatoid arthritis), interstitial keratitis, phthisis bulbi, long-standing glaucoma.
   Less common   Hypercalcemia (may be secondary to hyperparathyroidism, sarcoidosis, Paget's disease, vitamin D intoxication, etc.), gout, corneal dystrophy, chronic exposure to irritants (e.g., mercury fumes), renal failure, and others.

Work-up

1. History: Any chronic exposure to environmental irritants? Systemic disease? Chronic eye disease?
2. Slit-lamp examination, intraocular pressure measurement, and optic-nerve evaluation.
3. If no signs of chronic anterior segment disease or long-standing glaucoma are present and the band keratopathy cannot be accounted for, then consider the following work-up:
   a. Serum calcium, albumin, magnesium, phosphorus levels, BUN, and creatinine.
   b. Uric acid level if gout is suspected.

Treatment

MILD (i.e., foreign-body sensation)

Artificial tears (e.g., Refresh) 4-6×/day and artificial-tear ointment (e.g., Refresh PM) qhs.

SEVERE (obstruction of vision, irritation unrelieved with lubricants, or a cosmetic problem): Remove the calcium at the slit lamp.

1. Dilute a solution of 15% disodium EDTA (e.g., Endrate) by mixing 2 cc of the disodium EDTA with 8 cc of normal saline (0.9% NaCl). (This gives a 3% mixture).
2. Anesthetize the eye with a topical anesthetic (e.g., cocaine 4% or proparacaine).
3. Debride the corneal epithelium with a sterile scalpel or a sterile cotton-tipped applicator dipped in cocaine 4%.
4. Wipe a cellulose sponge or cotton swab saturated with the 3% disodium EDTA solution over the band keratopathy until the calcium clears (which may take 10-30 minutes).
5. Place an antibiotic ointment (e.g., erythromycin), a cycloplegic drop (e.g., cyclopentolate 2%), and a pressure patch on the eye for 24 hours.
6. Consider giving the patient an analgesic (e.g., acetaminophen +/− codeine).

Follow-up If surgical removal has been performed, then the patient needs to be followed every day with repatching, an antibiotic, and a cycloplegic until the epithelial defect heals. Surgical removal can be repeated if the band keratopathy recurs. Otherwise the patient may be followed every 3-12 months depending on the severity of the symptoms.

4.12 Infectious Corneal Infiltrate / Ulcer

Symptoms Red eye, mild-to-severe ocular pain, photophobia, decreased vision, and discharge.

Critical Signs Focal white opacity in the corneal stroma (infiltrate). An ulcer exists if there is an overlying epithelial defect which stains with fluorescein.

NOTE An examiner cannot see through an infiltrate/ulcer to the iris, whereas stromal edema and inflammation are more transparent.

Other Signs Conjunctival injection, corneal thinning, stromal edema and inflammation surrounding the infiltrate, folds in Descemet's membrane, anterior-chamber reaction, hypopyon, mucopurulent discharge, and/or upper eyelid edema. Posterior synechiae, hyphema, and glaucoma may occur in more severe cases.

Etiology

- Bacterial (Most common infectious etiology. In general, corneal infections are assumed to be bacterial until proven otherwise by laboratory studies or until a therapeutic trial is unsuccessful. Infections are occasionally treated as fungal from the outset in the southern United States, where fungal infections are more common.)
- Fungal (Must be considered after a traumatic corneal injury, particularly from vegetable matter [e.g., a tree branch]. Infiltrates commonly have feathery borders and may be surrounded by satellite lesions. Candida infections tend to occur in diseased eyes. Hyphae or yeast may be evident on Giemsa stain [although they are also seen with Gomori methenamine-silver stain]. Most fungi grow on Sabouraud's agar.)
- Acanthamoeba (An extremely painful stromal infiltrate usually in a soft-contact-lens wearer who practices poor lens hygiene or has a history of swimming with his contact lenses. In the late stages, the infiltrate assumes the shape of a ring. Acanthamoeba cysts may be seen on Giemsa stain, and the organism may be cultured on nonnutrient agar with E. coli overlay.)
- Herpes simplex virus (May have eyelid vesicles or corneal epithelial dendrites. A history of recurrent eye disease or known ocular herpes is common. Patients with chronic herpes simplex keratitis may develop bacterial superinfections.)

Differential Diagnosis

- Sterile ulcer (not infectious) (Dry eye syndrome, rheumatoid arthritis [or other collagen vascular diseases], vernal keratoconjunctivitis, neurotrophic keratopathy, vitamin A deficiency, others.) (Cultures negative, anterior-chamber inflammation minimal to none, eye may be white and comfortable.)
- Subepithelial infiltrates following viral conjunctivitis (epidemic keratoconjunctivitis) (Often bilateral. History of an acute, itchy red eye with discharge in the past several weeks to months.)
- Staphylococcal hypersensitivity (Peripheral corneal infiltrate[s], usually multiple, often bilateral, with a clear space between the infiltrate and the limbus. There is minimal-to-no anterior-chamber reaction.)
- Corneal infiltrates from an immune reaction to contact lenses/solutions (Generally multiple, small subepithelial infiltrates with an intact overlying epithelium and minimal to no anterior-chamber reaction. Usually a diagnosis of exclusion after ruling out an infectious process.)
- Residual corneal foreign body or rust ring (May be accompanied by corneal stromal inflammation, edema, and sometimes a sterile infiltrate. There may be a mild anterior-chamber reaction. The infiltrate and inflammation clear after removing the foreign body.)

Work-up

1. History: Contact-lens wear and lens-care regimen? Swim with lenses? Trauma or corneal foreign body? Eye care prior to visit (e.g., antibiotics or topical steroids)? Previous corneal disease? Systemic illness?
2. Slit-lamp examination: Stain with fluorescein to determine if there is epithelial loss overlying the infiltrate, document the size, depth, and location of the corneal infiltrate, assess the anterior-chamber reaction, and measure the intraocular pressure (IOP).
3. Swab the palpebral conjunctiva if a significant discharge is present and send the specimen for cultures.
4. Corneal scrapings for smears and cultures are performed as described below for infiltrates considered to be infectious and for all ulcers. Small, non-staining infiltrates are sometimes treated with regular-strength antibiotics without prior scraping.

Culture Procedure

EQUIPMENT

Slit lamp, sterile Kimura spatula or knife blade, culture media, micro slides, alcohol lamp.

PROCEDURE

• Anesthetize the cornea with topical drops (proparacaine is best as it appears to be less bacteriocidal than others.)
• At the slit lamp scrape the base and the leading edge of the infiltrate firmly with the spatula or blade and place the specimen on the culture medium or slide. Sterilize the spatula over the flame of the alcohol lamp between each separate culture or slide. Be certain that the spatula-tip temperature has returned to normal before touching the cornea again.

MEDIA

Routine:

1. Blood agar (most bacteria)
2. Sabouraud's medium without cyclohexamide (fungi) (place at room temperature)
3. Thioglycolate broth (aerobic and anaerobic bacteria)
4. Chocolate agar (Hemophilus, gonococcus) (place into a CO_2 jar)

Optional:

• Löwenstein-Jensen medium (mycobacteria, Nocardia)
• Nonnutrient agar with E. coli overlay (acanthamoeba)

SLIDES

Routine:

1. Gram's stain (bacteria, fungi)
2. Giemsa stain (bacteria, fungi, acanthamoeba)

Optional:

* Gomori methenamine-silver, PAS (fungi)
* Acid-fast (mycobacteria, Nocardia)
* Calcofluor white (acanthamoeba) (a fluorescent microscope is needed)

NOTE   When a fungal infection is suspected, deep scrapings into the base of the ulcer are essential. Sometimes a corneal biopsy is necessary to obtain diagnostic information.

In contact-lens wearers suspected of having an infectious ulcer, the contact lenses and case are cultured if at all possible. (It is explained to the patient that the cultured contact lenses can never be worn again.)

Treatment   As mentioned above, ulcers and infiltrates are generally treated as bacterial initially unless there is a high suspicion of another form of infection (see "Fungal Keratitis" (Section 4.13), "Acanthamoeba" (Section 4.14), and "Herpes Simplex Virus" (Section 4.15).

1. Cycloplegic (e.g., scopolamine 1/4% tid).
2. Topical antibiotics:
   a. Small nonstaining infiltrate with minimal to no anterior chamber reaction nor discharge:

      Non-contact-lens wearer   Broad-spectrum topical antibiotics (e.g., polymyxin B/bacitracin ointment qid).
      Contact-lens wearer   Tobramycin drops q 2-6 hours. Can add tobramycin ointment qhs.

   b. Large or staining infiltrate or moderate-to-severe anterior-chamber reaction or purulent discharge: Fortified tobramycin (15 mg/ml) every hour alternating with fortified cefazolin (50 mg/ml) every hour. This means that the patient will be placing one or the other drop in the eye every ½ hour. See Appendix 10 for directions on making fortified antibiotics.
3. Consider subconjunctival antibiotics (e.g., gentamicin 20-40 mg + cefazolin 100 mg) in very severe cases or when fortified antibiotics cannot be started within a short time period. See Appendix 8 describing the injection technique.

4. Eyes with corneal thinning may be protected by a shield without a patch (a patch is never placed over an eye considered to have an infection).
5. No contact-lens wear.
6. Oral pain medication as needed (e.g., acetaminophen).
7. Admission to the hospital may be necessary if:

- There is a severe sight-threatening infection.
- The patient is unable to give him or herself the antibiotics at the above frequency without difficulty.
- There is a likelihood of noncompliance.
- There is a possibility of being lost to follow-up.
- Systemic antibiotics are needed (e.g., corneal perforation, scleral extension of the infection, gonococcal or Hemophilus infection)

Follow-up

- The patient needs daily evaluations with repeat measurements of the size of the infiltrate and ulcer. The most important criteria in evaluating the response to treatment include the degree of eye pain, the size of the epithelial defect over the infiltrate, the size and depth of the infiltrate, and the anterior-chamber reaction. Less pain, a smaller epithelial defect and infiltrate, and a less-inflamed eye are all favorable responses. The IOP needs to be checked and glaucoma treated if present (see Section 10.4.)
- If the ulcer is improving, the antibiotic regimen is gradually tapered. Otherwise the antibiotic regimen is adjusted according to the culture and sensitivity results.
- If originally not cultured and now worsening, cultures, stains, and treatment with fortified antibiotics are needed. Hospitalization is (re)considered.
- Reculture the ulcer (with the addition of optional media and stains) if it does not seem to be responding to the current antibiotic regimen and the original cultures are negative.
- A corneal biopsy may need to be performed when the condition is worsening and infection is still suspected despite negative cultures.
- In an impending or completed corneal perforation, a corneal transplant or patch graft is considered. Cyanoacrylate glue may also work in a treated corneal ulcer.

NOTE   Outpatients are told to return immediately if the pain increases or the vision decreases.

4.13 Fungal Keratitis

Symptoms   Pain, photophobia, red eye, tearing, discharge, or a foreign-body sensation. A history of trauma, particularly with vegetable matter (e.g., a tree branch), or chronic eye disease is common.

Critical Signs   Corneal stromal gray-white opacity (infiltrate) with a feathery border. The epithelium over the infiltrate may be elevated above the remainder of the corneal surface or there may be an epithelial defect with stromal thinning (ulcer).

Other Signs   Satellite lesions surrounding the primary infiltrate, conjunctival injection, mucopurulent discharge, anterior-chamber reaction, and/or hypopyon.

Etiology

- Nonfilamentous fungi (typically Candida)   (Usually in previously unhealthy eyes.)
- Filamentous fungi (typically Fusarium or Aspergillus)   (Usually from trauma with vegetable matter.)

Differential Diagnosis   See Section 4.12.

Work-up   See Section 4.12 for a complete work-up and culture procedure.

NOTES

1. Be certain to obtain a Giemsa stain when a fungus is suspected (PAS and Gomori methenamine-silver stains can also be used), and scrape deep into the base of the ulcer for material.
2. If all cultures are negative, yet an infectious etiology is still suspected, consider a corneal biopsy to obtain further diagnostic information.

Treatment   In general, corneal infiltrates and ulcers of unknown etiology are treated as bacterial until proven otherwise by laboratory studies (see Section 4.12). If the stains and/or cultures indicate a fungal keratitis:

1. Admission to the hospital is usually necessary, unless you can be certain that the patient will be completely compliant with medications and follow-up.

2. Natamycin 5% (50 mg/ml) drops q 1-2 hours while awake, q 2 hours at night.
3. Cycloplegic (e.g., scopolamine 1/4% tid).
4. Treat glaucoma if present (see Section 10.4).
5. No topical steroids. If the patient is currently on steroids, they should be tapered rapidly.
6. No eye patch.
7. An eye shield, without a patch, may be advisable when the cornea is thinned.

- If the infection involves the deep corneal stroma or is worsening despite appropriate treatment, one or more of the following medications may be added:

    a. Amphotericin B 0.15% (1.5 mg/ml) drops q 1 hour. (May be especially effective in Candida infections.)
    b. Ketoconazole 200 mg po q day.
    c. Miconazole or clotrimazole 1% drops (10 mg/ml) q 1 hour. (May be especially effective in Aspergillus infections.)

A corneal transplant may be necessary for a progressive fungal infection on maximal medical therapy. A corneal transplant or patch graft may also be required in an impending or completed corneal perforation.

Follow-up   Daily, as per Section 4.12. The response to treatment is slower than in a bacterial infection. Lack of progression is a favorable sign.

4.14   Acanthamoeba

Corneal infection with acanthamoeba should be considered in any patient with a history of soft contact-lens use, poor contact-lens hygiene (e.g., using nonsterile homemade saline solutions to clean lenses and/or infrequent disinfection), and/or swimming with the contact lenses in.

Symptoms   Severe ocular pain, redness, and photophobia over a period of several weeks.

Critical Signs

Early   Less corneal and anterior segment inflammation than would be expected for the degree of pain the patient is experiencing, epithelial and subepithelial infiltrates (sometimes along corneal nerves, producing a radial keratitis), and pseudodendrites on the epithelium.

Late   A corneal stromal infiltrate in the shape of a ring.

NOTE   Cultures for bacteria are negative and the condition generally does not improve with antibiotic or antiviral medications.

Other Signs   Eyelid swelling, conjunctival injection, cells and flare in the anterior chamber. Generally no discharge nor corneal vascularization. Corneal ulceration may occur late in the course.

Differential Diagnosis

• Herpes simplex keratitis   (Often has a history of previous attacks in the same eye, typical branching corneal dendrites are common, much less painful than acanthamoeba, multinucleated giant cells may be seen on Giemsa stain.)
• Fungal ulcer   (May see hyphae on histologic staining, should grow on Sabouraud's medium.)
• Bacterial (e.g., pseudomonas) ulcer   (Much more acute course, over hours to days, should grow out on bacterial culture and respond to fortified antibiotic drops.)

Work-up   See Section 4.12 for a general work-up. The following are obtained when acanthamoeba is suspected.

1. Corneal scrapings for Giemsa and Gram's stains (Giemsa stain may show typical cysts).
2. Calcofluor white stain if available (requires a fluorescent microscope).
3. Culture on nonnutrient agar with *E. coli* overlay.
4. Consider a corneal biopsy if the stains and cultures are negative and the condition is not improving on the current regimen.

Treatment   The treatment of acanthamoeba is controversial and often ineffective. The following are modes of therapy which have been found to be successful in some cases.

One or more of the following are generally used in combination, usually in the hospital:

1. Polymyxin-neomycin-gramicidin (e.g., Neosporin) drops q ½ to 2 hours.
2. Propamidine isethionate 0.1% (e.g., Brolene) drops q ½ to 2 hours.
3. Clotrimazole 1% drops q 2 hours.
4. Ketoconazole 200 mg po bid.
Alternative therapy to clotrimazole includes miconazole 1% drops or paromomycin drops q 2 hours.

All patients:
5. Discontinue contact-lens wear.
6. Cycloplegic (e.g., atropine 1% tid).

7. Nonsteroidal antiinflammatory agent (e.g., sulindac 200 mg po bid) for pain.

• A corneal transplant may be indicated for medical failures, but can be complicated by recurrent infection.

Follow-up   Every day in the hospital until the condition is consistently improving. Medication may then be tapered judiciously and the patient followed as an outpatient. The required duration of therapy is not established, varying from 6 to 12 months.

NOTE   Brolene is available in England and may be obtained with FDA approval. Clotrimazole is not currently formulated as an ophthalmic suspension, but it can be formulated in artificial tears from a powder (with FDA approval). This solution must be shaken before each use.

4.15   Herpes Simplex Virus (HSV)

Symptoms   Usually unilateral red eye, pain, photophobia, tearing, decreased vision, and/or a skin (e.g., eyelid) rash. Previous episodes are common.

Signs   (Any or all of the following may be present.)

EYELID/SKIN INVOLVEMENT

Clear vesicles on an erythematous base which progress to crusting.

CONJUNCTIVITIS

Conjunctival injection with follicles and a palpable preauricular node.

CORNEAL EPITHELIAL DISEASE

May present as a superficial punctate keratitis, a stellate keratitis, a dendritic keratitis (a thin, linear, and branching lesion with club-shaped "terminal bulbs" at the end of each branch) or a geographic ulcer (a large amoeba-shaped corneal ulcer, with a dendritic edge). The edges of herpetic lesions are mildly heaped up with swollen epithelial cells which stain well with rose bengal, while the central ulceration stains well with fluorescein. Corneal sensitivity may be decreased. Scars may develop underneath the epithelial ulcers.

NEUROTROPHIC ULCER

A sterile ulcer with smooth margins over an area of stromal disease persisting despite antiviral therapy. May be associated with stromal melting and perforation.

CORNEAL STROMAL DISEASE

A. Disciform keratitis—Disc-shaped stromal edema with an intact epithelium. A mild iritis with localized granulomatous keratic precipitates is typical, and increased intraocular pressure (IOP) may be present. No necrosis nor corneal neovascularization is present.

B. Necrotizing interstitial keratitis—Multiple or diffuse whitish gray corneal stromal infiltrates often accompanied by stromal inflammation and neovascularization. Concomitant iritis, hypopyon, or glaucoma may be present. Bacterial superinfection must be ruled out.

UVEITIS

An anterior-chamber reaction may develop secondary to severe corneal stromal involvement. Less commonly it can develop without active corneal disease.

RETINITIS

Rare. In neonates it is usually associated with a severe systemic HSV infection and is often bilateral.

Differential Diagnosis   (Conditions which produce dendritic-appearing corneal lesions)

- Herpes zoster virus   (Frequently painful skin vesicles along a dermatomal distribution of the face, not crossing the midline, are present. [Note that pain may be present even without vesicles.] The dendrites in this condition do not have true terminal bulbs and do not stain well with fluorescein.)
- Recurrent corneal erosion   (A healing erosion often appears as a pseudodendrite. Patients frequently provide a history of a corneal abrasion in the involved eye or have underlying map-dot-fingerprint dystrophy. Pain frequently develops upon awakening from sleep.)
- Contact-lens-related pseudodendrites   (No skin involvement. Dendrites do not typically branch, do not have terminal bulbs, and stain minimally.)

Work-up

1. History: Previous episodes? History of corneal abrasion, contact-lens wear, or previous nasal, oral, or genital sores? Recent topical or systemic steroids? Immune deficiency state?
2. External examination: Note the distribution of skin vesicles if present.
3. Slit-lamp examination with IOP measurement.

Most cases of herpes simplex are diagnosed clinically and require no confirmatory laboratory tests. However, if the diagnosis is in doubt, any of the following tests may be supportive of the diagnosis:

4. Scrapings of a corneal or skin lesion (scrape the *edge* of a corneal ulcer or the *base* of a skin lesion) for Giemsa stain (shows multinucleated giant

cells). (A papanicolaou stain will show intranuclear eosinophilic inclusion bodies).
5. Viral culture: A sterile cotton-tipped applicator is used to swab the cornea, conjunctiva, or skin (after unroofing vesicles with a sterile needle) and is then placed into the viral transport medium.

NOTE   Smears and cultures for bacteria should be taken when the corneal condition suddenly gets worse. See Section 4.12.

Treatment

EYELID/SKIN INVOLVEMENT

1. Topical acyclovir ointment tid to the skin lesions (expensive and not proven to be effective; some physicians treat with an antibiotic ointment instead [e.g., erythromycin or bacitracin]).
2. Warm soaks to skin lesions tid.
3. If the eyelid margin is involved, add: trifluorothymidine 1% drops (e.g., Viroptic) or vidarabine 3% ointment (e.g., Vira-A) 5 × /day to the eye.
The above medications are continued for 7-14 days until resolution.

NOTE   Oral acyclovir 200 to 400 mg po 5 × /day for 7-14 days is given by some physicians to adults suspected of having primary herpetic disease ("flu-like" illness, fever, lymphadenopathy, etc.)

CONJUNCTIVITIS

Trifluorothymidine 1% drops (e.g., Viroptic) or vidarabine 3% ointment (e.g., Vira-A) 5 × /day. Stop the antiviral agent when the conjunctivitis has resolved after 7-14 days.

CORNEAL EPITHELIAL DISEASE

1. Trifluorothymidine 1% drops (e.g., Viroptic) 9 × /day or vidarabine 3% ointment (e.g., Vira-A) 5 × /day (rarely idoxuridine 0.5% ointment [e.g., Stoxil] 5 × /day is used when an allergic reaction develops to both of the other drugs).
2. Cycloplegic agent (e.g., scopolamine 1/4% tid) if an anterior-chamber reaction is present.
3. Patients on topical steroids should have them tapered in the presence of corneal epithelial disease.
4. Consider gentle debridement of the infected epithelium as an adjunct to the antiviral agents.
   Technique: After topical anesthesia (e.g., proparacaine), a sterile cotton-tipped applicator or semisharp instrument is used to carefully peal off the

lesions at the slit lamp. Following debridement, antiviral treatment should be instituted as above.

NOTE   Avoid debridement in children, in the presence of deep stromal lesions, or when a lesion has been previously treated with topical steroids.

In epithelial defects not resolving after several weeks, antiviral toxicity and/or a neurotrophic ulcer should be suspected. At that point the antiviral agent should be stopped and a nonpreserved artificial-tear ointment (e.g., Refresh PM) or an antibiotic ointment (e.g., erythromycin) should be used 2-4 × /day with or without a pressure patch for several days to watch for improvements.

NEUROTROPHIC ULCER

See Section 4.5.

CORNEAL STROMAL DISEASE

A. Disciform keratitis
  Mild   Cycloplegic (e.g., scopolamine 1/4% tid) alone.
  Severe and/or central   (i.e., vision is reduced)
  1. Cycloplegic (e.g., scopolamine 1/4% tid).
  2. Topical steroid (e.g., prednisolone acetate 1% qid).
  3. Antiviral drops (e.g., trifluorothymidine 1% tid).
  • Consider a corneal transplant if inactive postherpetic scars significantly affect vision.

NOTES

  1. Topical steroids are contraindicated in those with corneal epithelial disease.
  2. Rarely, a systemic steroid (e.g., prednisone 60-80 mg po q day tapered rapidly) is given to patients with severe stromal disease accompanied by an epithelial defect.

B. Necrotizing interstitial keratitis: Treated as severe disciform keratitis. A corneal transplant may be required if the cornea perforates.

NOTE   The persistence of an ulcer in the presence of stromal inflammation commonly is due to the underlying inflammation (requiring cautious steroid therapy); however, it may be due to antiviral toxicity. When an ulcer deepens, a new infiltrate develops, or the anterior-chamber reaction increases, smears and cultures should be taken for bacteria and fungi. See Section 4.12.

Follow-up   Patients are reexamined in 2-3 days to evaluate the response to treatment and then every 1-7 days, depending on the clinical findings. The following clinical parameters are evaluated: the size of the epithelial defect and ulcer, the corneal thickness and the depth to which the cornea is involved, the anterior-chamber reaction and the IOP (see Section 10.4 for glaucoma management). Antiviral medications for corneal dendrites and geographic ulcers should be continued 5-9×/day for 10-14 days. Topical steroids used for corneal stromal disease are tapered slowly (often over months to years). The initial concentration of the steroid (e.g., 1%) is eventually reduced (e.g., 1/8%). Prophylactic antiviral agents are used tid. No antiviral coverage is needed when the steroid is given once a day or less.

NOTE   The topical antivirals can cause a local allergic reaction (usually a papillary or follicular conjunctivitis). If an allergic reaction should occur, the antiviral should be replaced with another antiviral, as cross-reactivity is rare.

REFERENCE

LIESEGANG TJ. Ocular herpes simplex infection: pathogenesis and current therapy. *Mayo Clin Proc* 63:1092, 1988.

4.16   Herpes Zoster Virus (HZV)

Symptoms   Skin rash, headache, fever, malaise, blurred vision, eye pain, or red eye.

Critical Sign   Acute vesicular skin rash which follows a dermatome of the fifth cranial nerve and can progress to scarring. Characteristically the rash appears on one side of the forehead (obeying the midline) and involves the upper eyelid only.

Other Signs   Less commonly the rash involves the lower eyelid and cheek on one side and rarely one side of the jaw. Conjunctivitis, corneal involvement (pseudodendrites on the epithelium, superficial punctate keratitis, immune stromal keratitis, neurotrophic keratitis, etc.), uveitis, iris atrophy, scleritis, retinitis, choroiditis, optic neuritis, cranial-nerve palsy, and glaucoma can occur. Late postherpetic neuralgia may also occur.

NOTE   Corneal disease may follow the acute skin rash by many months to years. Rarely it can precede the skin rash.

Differential Diagnosis

• Herpes simplex virus (HSV) (The rash does not follow a dermatome nor obey the midline. Patients are typically younger. Corneal dendrites of HSV have true terminal bulbs and stain well with fluorescein; dendrites of herpes zoster virus (HZV) generally do not have true terminal bulbs and stain poorly with fluorescein.)

Work-up

1. History: Duration of rash and pain? Immunocompromised or risk factors for AIDS?
2. Complete ocular examination, including a slit-lamp evaluation with fluorescein staining, intraocular pressure (IOP) check, and dilated optic nerve and retinal examination.
3. Systemic evaluation:
   a. *Patients < 40 years old:* Medical evaluation to determine whether the patient may be immunocompromised.
   b. *Patients 40-60 years old:* None (unless immunodeficiency is suspected from the history).
   c. *Patients > 60 years old:* If systemic steroid therapy is to be instituted, obtain a steroid work-up (see Appendix 5).
   Immunocompromised patients should *not* receive systemic steroids.

Treatment See Section 14.1 for the treatment of zoster in immunocompromised patients.

SKIN INVOLVEMENT

A. *Adults with an acute moderate to severe skin rash less than 5-7 days old in which active skin lesions are present*
   1. Acyclovir[1] 600-800 mg po 5×/day for 7-10 days or if severe or the patient is systemically ill, hospitalize for acyclovir 5-10 mg/kg iv q 8 hours for 5-10 days.
   2. Bacitracin ointment to the skin lesions bid.
   3. Warm compresses tid to periocular skin (to keep it clean).

In patients > 60 years of age who are not immunocompromised and who do not have diabetes nor tuberculosis, consider adding the following to minimize postherpetic neuralgia:
   4. Prednisone 60 mg po × 3 days, then 40 mg po × 3 days, then 20 mg po × 4 days and then discontinue, plus:

[1]The dosage of acyclovir needs to be reduced in patients with renal insufficiency.

5. Anti-ulcer therapy (e.g., antacid or H_2 blocker) (Although it is un-proved, some physicians believe cimetidine relieves some of the discomfort from the acute skin rash. Thus, cimetidine 400 mg po bid may serve a dual purpose.)

B. *Adults with a skin rash of more than 5-7 days duration or no active skin lesions*
   1. Warm compresses tid to periocular skin.
   2. Bacitracin ointment to skin lesions bid.

C. *Children*
   Treat as in (B) unless there is evidence of systemic spread. For systemic spread, hospitalize and use acyclovir[1] 500 mg/m²/day in 3 divided doses for 7 days. The hospital pharmacy should have a conversion chart for height, weight, and surface area in square meters. The patient is usually transferred to the pediatric service.

OCULAR INVOLVEMENT

A. *Conjunctival involvement:* Cool compresses and erythromycin ointment to the eye bid.

B. *Corneal pseudodendrites or SPK:* Same as (A).

C. *Uveitis (with or without immune stromal keratitis):* Topical steroid (e.g., prednisolone acetate 1% qid), cycloplegic (e.g., cyclopentolate 2% qid), and erythromycin ointment qhs.

D. *Neurotrophic keratitis:* Treat mild epithelial defects with erythromycin ointment qid. If corneal ulceration occurs, obtain appropriate smears and cultures to rule out infection (see Section 4.12). If the ulcer is sterile, consider a tarsorrhaphy or conjunctival flap if there is no response to erythromycin ointment and patching. See Section 4.5.

E. *Scleritis:* Treat as any other scleritis (see Section 5.7).

F. *Retinitis, choroiditis, optic neuritis, or cranial-nerve palsy:* Acyclovir[1] 5-10 mg/kg iv q 8 hours × 1 week plus prednisone 60 mg po × 3 days tapering as described above.

G. *Glaucoma:* May be secondary to the uveitis or steroids. If uveitis is present, increase the frequency of the steroid administration for a few days. If the IOP remains elevated, change the prednisolone acetate to fluorometholone (e.g., FML) drops. Timolol 0.5% bid and a carbonic anhydrase inhibitor (e.g., methazolamide 25-50 mg po 2-3 × /day) will additionally help lower the IOP.

NOTE   Pain may be severe during the first two weeks, and analgesics (e.g., acetaminophen +/− codeine) may be required. An antidepressant (e.g., amitryptyline 25 mg po tid) may be beneficial, as depression frequently develops during the acute phase of HZV infection. Antidepressants may also help postherpetic neuralgia.

---

[1]The dosage of acyclovir needs to be reduced in patients with renal insufficiency.

Follow-up If ocular involvement is present, follow the patient every 1-7 days, depending on the severity. Patients without ocular involvement can be followed every 1-2 weeks. After the acute episode resolves, follow the patient every 3-6 months as relapses may occur months to years later, particularly as steroids are tapered. Systemic steroid administration requires collaboration with the patient's medical doctor.

NOTE   HZV is contagious for children and adults who have not had chicken pox—it can be spread by inhalation. Pregnant women who have not had chicken pox must be especially careful to avoid contact with a herpes zoster patient.

4.17   Contact-Lens-Related Problems

Symptoms Pain, photophobia, foreign-body sensation, decreased vision, and red eye. Itching may occur.

Signs See the distinguishing characteristics of each etiology below.

Etiology
- Corneal infiltrate/ulcer (bacterial, fungal, acanthamoeba) (White corneal lesion which may stain with fluorescein. Must always be ruled out in contact-lens patients with eye pain. See "Infectious Corneal Infiltrate/Ulcer" [Section 4.12], "Acanthamoeba" [Section 4.14], and "Fungal Keratitis" [Section 4.13].)
- Hypersensitivity/toxicity reactions to preservatives in solutions (Conjunctival injection and ocular irritation typically develop shortly after lens cleaning and insertion, but can be present chronically. A recent change from one type or brand of solution to another can often be elicited in the history. Commonly occurs in patients using preserved solutions [e.g., thimerosal or chlorhexidine as a component]. May be due to inadequate rinsing of lenses after enzyme use. Signs include superficial punctate keratitis [SPK], conjunctival injection, bulbar conjunctival follicles, and subepithelial or stromal corneal infiltrates.)
- Pseudo-superior limbic keratoconjunctivitis (Hyperemia and fluorescein staining of the superior bulbar conjunctiva, particularly at the limbus. Subepithelial infiltrates may be found on the superior cornea. This may represent a hypersensitivity or toxicity reaction to a solution or contact lens-related product (especially thimerosal). Unlike superior limbic keratoconjunctivitis

unassociated with contact lenses, there are no corneal filaments nor a papillary reaction, and there is no association with thyroid disease.)

- Giant papillary conjunctivitis   (Itching, mucus discharge, and lens intolerance in a patient with large superior tarsal conjunctival papillae. See Section 4.18.)
- Contact-lens deposits   (Multiple small deposits on the contact lens, leading to corneal and conjunctival irritation. The contact lens is often old and may not have been cleaned or enzymed properly in the past.)
- Tight-lens syndrome   (Symptoms may be severe and often develop within a day or two of being fit with the responsible contact lens. The lens does not move with blinking and appears "sucked-on" to the cornea. An imprint in the conjunctiva is often observed after the lens is removed. Corneal edema, SPK, an anterior chamber reaction, and sometimes a sterile hypopyon may develop.)
- Corneal warpage   (Seen predominantly in long-term polymethylmethacrylate [PMMA] hard-contact-lens wearers. Initially the vision becomes blurred with glasses, but remains good with contact lenses. Gradually, blurred vision and, sometimes, discomfort develop with contact lenses. There may or may not be SPK. Keratometry reveals distorted mires.)
- Corneal neovascularization   (Patients are often asymptomatic until the visual axis is involved. 1-2 mm of superficial corneal neovascularization is common and generally unalarming in aphakes, with the exception of corneal transplant eyes [which are at a greater risk for graft rejection]. Phakic [and corneal transplant] patients are generally treated.)
- Corneal epithelial changes   (Range from epithelial thickening to pseudodendritic changes. Not infectious in origin, but rather a toxic/traumatic reaction to the contact lens.)
- Others   (Contact lens inside out, corneal abrasion [see Section 3.2], poor lens fit, change in refractive error, others.)

Work-up

1. History: What is the main complaint . . . severe pain, mild discomfort, itching? What kind of contact lens does the patient wear (soft, hard, gas-permeable, daily-wear, extended-wear, or disposable)? How old are the lenses? For how many hours/days/weeks straight are the lenses worn? How are the lenses cleaned and disinfected? Are enzyme tablets used? Are the products preservative-free? Any recent changes in contact-lens habits?
2. In noninfectious conditions, while the contact lens is still in the eye evaluate its fit and examine its surface for deposits at the slit lamp.
3. Ocular examination, including a slit-lamp examination using fluorescein. (Remove the contact lens or the dye may temporarily stain it.) Evert the upper eyelids of both eyes, inspecting the superior tarsal conjunctiva for papillae.

4. Smears and cultures are taken when a corneal ulcer is suspected (see "Infectious Corneal Infiltrate/Ulcer" [Section 4.12], "Acanthamoeba" [Section 4.14], and "Fungal Keratitis" [Section 4.13]).

5. The contact lenses and lens case are cultured if possible when an infectious corneal process is suspected.

Treatment

I. When the diagnosis of infection cannot be ruled out, patients are treated as follows:

    A. Possible corneal ulcer (corneal infiltrate, epithelial defect, anterior chamber reaction, pain): Appropriate smears and cultures are obtained, fortified antibiotics and a cycloplegic are started, and contact-lens wear is discontinued (see Section 4.12).

    B. Small subepithelial infiltrates, corneal abrasion, or diffuse SPK

       1. Discontinue contact-lens wear.

       2. Topical antibiotic (e.g., tobramycin drops 4-8 × /day. Can also add tobramycin ointment qhs).

       3. No pressure patch.

II. When a specific contact-lens problem is suspected, it may be treated as follows (see "Contact lens-induced Giant Papillary Conjunctivitis" [Section 4.18] for treatment of this condition):

    A. Hypersensitivity/toxicity reaction

       1. Discontinue contact-lens wear.

       2. Preservative-free artificial tears (e.g., Refresh drops 4-6 × /day).

       3. New contact lenses and preservative-free solutions are used upon resolution of the condition, and appropriate lens hygiene is explained.[2]

       4. Patients are taught to rinse their lenses thoroughly after using enzymes.

    B. Pseudo-superior limbic keratoconjunctivitis: Treated as described for hypersensitivity/toxicity reactions. When a large subepithelial opacity extends toward the visual axis, topical steroids may be added (e.g., prednisolone acetate 1% q 6 hours), but are often ineffective.

    C. Contact-lens deposits

       1. Discontinue contact-lens wear.

       2. Replace with a new contact lens once the symptoms resolve. Consider changing the brand of contact lens.

---

[2]The following regimen for contact-lens care is one recommended system. We do not recommend extended-wear contact lenses to most patients; our experience with disposable extended-wear contact lenses, however, is limited at this time:

Daily cleaning regimen: Preservative-free daily cleaner (e.g., Miraflow), preservative-free saline (e.g., Unisol), disinfectant—preferably heat or hydrogen peroxide (4 hours).

Weekly: Enzyme tablets.

3. Teach proper contact-lens care, stressing weekly enzyme treatments.
D. Tight-lens syndrome
   1. Discontinue contact-lens wear.
   2. Consider a topical cycloplegic (e.g., scopolamine 1/4% tid or atropine 1% tid) in the presence of an anterior-chamber reaction.
   3. Patients should be refit with a flatter contact lens after the symptoms and signs resolve.

NOTE   Patients do not need to be cultured for their hypopyon when this syndrome is highly suspected.

E. Corneal warpage
   1. Discontinue contact-lens wear (it is explained to patients that vision may be poor for the following 2-4 weeks).
   2. A gas-permeable hard contact lens should be fit when the refraction and keratometric readings have returned to normal (obtain the original keratometric readings).
F. Corneal neovascularization
   1. Discontinue contact-lens wear.
   2. Consider a topical steroid (e.g., prednisolone acetate 1% qid) for extensive neovascularization.
   3. Consider refitting with a high-oxygen transmissible daily-wear contact lens which moves adequately over the cornea.
G. Corneal epithelial changes
   1. Discontinue contact-lens wear.
   2. Consider a new contact lens when the epithelial changes resolve, which may take weeks or months.
   3. Use preservative-free solutions.

Follow-up
- When a corneal infection cannot be ruled out, patients are reevaluated the following day. Eyes of contact lens patients are not patched. Treatment is maintained until the condition clears.
- In noninfectious conditions, patients are reevaluated in 1-4 weeks, depending on the clinical situation. Contact-lens wear is resumed when the condition resolves.

4.18   Contact-Lens-Induced Giant Papillary Conjunctivitis (GPC)

Symptoms   Itching, mucus discharge, decreased lens-wearing time, increased lens awareness, excessive lens movement.

Critical Sign Giant papillae on the superior tarsal conjunctiva. (NOTE: The upper eyelid must be everted to make the diagnosis.)

Other Signs Contact-lens coatings, high-riding lens, ptosis, mild conjunctival injection.

Work-up

1. History: Details of contact lens use, including age of lenses, cleaning and enzyming regimen.
2. Slit-lamp examination: Evert the upper eyelids and examine for papillae.

Treatment

MILD TO MODERATE

1. Replace the contact lens if it is older than 4-6 months or if it has numerous deposits. Refit with a new brand of soft contact lens or refit with a gas-permeable rigid contact lens.
2. Reduce contact-lens wearing time (switch extended-wear contact lens patients to daily wear).
3. Cromolyn sodium (e.g., Opticrom 4%) qid.
4. Have the patient clean the lenses more thoroughly—preferably using preservative-free solutions (e.g., Miraflow daily cleaner) and preservative-free saline (e.g., Unisol).
5. Increase enzyme use (use at least every week).

SEVERE

1. Discontinue contact-lens wearing.
2. Cromolyn sodium (e.g., Opticrom 4%) 4-6×/day.
3. Restart with a new contact lens in 1-4 months (when the condition clears).
4. Teach lens hygiene as above.

Follow-up In 2-4 weeks. Cromolyn sodium is tapered slowly.

NOTE GPC can also result secondary to an exposed suture or ocular prosthesis. Exposed sutures are removed. Otherwise, these entities are treated with cromolyn sodium as above.

4.19 Interstitial Keratitis (IK)

Acute symptomatic IK most commonly occurs within the first or second decade of life. Signs of old IK often persist throughout life.

Acute Phase

Symptoms   Pain, tearing, photophobia, red eye.

Critical Signs   Corneal stromal blood vessels and edema.

Other Signs   Anterior-chamber cells and flare, fine keratic precipitates on the corneal endothelium, conjunctival injection.

Signs of Old Disease

Deep corneal haze or scarring and often corneal stromal blood vessels containing no blood (ghost vessels), corneal stromal thinning.

Etiology

   More common   Congenital syphilis (usually affects both eyes within one year of each other).
   Less common   Acquired syphilis (unilateral—often sectorial), tuberculosis (unilateral—often sectorial), Cogan's syndrome (vertigo, tinnitus, hearing loss, negative FTA-ABS, often associated with polyarteritis nodosa), leprosy, herpes simplex virus.

Work-up   For active IK and old, previously untreated IK:

1. History: Venereal disease in the mother during pregnancy or in the patient? Difficulty hearing or tinnitus?
2. External examination: Look for "saddle nose," "Hutchinson's teeth," "frontal bossing," or other signs of congenital syphilis; hypopigmented or anesthetic skin lesions along with thickened skin folds, loss of the temporal eyebrow, and loss of eyelashes as in leprosy.
3. Slit-lamp examination: Note whether the corneal nerves are segmentally thickened like beads on a string and whether iris nodules are present (leprosy); look for patchy hyperemia of the iris with fleshy, pink nodules (syphilis).
4. Dilated fundus examination: Look for the classic "salt and pepper" chorioretinitis or optic atrophy of syphilis.
5. VDRL or RPR, FTA-ABS or MHA-TP.
6. PPD with anergy panel.
7. Chest x-ray if negative FTA-ABS (or MHA-TP) or positive PPD.
8. Consider ESR, ANA, rheumatoid factor.

Treatment

A. Acute disease
   1. Topical cycloplegic (e.g., atropine 1% tid).
   2. Topical steroid (e.g., prednisolone acetate 1% q 1-6 hours, depending on the degree of inflammation).
   3. Treat any underlying disease.
B. Old inactive disease: Corneal transplant surgery may improve vision when it is impaired from central corneal scarring.
C. Acute or old inactive disease
   • If (+) FTA-ABS and
   a. The patient has not been treated for syphilis in the past (or is unsure about treatment)
      or
   b. There are signs of active syphilitic disease (e.g., active chorioretinitis or papillitis)
      or
   c. The VDRL or RPR titer is positive and has not declined the expected amount after treatment (see ''Congenital Syphilis'' [Section 14.3] or ''Acquired Syphilis'' [Section 14.2])
   then treatment for syphilis is indicated (see ''Congenital Syphilis'' [Section 14.3] or ''Acquired Syphilis'' [Section 14.2])
   • If (+) PPD (> 10 mm of induration at 48-72 hours) and
   a. Patient < 35 years old and has not been treated for tuberculosis in the past
      or
   b. There is evidence of active systemic tuberculosis (e.g., (+) finding on chest x-ray)
   then refer the patient to a medical internist for treatment of tuberculosis.
   • If Cogan's syndrome is present then refer the patient to an ENT specialist.

Follow-up

A. *Acute disease* Every 3-7 days at first and then every 2-4 weeks. The frequency of steroid administration is slowly reduced as the inflammation subsides. Intraocular pressure is monitored closely and lowered with medication when it is thought to be dangerously high (e.g., > 30 mm Hg in a patient with a healthy optic nerve). (See ''Inflammatory Open-Angle Glaucoma'' [Section 10.4].)
B. *Old inactive disease* Routine follow-up every year unless treatment is required for an underlying etiology.

4.20   Peripheral Corneal Thinning

Symptoms   Pain and photophobia, but may be asymptomatic.

Critical Sign   Corneal thinning (seen best with a narrow slit of light from the slit lamp), may have a sterile infiltrate or ulcer.

Etiology

- Collagen vascular disease (e.g., rheumatoid arthritis, relapsing polychondritis, Wegener's granulomatosis, polyarteritis nodosa, systemic lupus erythematosus, and others)   (Peripheral, unilateral or bilateral corneal thinning/ulcers may progress circumferentially to involve the entire peripheral cornea. Perforation may occur. This may be the first manifestation of the systemic disease.)
- Terrien's degeneration   (Unilateral or bilateral slowly progressive thinning of the peripheral cornea superiorly, most often in men. The anterior chamber is quiet and the eye is typically white and not inflamed. A yellow line (lipid) may appear along with a fine pannus over the ulcerated area. The ulceration may slowly spread circumferentially. The epithelium usually remains intact, and perforation is rare.)
- Mooren's ulcer   (Unilateral or bilateral idiopathic painful corneal thinning and ulceration with inflammation, initially involving a focal area of peripheral cornea, but later extending circumferentially or centrally. An epithelial defect [i.e., stains with fluorescein], stromal thinning, and a leading undermined edge are present. Limbal blood vessels may grow into the ulcer and perforation can occur. This diagnosis can only be made after underlying systemic diseases are ruled out.)
- Pellucid marginal degeneration   (Painless, bilateral corneal thinning of the inferior peripheral cornea [usually from 4 to 8 o'clock]. There is no anterior-chamber reaction, conjunctival injection, lipid deposition, nor vascularization. The epithelium is intact. Corneal protrusion may be seen above the area of thinning. The thinning may slowly progress.)
- Furrow degeneration   (Corneal thinning just peripheral to an arcus senilis, typically in the elderly. There is no vascular infiltration, nor ocular inflammation, and perforation is rare. Usually nonprogressive and does not require treatment.)
- Dellen   (Oval-shaped corneal thinning secondary to drying adjacent to an abnormal conjunctival or corneal elevation.)
- Staphylococcal hypersensitivity (marginal keratitis)   (A peripheral white corneal infiltrate separated from the limbus by clear cornea, often multiple, may stain with fluorescein, may be mildly thinned, typically associated with blepharitis.)

- Dry eye syndrome   (Peripheral corneal ulcers may result from severe cases of dry eye. Patients may demonstrate a poor tear lake, a decreased tear break-up time, superficial punctate keratitis (SPK) inferiorly or centrally, and corneal filaments.)
- Exposure/neurotrophic keratopathy   (Typically, a sterile oval ulcer develops inferiorly on the cornea without signs of significant inflammation. An eyelid abnormality, a fifth- or seventh-cranial-nerve defect, or proptosis is common. It may become superinfected.)
- Sclerokeratitis   (Corneal ulceration is associated with severe ocular pain radiating to the temple and/or jaw due to accompanying scleritis. The sclera develops a blue hue, scleral vessels are engorged, and scleral edema with or without nodules is present. An underlying collagen vascular disease, especially Wegener's granulomatosis, must be ruled out.)
- Vernal keratoconjunctivitis   (Superior, shallow "shield-shaped" sterile corneal ulcer accompanied by giant papillae on the superior tarsal conjunctiva and/or limbal papillae. The conjunctivitis is usually bilateral, often occurs in children, and recurs during the summer months—but can occur anytime in warm climates.)
- Ocular rosacea   (Typically affects the inferior cornea in middle-aged patients. Erythema and telangiectasias of the eyelid margins, nose, forehead, and cheeks are characteristic. It can progress to rhinophyma.)
- Others   (Cataract surgery, inflammatory bowel disease and leukemia can rarely cause corneal thinning/ulceration.)

Differential Diagnosis

- Infectious infiltrate or ulcer   (A gray-white stromal infiltrate or ulcer [stains with fluorescein]. The conjunctiva is injected and an anterior chamber reaction is usually present. Often lesions are treated as infectious until cultures are noted to be negative. See Section 4.12.)

Work-up

1. History: Contact-lens wearer or previous herpes simplex keratitis (infectious)? Known collagen vascular disease or inflammatory bowel disease? Other systemic symptoms? Seasonal conjunctivitis with itching (vernal)?
2. External examination: Old facial scars of herpes zoster? Eyelid closure problem causing exposure? Blue tinge to the sclera? Rosacea facies?
3. Slit-lamp examination: Look for an infiltrate, hypopyon, uveitis, scleritis, old herpetic scarring, poor tear lake, SPK, blepharitis, giant papillae on the superior tarsal conjunctiva or limbal papillae, and measure the intraocular pressure (IOP).
4. Dilated fundus examination: Look for cotton wool spots consistent with collagen vascular disease.

5. Corneal scrapings and cultures when infection is suspected (see "Infectious Corneal Infiltrate/Ulcer," Section 4.12).
6. Serum ANA, rheumatoid factor, ESR, and CBC with differential to rule out collagen vascular disease and leukemia, if suspected.
7. Refer to an internist (or rheumatologist) when collagen vascular disease or leukemia is suspected.
8. Scleritis work-up when present (see Section 5.7).

Treatment The treatment of dellen, staphylococcal hypersensitivity, dry eye syndrome, exposure and neurotrophic keratopathies, scleritis, vernal conjunctivitis, and ocular rosacea are discussed elsewhere in this book.

A. Corneal thinning due to collagen vascular disease: Management is usually coordinated with a rheumatologist or internist.
   1. Antibiotic ointment (e.g., erythromycin ointment) and a pressure patch qhs.
   2. Ocular lubricants while awake (e.g., Refresh tears q 1 hour or Refresh PM ointment qid).
   3. Cycloplegic drops (e.g., atropine 1%) when an anterior-chamber reaction and/or pain are present.
   4. Systemic steroids (e.g., prednisone 60-100 mg po q day—the dosage is adjusted according to the response) + an H_2-blocker (e.g., ranitidine 150 mg po bid) are used for significant and progressive corneal thinning, but not for perforation.
   5. An immunosuppressive agent is usually required for Wegener's granulomatosis.
   6. Excision of adjacent conjunctiva is occasionally helpful when the condition progresses despite treatment.
   7. Punctal occlusion if dry eye syndrome is also present.
   8. Consider cyanoacrylate adhesive or corneal transplant surgery for an impending or actual corneal perforation. A conjunctival flap can also be used for an impending corneal perforation.
   9. Patients with significant corneal thinning should wear their glasses (or protective glasses [e.g., polycarbonate lens]) during the day and an eye shield at night.

NOTE Topical steroids are generally not used when significant corneal thinning is present because of the risk of perforation. Topical steroids should be gradually tapered if the patient is already on them. Corneal thinning due to relapsing polychondritis, however, seems to improve with topical steroids (e.g., prednisolone acetate 1% q 1-2 hours).

B. Terrien's degeneration: Correct astigmatism with glasses or contact lenses if possible.

C. Mooren's ulcer: Underlying systemic diseases must be ruled out before this diagnosis can be made. A stepwise approach to treatment is taken, utilizing any or all of the following therapeutic modalities. If the epithelial defect over the ulcer is not healing within a few days, more aggressive therapy is pursued. Some cases are resistant to all forms of treatment.
   1. Topical steroid (e.g., prednisolone acetate 1% q 1 hour).
   2. Systemic steroid (prednisone 60-100 mg po q day) + an H_2-blocker (e.g., ranitidine 150 mg po bid).
   3. Immunosuppressive agents (e.g., cyclophosphamide or methotrexate) after consultation with a medical physician familiar with these agents.
   4. Consider conjunctival excision, a conjunctival flap, or cryotherapy if the ulceration progresses.
   5. Consider cyanoacrylate adhesive or corneal surgery to prevent or treat a corneal perforation.
   All patients are given the following:
   6. Topical antibiotic drops (e.g., gentamicin qid) to prevent secondary bacterial infection.
   7. Cycloplegic (e.g., atropine 1% tid).
   8. Glasses during the day and an eye shield at night because of the risk of perforation with minor trauma.
D. Pellucid marginal degeneration: See "Keratoconus," Section 4.23.
E. Furrow degeneration: No treatment is required.

NOTE   If systemic steroid therapy is to be instituted, obtain a steroid work-up (see Appendix 5).

Follow-up   Patients with severe disease are followed daily in the hospital or as outpatients; those with milder conditions are followed less frequently. Watch carefully for signs of superinfection (increased pain, stromal infiltration, anterior-chamber cells and flare, conjunctival injection), increased IOP, and progressive corneal thinning. Treatment is maintained until the epithelial defect over the ulcer heals. Therapy is then gradually tapered. As long as an epithelial defect is present, there is a risk of progressive thinning and perforation.

4.21   Dellen

Symptoms   Usually asymptomatic. Irritation and foreign-body sensation may occur.

Critical Sign Corneal thinning usually at the limbus, often in the shape of an ellipse, accompanied by an adjacent focal conjunctival or corneal elevation.

Other Signs Fluorescein pooling in the area, but minimal staining. No infiltrate, no anterior-chamber reaction, no hyperemia.

Etiology Poor spread of the tear film over a focal area of cornea due to an adjacent surface elevation (e.g., chemosis, conjunctival hemorrhage, filtering bleb from glaucoma surgery, pterygium, tumor, or following muscle surgery).

Differential Diagnosis See "Peripheral Corneal Thinning," Section 4.20.

Work-up

1. History: Previous eye surgery?
2. Slit-lamp examination with fluorescein staining. Look for an adjacent area of elevation.

Treatment

1. Lubricating or antibiotic ointment (e.g., Refresh PM or erythromycin ointment) and a pressure patch for 24 hours.
2. Lubricating ointment qhs to follow the removal of the pressure patch. Maintain the ointment until the adjacent elevation is eliminated.
3. If the cause cannot be removed (e.g., filtering bleb), lubricating ointment should be applied nightly and artificial tear drops (e.g., Refresh) used 4-8 ×/day chronically. (Most conjunctival elevations will regress with patching.)

Follow-up Unless there is severe thinning, reexamination can be performed in 1-7 days, at which time the cornea can be expected to be of normal thickness. If it is not, full-time patching and lubrication should again be instituted.

4.22 Staphylococcal Hypersensitivity

Symptoms Acute photophobia, mild pain, and red eye; chronic eyelid crusting and itching. A history of recurrent acute episodes is common.

Critical Signs Usually multiple peripheral corneal stromal infiltrates with a clear space between the infiltrates and the limbus, and minimal-to-no staining with fluorescein. The anterior chamber is usually quiet and only a sector of the conjunctiva is typically injected.

Other Signs Blepharitis, inferior superficial punctate keratitis, phlyctenule (a wedge-shaped, raised infiltrate near the limbus), and peripheral scarring and corneal neovascularization in the fellow eye.

Etiology Staphylococcal blepharitis (Infiltrates are a noninfectious reaction of the host's antibodies to the staphylococcal antigens.)

NOTE Patients with ocular rosacea (telangiectasias of the eyelids, nose, cheeks, and forehead which may progress to rhinophyma) are especially susceptible to this condition.

Differential Diagnosis

- Infectious corneal infiltrates (A white-gray stromal infiltrate, often more central and painful and associated with a more marked anterior-chamber reaction. Not usually multiple and recurrent.)
- See Section 4.20 for other causes of marginal thinning/infiltrates.

Work-up

1. History: Recurrent episodes? Contact-lens wearer (a risk of infection)?
2. Slit-lamp examination. Examine with fluorescein staining.
3. If an infectious infiltrate is being considered, then corneal scrapings for culture and smears should be obtained. (See Section 4.12).

Treatment

MILD

Warm compresses, eyelid hygiene, and erythromycin or bacitracin ointment qhs (see ''Blepharitis/Meibomianitis'' treatment [Section 5.10]).

MODERATE-TO-SEVERE

Treat as above and add a topical steroid (e.g., prednisolone acetate 1/8% qid) or a combination antibiotic/steroid (e.g., prednisolone acetate 1%/gentamicin qid). Maintain until the symptoms improve, then slowly taper.

If recurrent episodes are not prevented by eyelid hygiene, consider systemic tetracycline 250 mg po qid × 1 month then bid × 3 months and then q day until the ocular disease is controlled for several months. Tetracycline may have to be maintained indefinitely.

NOTE   Tetracycline is contraindicated in children, pregnant women, and breast-feeding mothers. Erythromycin in the same dose may be substituted.

Follow-up   In 2-7 days depending on the clinical picture. The intraocular pressure is monitored while patients are on topical steroids.

4.23   Keratoconus

Symptoms   Progressive decreased vision usually beginning in the adolescent years and continuing into middle age. Acute corneal hydrops can cause a sudden decrease in vision, pain, photophobia, and profuse tearing.

Critical Signs   Slowly progressive irregular astigmatism secondary to paracentral thinning and bulging of the cornea (maximal thinning near the apex of the protrusion), vertical tension lines in the posterior cornea, an irregular corneal retinoscopic reflex, and egg-shaped mires on keratometry. Usually bilateral but often asymmetric.

Other Signs   Fleischer's ring (epithelial iron deposits at the base of the cone), bulging of the lower eyelid when looking downward (Munson's sign), superficial corneal scarring. *Corneal hydrops* (sudden development of corneal edema) results from a rupture in Descemet's membrane.

Associations   Keratoconus is frequently seen in Down's syndrome, Marfan's disease, atopic disease, and others. It may be related to chronic eye rubbing.

Differential Diagnosis

- Pellucid marginal degeneration   (Corneal thinning in the inferior periphery. The cornea protrudes above the band of thinning.)
- Keratoglobus   (Rare. Uniform circularly thinned cornea with maximal thinning in the mid-periphery of the cornea. The cornea protrudes above the area of the thinning.)

Treatment for these two conditions is the same as keratoconus, except corneal transplants are not as readily performed as they are technically more difficult and have a higher failure rate.

Work-up

1. History: Duration and rate of decreased vision? History of eye rubbing? Medical problems?

2. Slit-lamp examination. (NOTE The Fleischer ring is best seen with the blue light of the slit lamp.)
3. Retinoscopy and refraction (look for irregular astigmatism and a "water drop" or "scissors" red reflex).
4. Keratometry (can show irregular mires with central and inferior steepening).

Treatment

1. Patients are instructed not to rub their eyes.
2. Correct refractive errors with glasses (for mild cases) or rigid gas permeable contact lenses (successful in most cases).
3. Corneal transplant surgery is usually indicated when contact lenses cannot be tolerated or no longer produce satisfactory vision because of corneal scarring.
4. Thermokeratoplasty, epikeratophakia, and lamellar keratoplasty are occasionally used.

CORNEAL HYDROPS

1. Cycloplegic agent (e.g., scopolamine 1/4%), sodium chloride 5% ointment, and a pressure patch.
2. Patients are instructed to remove the pressure patch in 24-48 hours and start sodium chloride 5% ointment bid until resolved (usually several weeks).

NOTE Acute hydrops does not cause corneal perforation and is not an indication for an emergent corneal transplant.

Follow-up Every 3-12 months depending on the progression of symptoms. After an episode of hydrops, follow the patient every 1-2 weeks until resolved.

4.24 Corneal Dystrophies

Bilateral, inherited corneal disorders showing no signs of inflammation or corneal vascularization.

Anterior Corneal Dystrophies

Anterior Basement Membrane Dystrophy (Map-Dot-Fingerprint Dystrophy)

Diffuse gray patches (maps), large or tiny cysts (dots), or fine refractile lines (fingerprints) in the corneal epithelium, best seen with retroillumination or a broad slit-lamp beam angled from the side; spontaneous corneal epithelial defects (erosions) and associated pain and photophobia may develop, particularly upon opening the eyes from sleep. See Section 4.6 for treatment.

Meesmann's Dystrophy

Rare, autosomal dominant, epithelial dystrophy, which presents in the first years of life, but is usually asymptomatic until middle age. Retroillumination shows discrete tiny epithelial vesicles diffusely involving the cornea, but concentrating in the palpebral fissure. Although treatment is usually not required, a superficial keratectomy or a lamellar corneal transplant may be beneficial if visual acuity is severely affected.

Reis-Bücklers' Dystrophy

Autosomal dominant, progressive dystrophy that appears early in life. Superficial, gray reticular opacities are noted primarily in the central cornea. Painful episodes from recurrent erosions are relatively common, and require treatment. Corneal transplant surgery may be necessary to improve vision, but the dystrophy often recurs in the graft. Superficial lamellar keratectomy may be adequate treatment in some cases.

Corneal Stromal Dystrophies

Patients with reduced vision from these conditions usually benefit from a corneal transplant.

Lattice Dystrophy

Refractile lines, white dots, and scarring of the corneal stroma centrally, best seen in retroillumination. Recurrent erosions are common (see Section 4.6). The corneal periphery is clear. Autosomal dominant.

Granular Dystrophy

White, anterior stromal deposits in the central cornea separated by discrete clear intervening spaces. The corneal periphery is typically spared. Appears in the first decade, but rarely becomes symptomatic before mid-life. Autosomal dominant.

Macular Dystrophy

Gray-white stromal opacities with ill-defined edges extending from limbus to limbus with cloudy intervening spaces. Can involve full thickness stroma. Autosomal recessive.

Central Crystalline Dystrophy (of Schnyder)

Fine yellow-white stromal crystals located in the central cornea. Can be associated with hyperlipidemia and hypercholesterolemia. Autosomal dominant. Workup includes fasting serum cholesterol and triglyceride levels.

Corneal Endothelial Dystrophies

Fuchs' Dystrophy   See Section 4.25.

Posterior Polymorphous Dystrophy

Changes at the level of Descemet's membrane, including vesicles arranged in a linear or grouped pattern, gray haze, or broad bands with irregular scalloped edges. Iris abnormalities, including iridocorneal adhesions and a decentered pupil may be present. Glaucoma may occur. Usually autosomal dominant. See "Developmental Anterior Segment Abnormalities" (Section 9.11) for a differential diagnosis.

Congenital Hereditary Endothelial Dystrophy (CHED)

Bilateral corneal edema. Normal corneal diameter, normal intraocular pressure, no guttata.

Types

- Autosomal recessive: Present at birth, nonprogressive, nystagmus present.
- Autosomal dominant: Presents during childhood, slowly progressive, no nystagmus, but pain, tearing, and photophobia are common.

See "Congenital Glaucoma," Section 9.9, for a differential diagnosis.
Some patients may benefit from a corneal transplant.

4.25 Fuchs' Endothelial Dystrophy

Symptoms Glare and blurred vision, especially upon awakening. It may progress to severe pain. Symptoms rarely develop before age 50 years. May be autosomal dominant.

Critical Signs Corneal guttata plus corneal stromal edema. The disease is bilateral, but may be asymmetric.

NOTE Central corneal guttata without stromal edema is called *endothelial dystrophy*, which may progress to Fuchs' dystrophy.

Other Signs Fine pigment dusting on the endothelium, central epithelial edema and bullae, folds in Descemet's membrane, subepithelial scar tissue.

Differential Diagnosis

- Aphakic or pseudophakic bullous keratopathy (History of cataract surgery, unilateral.)
- Congenital hereditary endothelial dystrophy (Bilateral corneal edema at birth.)
- Posterior polymorphous dystrophy (Autosomal dominant, presents early in life; corneal endothelium shows either grouped vesicles, geographic-shaped gray lesions, or broad bands. Iridocorneal adhesions and pupillary abnormalities may be present.)

Work-up

1. History: Previous cataract surgery?
2. Slit-lamp examination: Guttata are often best seen with retroillumination. Fluorescein staining may demonstrate ruptured bullae.
3. Measure the intraocular pressure (IOP).
4. Consider corneal pachymetry to determine the central corneal thickness.

Treatment

1. Topical sodium chloride 5% drops qid and ointment qhs.
2. May gently blow warm air from a hair dryer toward the eyes for 5-10 minutes every morning to dehydrate the cornea.
3. Reduce the IOP with antiglaucoma medications if > 20-22 mm Hg (e.g., topical beta-blocker such as timolol 1/4-1/2% bid or levobunolol 1/2% bid).

4. Ruptured corneal bullae are painful and should be treated as a corneal abrasion (see Section 3.2).
5. Corneal transplant surgery is usually indicated when visual acuity falls or the disease becomes advanced and painful.

Follow-up   Every 3-4 months to check IOP and assess corneal edema. The condition progresses very slowly, and visual acuity remains good until epithelial edema develops.

4.26   Wilson's Disease (Hepatolenticular Degeneration)

Symptoms   Typically, no ocular complaints. Patients experience symptoms of cirrhosis, renal disease, or neurologic dysfunction (motor, but not sensory dysfunction). Age usually less than 40 years at the onset of clinical manifestations.

Critical Signs   Typically, a greenish-brown band (Kayser-Fleischer ring) in the corneal periphery (although it may appear red), 1-3 mm in width, at the level of Descemet's membrane (deep in the cornea). It first appears superiorly, but eventually forms a ring that involves the entire corneal periphery. The ring usually extends to the limbus, without clear cornea interspersed. Serum and urine copper levels are elevated and the serum ceruloplasmin level is low.

Other Ocular Signs   Anterior subcapsular cataract.

Inheritance   Autosomal recessive.

Differential Diagnosis

- Other rare causes of a Kayser-Fleischer ring   (Primary biliary cirrhosis, chronic active hepatitis, progressive intrahepatic cholestasis, and rarely multiple myeloma.) (Normal serum ceruloplasmin levels, no neurologic symptoms.)
- Arcus senilis   (Corneal stromal lipid deposition, first seen inferiorly and superiorly before it extends around the corneal periphery. Appears white, typically with a clear zone of cornea separating the edge of the arcus from the limbus. In patients less than 40 years of age, a lipid profile with lipoprotein electrophoresis and serum cholesterol should be obtained to rule out hyperlipidemia, hyperlipoproteinemia, and hypercholesterolemia.)

Work-up

1. Slit-lamp examination: Narrow the beam of light to a thin slit and determine the level at which the deposition is located.
2. Gonioscopy if the Kayser-Fleischer ring is not evident on slit-lamp examination (pigment may be noted in peripheral Descemet's membrane before it is apparent on slit-lamp examination).
3. Serum copper and ceruloplasmin levels.
4. Urine copper level.
5. Serum protein electrophoresis when ceruloplasmin levels are normal.
6. Referral to an internist and neurologist.

Treatment   Systemic therapy is instituted by an internist. The ocular manifestations usually require no treatment.

Follow-up

- In conjunction with an internist and neurologist who manage systemic therapy and monitor blood cell counts.
- Successful treatment should lead to reabsorption of the corneal copper deposition and clearing of the Kayser-Fleischer ring (although residual corneal changes may remain). There are no ocular complications of a Kayser-Fleischer ring.

4.27   Corneal Graft Rejection

Symptoms   Decreased vision, redness, and photophobia in an eye which has undergone a prior corneal transplant, usually several weeks to years previously.

Critical Signs   (Any of the following suggest corneal graft rejection)   New keratic precipitates or a fine line of white blood cells on the corneal endothelium (endothelial rejection line), stromal edema or cellular infiltration, subepithelial infiltrates, epithelial edema, or an irregularly elevated epithelial line (epithelial rejection line).

Other Signs   Conjunctival injection, particularly circumcorneal injection, anterior-chamber cells and flare, neovascularization growing up to or extending onto the graft (typically the rejection starts near a blood vessel adjacent to the graft wound). Tearing may occur, but discharge is not present.

Etiology   Immune response.

Differential Diagnosis

- Suture abscess or corneal infection (May have a corneal infiltrate, hypopyon, or a purulent discharge. Cultures must be taken, including a culture of the suture [which should be removed]. Steroid frequency is usually reduced slowly rather than increased. Patients are often hospitalized and treated with fortified topical antibiotics. See Section 4.12.)
- Uveitis (May produce anterior-chamber cells and flare with keratic precipitates. Often a previous history of uveitis can be obtained. It is best to treat as if it were a graft rejection.)
- Increased intraocular pressure (IOP) (A markedly elevated IOP may produce epithelial corneal edema, but few-to-no other signs of graft rejection are present and the edema often clears after the IOP is lowered.)
- Other causes of graft failure (Corneal endothelial decompensation in the graft, recurrent disease in the graft [e.g., herpes keratitis, corneal dystrophy].)

Work-up

1. History: Time period since the corneal transplant? Current eye medications? Recent change in topical steroid regimen? Previous ocular disease leading to the corneal transplant?
2. Slit-lamp examination, looking for the critical signs listed above. Look carefully for keratic precipitates and subepithelial infiltrates.

Treatment

1. Topical steroids (e.g., prednisolone acetate 1% q 1 hour if severe, q 2-6 hours if only subepithelial infiltrates or an epithelial rejection is present). Note that many patients are on low-dose topical steroids at the time of the graft rejection; their frequency should be increased.
2. Consider systemic steroids (e.g., prednisone 40-60 mg po q day) or subconjunctival steroids (e.g., betamethasone 3 mg in 0.5 ml) to be used additionally when the graft rejection does not respond to topical steroids alone.
3. Control IOP if elevated (see "Inflammatory Open-Angle Glaucoma," [Section 10.4]).

Follow-up Treatment must be instituted immediately to maximize the likelihood of graft survival. Follow the patient every 3-7 days. Once improvement is noted, the steroids are tapered very slowly and may need to be maintained at low doses for months to years. ICP needs to be followed in patients on topical steroids.

4.28 Aphakic Bullous Keratopathy (ABK) / Pseudophakic Bullous Keratopathy (PBK)

Symptoms Decreased vision, pain, tearing, photophobia, and red eye. History of cataract surgery in the involved eye.

Critical Sign Corneal edema in an eye in which the natural lens has been removed.

Other Signs Corneal bullae, corneal neovascularization, or preexisting endothelial guttata. Cystoid macular edema may be present.

Etiology Often results from a combination of the following factors: corneal endothelial damage, intraocular inflammation, or vitreous or subluxed intraocular lens touching (or intermittently touching) the cornea.

Work-up

1. Slit-lamp examination: Stain the cornea with fluorescein to check for denuded epithelium, check the position of the intraocular lens if present, determine whether vitreous is touching the corneal endothelium, and evaluate the eye for inflammation. Evaluate the fellow eye for corneal endothelial dystrophy.
2. Check the intraocular pressure (IOP).
3. Dilated fundus examination, looking for cystoid macular edema and vitreous inflammation.
4. Consider a fluorescein angiogram to help detect cystoid macular edema.

Treatment

1. Topical sodium chloride 5% drops qid and ointment qhs if epithelial edema is present.
2. Reduce the IOP with antiglaucoma medications if elevated (e.g., > 20 mm Hg). (Avoid epinephrine derivatives if possible due to the risk of cystoid macular edema.) (See "Primary Open-Angle Glaucoma," Section 10.1).
3. Ruptured epithelial bullae (producing corneal epithelial defects) may be treated with an antibiotic ointment (e.g., erythromycin), a cycloplegic (e.g., scopolamine 1/4%), and pressure patching for 24-48 hours.

4. Corneal transplant surgery (possibly including intraocular lens repositioning, replacement, or removal) is indicated when the vision fails or the disease becomes advanced and painful.

NOTE   Poor vision may be due to cystoid macular edema or corneal disease, and the role of each may be difficult to determine.

Follow-up   In 24-48 hours if the patient is being patched. Otherwise, every 2-6 months, depending on the symptoms.

5

Conjunctiva/ Sclera/External Disease

5.1   Acute Conjunctivitis

Characterized by a discharge and/or eyelid sticking (worse in the morning), a red eye (due to conjunctival injection), and a foreign-body sensation of less than 3 weeks' duration. Superficial punctate keratitis (SPK) may be present. Specific signs and symptoms of the individual entities are noted below. See "Red Eye" in Chapter 1 for other diseases which may present similarly.

Hyperacute onset (within 12 hours)

Gonococcal (GC)

Critical Sign   Severe purulent discharge.

Other Signs   Subconjunctival hemorrhage, conjunctival papillae, chemosis.

Work-up   Conjunctival scrapings for culture and sensitivities (blood agar, chocolate agar [37°, 10% CO_2], and Thayer-Martin plate, if available) and immediate Gram's stain.

Treatment   Initiated if the Gram's stain shows gram negative intracellular diplococci or there is a high suspicion of GC clinically. Our therapeutic regimen is as follows:

1. Hospitalize.
2. Topical bacitracin or erythromycin ointment qid.
3. Eye irrigation with saline qid until the discharge is eliminated.
4. Ceftriaxone 1 g iv q 12 hours for at least 3 days (the duration of treatment depends on the clinical response).
5. Tetracycline or erythromycin 250-500 mg po qid or doxycycline 100 mg po bid × 2-3 weeks (treatment for chlamydia, which may also be present).

NOTE   If the patient is penicillin/cephalosporin allergic, an infectious disease consult is obtained.

Follow-up   The patient needs to be followed every day until consistent improvement is noted, at which point reexamination is performed every 2-3 days until the condition resolves. The patient and sexual partners need to be evaluated by their medical doctors for other sexually transmitted diseases.

Acute onset

Viral (usually adenoviral)

A recent upper respiratory tract infection or contact with someone with a red eye is common. It generally starts in one eye and a few days later involves the other eye.

Critical Sign   Tarsal conjunctival follicles.

Other Signs   Watery/mucus discharge, red and edematous eyelids, palpable preauricular node (PAN), pinpoint subconjunctival hemorrhages, membrane/pseudomembrane, or subepithelial infiltrates which may develop several weeks after the onset of the conjunctivitis.

Treatment

1. Artificial tears 4-8 ×/day for 1-3 weeks.
2. Cool compresses several ×/day for 1-2 weeks.
3. Vasoconstrictor/antihistamine (e.g., naphazoline/pheniramine) qid, if the itching is severe.

• In cases of severe discomfort, topical steroids (e.g., fluorometholone or prednisolone acetate 1% qid) may be given. Therapy is maintained for 1 week and then tapered over one week.

• If a membrane/pseudomembrane is present, it can be gently peeled and a topical steroid can be started as described above. If a symblepharon is forming then the membrane/pseudomembrane should be peeled.

Follow-up   In 1-3 weeks, but sooner if the condition worsens significantly.

NOTE   Viral conjunctivitis typically gets worse for the first 4-7 days after onset and may not resolve for 2-3 weeks.

Variants (treated the same as above)

• Pharyngoconjunctival fever—As above, but associated with pharyngitis and fever.
• Acute hemorrhagic conjunctivitis—As above, but associated with a large subconjunctival hemorrhage.

NOTE   Viral conjunctivitis is very contagious, usually for 10-12 days from the day of onset. Patients should avoid touching their eyes, shaking hands with other people, sharing towels, etc. No school or camp as long as the eyes are red and weeping.

Herpes Simplex Virus

Patients may have a known history of ocular herpes simplex.

Critical Signs   Same as for "Viral," but occasionally concurrent herpetic skin vesicles along the eyelid margin or periocular skin are present.

Treatment   (If the cornea or skin is involved, see "Herpes Simplex Virus," Section 4.15)

1. Antiviral therapy (e.g., trifluorothymidine 1% (e.g., Viroptic) drops 5 ×/day or vidarabine 3% ointment (e.g., Vira-A) 5×/day).
2. Cool compresses several ×/day.

Follow-up   Every 2-3 days at first to monitor for corneal involvement, then every 1-2 weeks until resolved.

Allergic (e.g., hayfever)

Itching, watery discharge, and a history of allergies is typical.

Critical Signs   Chemosis, red edematous eyelids, conjunctival papillae, no PAN.

Treatment

1. Eliminate the inciting agent.
2. Cool compresses several times a day.
3. Topical drops, depending on the severity.
   a. Mild: Artificial tears (e.g., Refresh) 4-8 × /day.
   b. Moderate: Vasoconstrictor/antihistamine qid (e.g., naphazoline/phen-iramine); these should only be used for several days at a time, as rebound vasodilation occurs after prolonged use.
   c. Severe: Mild topical steroid (e.g., fluorometholone qid × 1-2 weeks).
4. Consider an antihistamine (e.g., diphenhydramine 25 mg po 3-4 × /day) in moderate-to-severe cases.

Follow-up In 1-2 weeks as needed. If topical steroids are being used, patients should be followed weekly.

Vernal/Atopic

Same as allergic except seasonal (spring/summer) recurrences are noted and a history of atopy may be elicited.

Critical Signs Large conjunctival papillae under the upper eyelid or along the limbus (limbal vernal). The upper eyelid often needs to be everted to make the diagnosis.

Other Signs A superior corneal shield ulcer (a sterile, well-delineated super-ficial corneal thinning, typically with heaped-up margins).

Treatment

- If no shield ulcer is present, treat as "allergic" except add topical cromolyn sodium 4% qid.
- If a shield ulcer is present:

1. Topical steroid (e.g., fluorometholone or prednisolone acetate 1%) 4-6 × /day.
2. Topical antibiotic (e.g., erythromycin ointment tid or sulfacetamide drops qid).
3. Cycloplegic agent (e.g., scopolamine 1/4% tid).
4. Cromolyn sodium 4% qid.
5. Cool compresses qid.

Follow-up Every 1-3 days in the presence of a shield ulcer; otherwise, every few weeks. Topical medications are tapered slowly as improvement is noted.

Cromolyn sodium is maintained for the duration of the season and often reinitiated a few weeks before the next spring.

Bacterial

Critical Sign   Purulent discharge of mild-to-moderate degree.

Other Signs   Conjunctival papillae, subconjunctival hemorrhage, chemosis.

Work-up   Conjunctival swab for routine cultures and sensitivities (blood and chocolate agars) and Gram's stain.

NOTE   If suspect GC then see hyperacute onset (above).

Treatment   Topical antibiotic therapy (e.g., erythromycin ointment qid, sulfacetamide drops or ointment qid, or bacitracin ointment qid) for 5-7 days.

Follow-up   Every 1-2 days at first, then every 2-5 days until resolved. Antibiotic therapy is adjusted according to culture and sensitivity results if the condition does not respond.

Pediculosis (lice, crabs)

Typically develops from contact with pubic lice (usually sexually transmitted).

Critical Sign   Adult lice, nits, and blood-tinged debris on the eyelids and eyelashes.

Other Signs   Conjunctival follicles.

Treatment
1. Mechanical removal of lice and eggs with jewelers forceps, if feasible.
2. Physostigmine (e.g., Eserine) ointment, white petroleum jelly, or any ophthalmic ointment to the eyelids tid × 10 days to smother the lice and nits.
3. Lindane (e.g., Kwell) lotion and shampoo as directed to *non*ocular areas for patient and close contacts.
4. Thoroughly wash all clothes, sheets, etc.

Chlamydial   See "Chronic Conjunctivitis," Section 5.2.

Toxic   See "Chronic Conjunctivitis," Section 5.2.

Molluscum Contagiosum   See "Chronic Conjunctivitis," Section 5.2.

Neonatal Conjunctivitis   See "Ophthalmia Neonatorum," Section 9.7.

Stevens-Johnson Syndrome   See "Stevens-Johnson Syndrome," Section 14.9.

Ocular Pemphigoid   See "Ocular Cicatricial Pemphigoid," Section 5.9.

NOTE   Many systemic diseases can cause a nonspecific conjunctivitis (e.g., measles, mumps, influenza, etc.). The underlying disease should be managed appropriately; the eyes are treated with artificial-tear drops 4-8 ×/day or artificial-tear ointment 2-3 ×/day as needed.

REFERENCE

ULLMAN S, ROUSSEL TJ, FORSTER RK: Gonococcal keratoconjunctivitis. *Surv Ophthalmol* 32:199-208, 1987.

5.2   Chronic Conjunctivitis

Discharge or eyelid sticking, red eye (due to conjunctival injection), and ocular irritation of greater than 3 weeks' duration. Superficial punctate keratitis (SPK) may be present.

Chlamydial Inclusion Conjunctivitis

Sexually transmitted, typically in teenagers and young adults. A history of vaginitis, cervicitis, or urethritis may be noted.

Signs   Inferior tarsal conjunctival follicles, corneal pannus, palpable preauricular node (PAN), and/or tiny gray-white subepithelial infiltrates.

Work-up

1. History: (Duration of red eye? Prior treatment? Concomitant vaginitis, cervicitis, or urethritis? Sexual contacts with chlamydia?)
2. Slit-lamp examination
3. Direct chlamydial immunofluorescence test (slide) and/or chlamydial culture of conjunctiva.

4. Conjunctival scraping for Giemsa stain: shows basophilic intracytoplasmic inclusion bodies in epithelial cells, polymorphonuclear leukocytes, and lymphocytes.

Treatment

1. Tetracycline 250-500 mg po qid or doxycycline 100 mg po bid or erythromycin 250-500 mg po qid for 3-6 weeks is given to the patient and sexual partners.[1]
2. Erythromycin, tetracycline, or sulfacetamide ointment 2-3 ×/day for 2-3 weeks.

Follow-up 1-3 weeks depending on the severity. The patient and sexual partners should be evaluated by their medical doctors for other sexually transmitted diseases.

Trachoma

Principally occurs in underprivileged countries.

Signs

Stages 1 and 2 Similar to inclusion conjunctivitis; however, follicles (along with papillae in stage 2) are more prominent on the superior palpebral conjunctiva.
Stage 3 Follicles and scarring of superior tarsal conjunctiva.
Stage 4 No follicles, extensive conjunctival scarring.
Late complications Severe dry eyes, trichiasis, entropion, keratitis, corneal scarring, superficial fibrovascular pannus, limbal follicles (scar to form Herbert's pits), corneal bacterial superinfection, and ulceration.

Work-up Same as for chlamydial inclusion conjunctivitis, see above.

Treatment

1. Tetracycline or erythromycin 250-500 mg po qid × 3-4 weeks.[1]
2. Tetracycline, erythromycin, or sulfacetamide ointment 2-4 ×/day for 3-4 weeks.

---

[1]The tetracyclines are contraindicated in children less than 8 years old, pregnant women, and breast-feeding mothers.

Follow-up   Every 2-3 weeks at first, then as needed. While the above treatment ~~is usually curative, reinfection is common if hygienic conditions do not im-~~ prove.

Molluscum Contagiosum

Critical Sign   Dome-shaped, usually multiple, umbilicated shiny nodules on the eyelid or eyelid margin.

Other Signs   The conjunctivitis may appear similar to chlamydial inclusion conjunctivitis or trachoma.

Treatment   Removal of lesions by simple excision, incision and curettage, or cryosurgery.

Follow-up   Every 2-4 weeks until the conjunctivitis resolves.

Toxic (eye drops)

Many eye drops can cause a conjunctivitis (classically atropine, epinephrine, dipivefrin, pilocarpine, aminoglycoside antibiotics, antiviral agents, and physostigmine).

Signs   Conjunctival follicles and/or papillae.

Treatment   Discontinue the offending eye drop and treat as allergic conjunctivitis, see Section 5.1.

Follow-up   Same as allergic conjunctivitis, see Section 5.1.

Papilloma

See "Conjunctival Tumors," Section 8.1.

Silent Dacryocystitis

See "Acute Dacryocystitis," Section 6.9.

Parinaud's Oculoglandular Conjunctivitis

See "Parinaud's Oculoglandular Conjunctivitis," Section 5.3.

5.3 Parinaud's Oculoglandular Conjunctivitis

Symptoms   Red eye, mucopurulent discharge, foreign-body sensation.

Critical Signs   Granulomatous nodule(s) on the palpebral conjunctiva, visibly swollen preauricular or submandibular lymph node on the same side.

Other Signs   Same as other forms of conjunctivitis, but may be associated with fever and a rash.

Etiology

- Cat scratch disease   (History of being scratched or licked by a cat within two weeks prior to the onset of symptoms.)
- Tularemia   (History of contact with rabbits, other small wild animals, or ticks. Patients have a severe headache, fever, and other systemic manifestations.)
- Tuberculosis and other mycobacteria
- Syphilis
- Others   (Leukemia, lymphoma, mumps, mononucleosis, fungi, sarcoidosis, etc.)

Work-up   (Initiated when the etiology is not known [e.g., no recent cat scratch])

1. Conjunctival biopsy with scrapings for Gram's, Giemsa, and acid-fast stains.
2. Blood, Lowenstein-Jensen, Sabouraud's, and thioglycolate cultures.
3. CBC, RPR, FTA-ABS, and, if the patient is febrile, blood cultures.
4. Chest x-ray, PPD, and anergy panel.
5. If suspect tularemia, serologic titers are needed.

Treatment

1. Warm compresses for tender lymph nodes.
2. Antipyretics prn.
3. Specifically:

   Cat scratch disease The disease generally resolves spontaneously in 6 weeks. Consider tetracycline 250 mg qid × 2 weeks plus a topical antibiotic (e.g., bacitracin/polymyxin B ointment or gentamicin drops qid) × 2 weeks.

   Tularemia Streptomycin 1 gram im 8 day × 7 days plus gentamicin drops q 2 h × 1 week then 5×/day until resolved. Refer to a medical internist for systemic management.

   Tuberculosis Refer to an internist for antituberculous medication (e.g., isoniazid and rifampin).

   Syphilis Systemic penicillin (dose depending on the stage of the syphilis) plus topical tetracycline ointment. See Section 14.2.

Follow-up Repeat the ocular examination in 1-2 weeks.

5.4 Subconjunctival Hemorrhage

Symptoms Red eye, may have mild irritation.

Critical Sign Blood underneath the conjunctiva, often in a sector of the eye. Following trauma, the entire view of the sclera may be obstructed by blood.

Etiology

- Valsalva (e.g., coughing or straining)
- Traumatic (May be isolated or associated with a retrobulbar hemorrhage or ruptured globe.)
- Hypertension
- Bleeding disorder
- Idiopathic

Differential Diagnosis

- Kaposi's sarcoma (Red or purple lesion beneath the conjunctiva, usually elevated slightly. These patients should be evaluated for AIDS.)
- Other conjunctival neoplasms (e.g., lymphoma) with secondary hemorrhage.

Work-up

1. History: Bleeding or clotting problems? Eye rubbing, trauma, heavy lifting or Valsalva? Recurrent subconjunctival hemorrhage? Recent URI or "cold"?
2. Ocular examination, ruling out a conjunctival lesion and checking the intraocular pressure. In traumatic cases, rule out a ruptured globe (abnormally deep anterior chamber, significant subconjunctival edema, hyphema, vitreous hemorrhage, and/or limitation of extraocular motility) and a retrobulbar hemorrhage (associated with proptosis, increased intraocular pressure, and occasionally conjunctival swelling).
3. Blood pressure check.
4. If the patient has recurrent subconjunctival hemorrhages or a history of bleeding problems, a bleeding time, PT, PTT, and CBC with platelets should be obtained and a medical consultation considered.

Treatment   None required. Artificial-tear drops (e.g., Refresh) qid can be given if mild ocular irritation is present.

Follow-up   This condition usually clears spontaneously within 1-2 weeks. Patients are told to return if the blood does not fully resolve, or if they suffer a recurrence. Referral to an internist or family physician should be made as indicated for hypertension or a bleeding diathesis.

5.5   Superior Limbic Keratoconjunctivitis (SLK)

Symptoms   Red eye, burning, foreign-body sensation, pain, tearing, and mild photophobia. The course may be chronic with exacerbations and remissions.

Critical Sign   Thickening and inflammation of the superior bulbar conjunctiva, especially at the limbus.

Other Signs   Papillae on the superior palpebral conjunctiva; fine punctate fluorescein staining on the superior cornea, limbus and conjunctiva; superior corneal micropannus and filaments. Usually bilateral.

Work-up

1. History: Recurrent episodes?
2. Slit-lamp examination with fluorescein staining, particularly of the superior cornea and adjacent conjunctiva. The upper eyelid often needs to be lifted

by the examiner to see the superior limbal area, and then should be everted to visualize the tarsus. Sometimes the localized thickening, inflammation, and staining of the superior bulber conjunctiva is best appreciated by direct inspection without a slit lamp.

3. Thyroid function tests (T3, T4, TSH). (50% have associated dysthyroid disease).

Treatment

MILD

1. Artificial tears (e.g., Refresh) 4-8 ×/day.
2. Artificial-tear ointment (e.g., Refresh PM) qhs.

MODERATE-TO-SEVERE

1. Silver nitrate 0.5-1.0% *solution* (from wax ampules) applied on a cotton-tipped applicator for 10-20 seconds to the superior tarsal and superior bulbar conjunctiva after topical anesthesia (e.g., proparacaine). Then antibiotic ointment (e.g., erythromycin) qhs for 1 week.

NOTE   Do *not* use the silver nitrate cautery sticks.

2. If significant mucus or filaments are present then acetylcysteine 20% drops (e.g., Mucomyst) 3-5 ×/day are usually added.
3. If 3-4 separate silver nitrate solution applications are unsuccessful then consider mechanical scraping, cryotherapy, cautery, or surgical resection or recession of the superior bulbar conjunctiva.
4. Dry eye syndrome and/or blepharitis need to be treated if present (see the appropriate sections).

Follow-up   Every week during an exacerbation. If signs and symptoms persist, a reapplication of silver nitrate solution as described above may be performed at the weekly follow-up visit.

5.6   Episcleritis

Symptoms   Acute onset of redness and mild pain in one or both eyes, typically in young adults. A history of recurrent episodes is common.

Critical Signs   Sectorial (and less commonly diffuse) redness of one or both eyes, mostly due to engorgement of the episcleral vessels. These vessels are large, run in a radial direction, and can be seen beneath the conjunctiva. (The conjunctiva can be moved above the episcleral vessels with a cotton-tipped applicator.) The episcleral vessels blanch with topical phenylephrine 2.5%.

Other Signs   Tenderness over the area of episcleral injection or a nodule which can be moved slightly over the underlying sclera may be seen. The cornea is rarely affected and there are no aqueous cells nor flare. Vision is normal.

Etiology

- Idiopathic   (Most common.)
- Collagen vascular disease (e.g., rheumatoid arthritis, polyarteritis nodosa, systemic lupus erythematosus, Wegener's granulomatosis, etc.)
- Gout   (Serum uric acid elevated.)
- Herpes zoster virus   (Scars from an old facial rash may be present.)
- Syphilis   ([+] FTA-ABS.)

Differential Diagnosis

- Scleritis   (The pain is deep, severe, and often radiates to the ipsilateral side of the head or face. The sclera may have a bluish hue when observed in natural light. Scleral [and deep episcleral] vessels, as well as conjunctival and superficial episcleral vessels, are injected. The scleral vessels do not blanch to topical phenylephrine 2.5%. Corneal involvement may be present.)
- Iritis   (Cells and flare are present in the anterior chamber. May be present with scleritis.)
- Conjunctivitis   (Characterized by a discharge, eyelids sticking together in the morning, and inferior tarsal conjunctival follicles or papillae.)

Work-up

1. History: Rash? Arthritis? Venereal disease? Recent viral illness? Medical problems?
2. External examination in natural light: Look for the bluish hue of scleritis.
3. Slit-lamp examination: Anesthetize (e.g., topical proparacaine) and move the conjunctiva with a cotton-tipped applicator to determine the depth of the injected blood vessels. Determine whether there is any corneal or anterior-chamber involvement. Check the intraocular pressure (IOP).
4. Place a drop of phenylephrine 2.5% in the affected eye and reexamine the vascular pattern 10-15 minutes later. Episcleral vessels should blanch.
5. If the history suggests an underlying etiology, the appropriate laboratory tests should be obtained (e.g., ANA, rheumatoid factor, ESR, serum uric acid level, RPR, FTA-ABS).

Treatment

- If mild, treat with artificial tears (e.g., Refresh) qid or a topical vasoconstrictor/antihistamine (e.g., naphazoline/pheniramine) qid.

- If moderate to severe, a topical steroid (e.g., fluorometholone) qid often relieves the discomfort. Rarely, more frequent topical steroid application is necessary.
- In the very rare cases where topical steroids do not provide relief, oral nonsteroidal antiinflammatory drugs may help (e.g., ibuprofen 200-600 mg po 3-4 × /day or aspirin 325-1000 mg po 3-4 × /day, with food and/or antacids).

Follow-up   Patients placed on topical steroids are checked weekly (including an IOP check) until their symptoms have resolved. The frequency of steroid administration is then tapered. Patients treated with artificial tears or a topical vasoconstrictor/antihistamine need not be seen for several weeks for their episcleritis unless it worsens or continues to bother them. Patients are informed that episcleritis may recur in the same or fellow eye.

5.7   Scleritis

Symptoms   Severe and boring eye pain (most prominent feature) which may radiate to the forehead, brow, or jaw and may awaken the patient at night. Gradual onset in most cases. Red eye, tearing, photophobia, or insidious decrease in vision. Recurrent episodes are common. No discharge.

Critical Signs   Inflammation of *scleral*, episcleral, and conjunctival vessels (scleral vessels are deep, large vessels which cannot be moved with a cotton swab and which do not blanch with topical phenylephrine)—can be sectorial or diffuse. The sclera has a characteristic bluish hue (best seen in natural light by gross inspection) and may be thin or edematous.

Other Signs   Scleral nodules, corneal changes (peripheral keratitis, limbal guttering, and/or keratolysis), glaucoma, subretinal granuloma, uveitis, exudative retinal detachment (RD), cataract, proptosis (posterior scleritis), or rapid onset hyperopia (posterior scleritis).

NOTE   The patient needs to be examined in all directions of gaze in daylight or at least room illumination without a slit lamp.

Classification

Diffuse anterior scleritis:
- Widespread inflammation of the anterior segment.

Nodular anterior scleritis:
- Immovable inflamed nodule(s).

Necrotizing anterior scleritis with inflammation:
- Extreme pain.
- The sclera becomes transparent (choroidal pigment visible by daylight) secondary to the inflammation.
- High mortality rate due to a systemic inflammatory disease.

Necrotizing anterior scleritis without inflammation (scleromalacia perforans):
- Almost complete lack of symptoms.
- Almost exclusively in patients with long-standing rheumatoid arthritis (RA).

Posterior scleritis:
- May start posteriorly or be an extension of anterior scleritis.
- May simulate an amelanotic choroidal mass.
- Exudative RD, disc swelling, retinal hemorrhage, choroidal folds.
- Restricted extraocular movements.
- Proptosis, pain, and tenderness.
- Usually unrelated to systemic disease.

Etiology 50% of patients with scleritis have an associated systemic disease identified.

More common Connective tissue disease (e.g., RA, anklylosing spondylitis, systemic lupus erythematosus, polyarteritis nodosa, Wegener's granulomatosis), post herpes zoster ophthalmicus, syphilis, and gout.
Less common Tuberculosis (TB), other bacteria (pseudomonas), hypertension, foreign body, and parasite.

Differential Diagnosis

- Episcleritis   (Sclera not involved. Blood vessels blanch with topical phenylephrine.)

Work-up

1. History: Previous episodes? Medical problems?
2. Examine the sclera in natural light, or at least room light.
3. Slit-lamp examination with the red free filter (green light) to determine whether avascular areas of the sclera exist.
4. Dilated fundus examination to rule out posterior involvement.
5. Complete physical examination (especially joints, skin, cardiovascular and respiratory system, often performed by an internist or rheumatologist).
6. CBC, ESR, uric acid, RPR, FTA-ABS, rheumatoid factor, ANA, and fasting blood sugar.
7. If a connective tissue disease is suspected: serum protein electrophoresis

(SPEP), circulating immune complexes, and C reactive protein are obtained.

8. Other tests if clinical suspicion warrants additional work-up: PPD with anergy panel, chest x-ray, x-ray of sacroiliac joints, x-rays of other joints as indicated by the physical examination, B-scan ultrasonography to detect posterior scleritis, MRI or CT scan if indicated.

Treatment

1. *Symptomatic scleritis*: One or more of the following may be required. (An antacid or H_2-blocker (e.g., ranitidine 150 mg po bid) is often used in conjunction.)
   a. Nonsteroidal antiinflammatory drug (NSAID) (e.g., ibuprofen 400-600 mg po qid or indomethacin 25 mg po tid for at least 1 week)
   b. Systemic steroids: Highly recommended in the presence of severe or necrotizing scleritis, pronounced uveitis, or areas of vascular closure by slit-lamp examination or fluorescein angiogram or after no response to the NSAID (e.g., prednisone 60-80 mg po q day for several days, then tapering slowly. The addition of a NSAID often facilitates the tapering of the steroid.) See Appendix 5 for a systemic steroid work-up.
   c. Immunosuppressive therapy (e.g., cyclophosphamide): Particularly useful in patients with systemic vasculitis, polyarteritis nodosa, and Wegener's granulomatosis. It can be used as an adjunct when high-dose steroids alone cannot improve the disease—use in collaboration with an internist or rheumatologist.
   d. Surgery: Only when persistence of scleritis is thought to be due to production of local antibodies following a local ocular problem (e.g., foreign body, parasite, or catapillar hair).
2. *Scleromalacia perforans*: No ocular treatment is available. Patients are referred to a rheumatologist for systemic treatment and consideration of immunosuppression, as the associated systemic disease is often severe.

NOTE   Glasses or an eye shield should be worn at all times if there is significant corneal thinning and a risk of perforation with minor trauma.

Follow-up   Depends on the severity of the symptoms and corneal thinning.

NOTES

1. Decreased pain is a sign of response to treatment, even if inflammation appears unchanged.
2. Topical steroids are rarely indicated in scleritis and are not effective. (A trial of topical steroids can be given to distinguish between episcleritis and scleritis since the former will often respond.)
3. Subconjunctival steroids are *contraindicated* in scleritis and may lead to scleral thinning and perforation at the injection sites.

5.8   Ocular Rosacea

Symptoms   Bilateral chronic ocular irritation, redness, burning, and foreign-body sensation. Patients are typically middle-aged adults.

Critical Signs   Telangiectasias, pustules, papules, and/or erythema of the cheeks, forehead, and nose (the findings may be subtle and are often best seen in natural light). Superficial or deep corneal vascularization, particularly in the inferior cornea, is sometimes seen, and it may extend into a stromal infiltrate.

Other Signs   Rhinophyma of the nose occurs in the late stages. Blepharitis (telangiectasias of the eyelid margin with inflammation) and chalazia are common. Conjunctival injection, superficial punctate keratitis, iritis, or even corneal perforation may occur.

Differential Diagnosis

- Herpes simplex keratitis   (Usually unilateral. The keratitis is often dendritic, but may appear similar. The typical facial lesions of rosacea are absent.)
- See "Superficial Punctate Keratitis," Section 4.1, for further differential diagnosis.

Work-up

1. External examination: Look at the face for the characteristic skin findings and inspect the eyelids for chalazia.
2. Slit-lamp examination: Look for telangiectasias of the eyelid margins; conjunctival injection; and corneal vascularization, in particular, inferiorly.

Treatment

1. Tetracycline 250 mg po qid × 3-6 weeks, tapering the dose slowly once relief of symptoms is obtained. Some patients are maintained on low-dose tetracycline (e.g., 250 mg q day) indefinitely if active disease recurs off of medication. Erythromycin, in the same dose as tetracycline, may be substituted if tetracycline cannot be used (e.g., pregnant woman or a nursing mother).

   NOTE   Patients diagnosed with ocular rosacea who are asymptomatic and who do not demonstrate progressively worsening eye disease need not be treated with oral antibiotics.

2. Warm compresses and eyelid hygiene for blepharitis or meibomianitis (see Soction 5.10).
3. Treat chalazia as needed (see Section 6.1).
4. Corneal perforations may be treated with cyanoacrylate adhesive if small, while larger ones may require surgical correction. (Tetracycline is usually administered in the pre- and postoperative periods.)
5. If infiltrates stain with fluorescein, smears, cultures, and antibiotic treatment may be necessary (see Section 4.12).

Follow-up Variable, depending on the severity of disease. Patients without corneal involvement are seen weeks to months later. Those with corneal disease are followed more closely.

NOTE Tetracycline should not be given to pregnant women, breast-feeding women, or children less than 8 years old. Patients should be told to take the medicine on an empty stomach and be warned of susceptibility to sunburn while on tetracycline.

5.9 Ocular Cicatricial Pemphigoid

Symptoms Insidious onset of redness, foreign-body sensation, tearing, and photophobia. Bilateral involvement. The course is characterized by remissions and exacerbations. Age is usually >55 years.

Critical Signs Inferior symblepharon (linear folds of conjunctiva connecting the palpebral conjunctiva of the lower eyelid to the inferior bulbar conjunctiva), foreshortening and tightness of the lower fornix.

Other Signs Superficial punctate keratitis, secondary bacterial conjunctivitis, and corneal ulcer. Later, poor tear film, entropion, trichiasis, corneal opacification with pannus and keratinization, and obliteration of the fornices with eventual limitation of ocular motility can occur. Open-angle glaucoma may be present also.

Systemic Signs Mucous membrane (nose, oral cavity, pharynx, larynx, esophagus, anus, vagina, urethra) vesicles; ruptured or formed bullae; denuded epithelium; and scarring, which can lead to strictures of the esophagus, anus, vagina, or urethra. In the mouth a desquamative gingivitis is common. Vesicles and bullae may also be noted on the skin, sometimes with erythematous plaques or scars near affected mucous membranes.

Differential Diagnosis

- Stevens-Johnson syndrome (erythema multiforme major) (Acute onset, usually with fever and malaise. Similar ocular involvement as ocular pemphigoid. The lips are typically swollen and crusted and "target lesions" of the skin [red centers surrounded by a pale zone] are often found.)
- Membranous conjunctivitis with scarring (Usually adenovirus or beta-hemolytic strep. Symblepharon can follow severe membranous/pseudomembranous conjunctivitis.)
- Severe chemical burn.
- Chronic topical medicine (e.g., epinephrine, pilocarpine, antiviral agents).

Work-up

1. History: Chronic topical medications? Acute onset of severe systemic illness in the past?
2. Skin and mucous membrane (especially the mouth) examination.
3. Slit-lamp examination, especially examining for inferior symblepharon. (Pull down the lower eyelid and have the patient look up.) Check the intraocular pressure.
4. Dermatology, ENT, GI, and pulmonary consults if needed.
5. Gram's stain and culture of the conjunctiva if secondary bacterial infection is suspected.
6. Consider a conjunctival biopsy for immunofluorescence studies.

Treatment (Often needs to be coordinated with an internist and/or dermatologist.)

1. Artificial tears (e.g., Refresh drops) 4-10×/day. Can add an artificial-tear ointment (e.g., Refresh PM) 2-4×/day and qhs.
2. Treat any blepharitis vigorously with eyelid hygiene, warm compresses, and antibiotic ointment (e.g., bacitracin tid), see "Blepharitis/Meibomianitis," Section 5.10.
3. Goggles or glasses with sides to provide a moist surrounding for the eyes.
4. Topical steroids (e.g., prednisolone acetate 1% qid) may help in suppressing acute exacerbations.
5. Systemic steroids (e.g., prednisone 60 mg po q day) may additionally help in suppressing acute exacerbations.
6. Immunosuppressive agents (e.g, cyclophosphamide) and dapsone are occasionally used for progressive disease.
7. Consider surgical correction of entropion and cryotherapy and electrolysis of trichiasis. (May be necessary, but carries a risk of further scarring and of provoking an acute exacerbation.)
8. Consider a keratoprosthesis in an endstage eye with apparently good macular function.

NOTE Surgery should be avoided if possible due to the risk of exacerbating the condition.

Follow-up Every 1-2 weeks during acute exacerbations, every 1-3 months during remissions.

5.10 Blepharitis/Meibomianitis

Symptoms Itching, burning, mild pain and foreign-body sensation, tearing, crusting around the eyes upon awakening.

Critical Sign Crusty, red, thickened eyelid margins with prominent blood vessels (blepharitis) and/or inspissated oil glands at the eyelid margins (meibomianitis).

Other Signs Conjunctival injection, swollen eyelids, mild mucus discharge, superficial punctate keratitis. Acne rosacea may be present.

Treatment (See Section 5.8 in the presence of acne rosacea.)

1. Scrub the eyelid margins with mild shampoo (e.g., Johnson's baby shampoo or I-Scrub) 2×/day on a cotton-tipped applicator or a wash cloth.
2. Warm compresses for 15 minutes qid.
3. If associated with dry eyes then use artificial tears (e.g., Refresh) 4-8 ×/day.
4. If moderately severe then add erythromycin or bacitracin ointment to the eye qhs.
5. Recurrent meibomianitis can be treated with tetracycline 250 mg po qid × 6 weeks; then taper slowly.

NOTE Tetracycline should not be used in pregnant women, breast-feeding mothers, or children less than 8 years old. Erythromycin 250 mg po qid can be used instead.

Follow-up Follow-up in 3-4 weeks as needed. Eyelid cleaning and warm compresses may be reduced to once a day as the condition improves. They often need to be maintained indefinitely.

NOTE Rarely, intractable, unilateral or asymmetric blepharitis is the only manifestation of sebaceous-gland carcinoma.

5.11 Contact Dermatitis

Symptoms   Sudden onset of a periorbital rash or eyelid swelling, mild watery discharge.

Critical Signs   Periorbital edema, erythema, vesicles, and lichenification of the skin.

Other Signs   Conjunctivitis, watery discharge. Crusting of the skin may develop when secondary infection arises.

Etiology   Most commonly eye drops and cosmetics, including nail polish.

Treatment

1. Avoid the offending agent (or the several potential agents).
2. Cool compresses 4-6×/day.
3. Consider a mild steroid cream (e.g., dexamethasone cream 0.05%) to the periocular area 2-3×/day for 4-5 days.
4. Consider an oral antihistamine (e.g., diphenhydramine [e.g., Benadryl] 25-50 mg po 3-4×/day) for several days.

Follow-up   Reexamine within 1 week.

6

Eyelid

6.1 Chalazion / Hordeolum

Symptoms   Eyelid lump, swelling, pain, tenderness, or erythema.

Critical Signs   Visible or palpable, well-defined subcutaneous nodule within the eyelid (in some cases, a nodule cannot be identified).

Other Signs   Blocked meibomian orifice, eyelid swelling and erythema, localized eyelid tenderness, and a palpable preauricular node. There may be associated blepharitis or acne rosacea.

Differential Diagnosis

- Preseptal cellulitis   (Eyelid erythema, edema, and warmth. Often there is a periorbital skin abrasion, laceration, or site of infection. Patients may be febrile.)
- Sebaceous cell carcinoma   (Should be suspected in a recurrent chalazion, thickening of both the upper and lower eyelids, and a chalazion associated with loss of the eyelashes. It usually develops in older patients. A biopsy along with frozen sections can establish the diagnosis. A special request must be made for lipid stains on frozen sections.)
- Adenovirus conjunctivitis   (Eyelid swelling and erythema along with a palpable preauricular node accompanying an acute conjunctivitis. Inferior tarsal conjunctival follicles are usually abundant. Patients typically complain of eyelids sticking together upon awakening from sleep.)

- Pyogenic granuloma   (Deep red, pedunculated lesion which may be associated with a chalazion/hordeolum or develop after trauma or surgery to the conjunctiva or skin. If associated with a chalazion/hordeolum, it may be excised or treated with a topical antibiotic-steroid combination (e.g., gentamicin/prednisolone acetate qid for 1-2 weeks).)

Work-up

1. History: Previous chalazion excision?
2. Palpate the involved eyelid, feeling for a nodule.
3. Slit-lamp examination: Evaluate the meibomian glands and evert the involved eyelid (this may allow better visualization of the nodule).

Treatment

1. Warm compresses for 15-20 minutes qid.
2. Consider a topical antibiotic (e.g., bacitracin or erythromycin ointment bid).
3. Light massage over the lesion several times a day may help.

If the chalazion does not disappear after 3-4 weeks of appropriate medical therapy and the patient would like to have it removed, incision and curettage are performed. Rarely, an injection of steroids into the lesion is performed instead of minor surgery, especially if the chalazion is near the lacrimal apparatus (e.g., 0.2-1.0 ml of triamcinolone 40 mg/ml is injected into and around the chalazion; the total dosage depends on the size of the lesion. NOTE A steroid injection can lead to permanent depigmentation of the skin at the injection site.)

Follow-up   Patients are not reseen after instituting medical therapy unless the lesion persists beyond 3-4 weeks. Patients having had incision and curettage are reexamined in one week.

6.2   Ectropion

Symptoms   Asymptomatic, tearing, or eye or eyelid irritation.

Critical Sign   Outward turning of the eyelid margin.

Other Signs   Superficial punctate keratitis (SPK) (may result from exposure keratopathy), conjunctival injection and eventually keratinization (may result from conjunctival drying).

Etiology

- Congenital
- Paralytic   (Seventh-cranial-nerve palsy.)
- Involutional   (Aging.)
- Cicatricial   (e.g., from a chemical burn, surgery, eyelid laceration scar.)
- Mechanical   (e.g., herniated orbital fat, eyelid tumor.)
- Allergic   (Contact dermatitis.)

Work-up

1. History: Previous surgery, trauma, chemical burn, or seventh-nerve palsy?
2. External examination: Check orbicularis oculi function, look for an eyelid tumor, eyelid scarring, herniated orbital fat, etc.
3. Slit-lamp examination: Check for SPK due to exposure and evaluate conjunctival integrity.

Treatment

1. Treat exposure keratopathy with lubricating agents (see Section 4.4).
2. Treat an inflamed, exposed eyelid margin with warm compresses and antibiotic ointment (e.g., bacitracin or erythromycin tid).
3. Taping the eyelids into position with adhesive tape may be a temporizing measure.
4. Definitive treatment usually requires surgery. Surgery is delayed for 3-6 months in patients with a seventh-nerve palsy, as it may resolve spontaneously.

Follow-up   Patients with signs of corneal or conjunctival drying are reevaluated in 1-2 weeks to evaluate the efficacy of therapy. Otherwise follow-up is not urgent.

6.3   Entropion

Symptoms   Ocular irritation or foreign-body sensation, tearing, red eye.

Critical Sign   Inward turning of the eyelid margin.

Other Signs   Superficial punctate keratitis (SPK) (from eyelashes contacting the globe), conjunctival injection.

Etiology

- Involutional (Aging.)
- Cicatricial (Due to conjunctival scarring in ocular pemphigoid, Stevens-Johnson syndrome, chemical burns, trauma, trachoma, and others.)
- Spastic (Due to surgical trauma, ocular irritation, or blepharospasm.)
- Congenital

Work-up

1. History: Previous surgery, trauma, chemical burn, severe eye disease?
2. Slit-lamp examination: Check for SPK, conjunctival and eyelid scarring.

Treatment See Section 6.6 if blepharospasm is present.

1. Antibiotic ointment (e.g., erythromycin or bacitracin tid) for SPK.
2. Everting the eyelid margin away from the globe and taping it in place with adhesive tape may be a temporizing measure.
3. Surgery is often required for permanent correction (spastic entropion may respond to the above measures and not require surgery).

Follow-up If the cornea is relatively healthy, the condition does not require urgent attention. If the cornea is significantly damaged, aggressive treatment is indicated (see "Superficial Punctate Keratitis," Section 4.1).

6.4 Trichiasis

Symptoms Ocular irritation or foreign-body sensation, tearing, red eye.

Critical Sign Misdirected eyelashes are found to be rubbing against the globe.

Other Signs Superficial punctate keratitis (SPK), conjunctival injection.

Etiology

- Chronic blepharitis (Thickened, erythematous, inflamed eyelid margin with excess secretions and telangiectatic blood vessels running across it.)
- Entropion (Inward turning of the eyelid margin. May be due to Stevens-Johnson syndrome, ocular pemphigoid, chemical burns, trachoma, or others.)
- Idiopathic

Work-up

1. History: Recurrent episodes? Severe systemic illness in the past?
2. Slit-lamp examination with fluorescein staining (evert the eyelids and inspect the palpebral conjunctiva).

Treatment   See Sections 6.3 and 5.10 for treatment of entropion and blepharitis.

1. Remove the misdirected lashes.
   a. A few misdirected lashes: Remove them at the slit lamp with fine forceps (recurrence is common).
   b. Diffuse, severe, or recurrent trichiasis: Can attempt to remove the misdirected lashes as above; however, definitive therapy generally requires electrolysis, cryotherapy, or surgery.
2. Treat the SPK with antibiotic ointment (e.g., erythromycin or bacitracin tid) × several days.

Follow-up   As needed.

6.5 Floppy Eyelid Syndrome

Symptoms   Chronically red, irritated eye, often worst upon awakening from sleep, and a mild mucus discharge. Patients are typically obese.

Critical Signs   An upper eyelid which can be everted easily, without an accessory finger or cotton-tipped applicator exerting counter pressure.

Other Signs   A soft and rubbery superior tarsal plate, a superior tarsal papillary conjunctivitis, superficial punctate keratitis (SPK).

NOTE   The symptoms are thought to result from spontaneous eversion of the upper eyelid during sleep, allowing the superior palpebral conjunctiva to rub against a pillow or mattress.

Differential Diagnosis   All of the following may produce a superior tarsal papillary conjunctivitis, but none of them has easily everted eyelids as described above.

- Vernal conjunctivitis   (Seasonal itching).
- Giant papillary conjunctivitis   (Often related to contact-lens wear or an exposed suture.)

- Superior limbic keratoconjunctivitis   (Hyperemia and thickening of the superior bulbar conjunctiva.)
- Toxic keratoconjunctivitis   (Papillae and/or follicles are usually more abundant on the inferior tarsal conjunctiva in a patient using eyedrops.)

Work-up

1. Pull the skin of the upper eyelid toward the patient's forehead and watch to see if the eyelid spontaneously everts or is abnormally lax.
2. Slit-lamp examination of the cornea and conjunctiva, with fluorescein staining.

Treatment

1. Topical antibiotics or lubricants for any mild corneal or conjunctival abnormality (e.g., erythromycin ointment 2-3 × /day for SPK, then Refresh PM ointment qhs when corneal pathology resolves.)
2. The eyelids are taped closed during sleep and/or an eye shield is worn to protect the eyelid from rubbing against the pillow or bed. Sometimes an eyelid-tightening surgical procedure is performed.
3. Patients are asked to refrain from sleeping face down on their pillow or mattress.

Follow-up   Every 2-7 days at first, then every few weeks to months as the condition stabilizes.

6.6   Blepharospasm

Symptoms   Uncontrolled blinking, twitching, or closure of the eyelids; decreased vision, always bilateral.

Critical Sign   Episodic involuntary contractions of the orbicularis oculi muscles.

Other Signs   Disappears during sleep, may have uncontrollable orofacial and head and neck movements.

Differential Diagnosis

- Hemifacial spasm   (Unilateral, contractures involve the entire side of the face, does not disappear during sleep, damage to the seventh nerve at the

level of the brainstem is the most common etiology. Treated similarly to blepharospasm.)
- Ocular irritation (e.g., corneal or conjunctival foreign body, trichiasis, blepharitis, dry eye)
- Tourette's syndrome (Multiple compulsive muscle spasms associated with utterances of bizarre sounds or vile words.)
- Tic douloureux (trigeminal neuralgia) (Acute episodes of pain in the distribution of the fifth cranial nerve, often causing a wince or tic.)
- Tardive dyskinesia (Oral-facial dyskinesia often with restlessness and dystonic movements of the trunk and limbs, typically from long-term use of antipsychotic medications.)
- Eyelid myokymia (Eyelid twitches, often brought on by stress.)

Work-up

1. History: Unilateral or bilateral? Are the eyelids alone involved or are the facial and limb muscles also involved? Medications?
2. Slit-lamp examination, searching for a local ocular disorder.
3. Neuro-ophthalmic examination to rule out other accompanying abnormalities.
4. CT scan (axial and coronal views) and/or MRI of the posterior fossa in atypical cases.

Treatment

1. Treat any underlying eye disorder (e.g., treat dry eye/blepharitis with eyelid hygiene and artificial tears 4-6 × /day).
2. Consider botulinum toxin injections into the orbicularis muscles around the eyelids if the blepharospasm is severe.
3. If the spasm is not relieved with botulinum toxin injections, consider surgical excision of the orbicularis muscle from the upper eyelids and brow.

Follow-up Not an urgent condition, but with severe blepharospasm patients can be functionally blind.

6.7 Canaliculitis

Symptoms Tearing or discharge, red eye, mild tenderness over the nasal aspect of the lower (or upper) eyelid.

Critical Signs   Erythematous pouting punctum, erythema of the skin surrounding the punctum. Mucopurulent discharge or concretions may be expressed from the punctum when pressure is applied over the nasal corner of the lower eyelid (the lacrimal sac).

Other Signs   A conjunctivitis confined to the nasal aspect of the eye, a gritty sensation upon probing of the canaliculus.

Etiology

- Actinomyces israelii (streptothrix)   (Most common.) (Gram positive rod with fine branching filaments seen on Gram's stain.)
- Fungal (e.g., Candida, Fusarium, Aspergillus)
- Viral (e.g., herpes simplex and varicella-zoster)
- Other bacteria (e.g., Fusobacterium, Nocardia)

Differential Diagnosis

- Dacryocystitis   (Much more swelling, tenderness, and pain. Swelling of the skin is more prominent than pouting of the punctum.)
- Nasolacrimal duct obstruction   (Tearing, minimal to no erythema nor tenderness around the punctum.)
- Conjunctivitis   (Conjunctival follicles and/or papillae, discharge. No pouting punctum nor punctal discharge.)

Work-up

1. Apply gentle pressure over the lacrimal sac with a cotton swab and roll it toward the punctum; observe for a punctal discharge.
2. Smears and cultures of the material expressed from the punctum: Gram's stain, Giemsa stain, and a KOH smear if available (1 drop of KOH 10-20% is placed on a slide, the discharge is added to the drop with a spatula, and a cover-slip is placed over the mixture before microscopic examination); consider thioglycolate and Sabouraud's cultures.

Treatment

1. Remove obstructing concretions—Can try expressing the concretions through the punctum at the slit lamp, but it usually requires a surgical canaliculotomy (with marsupialization of the canaliculus) to remove them all.
2. After removing the concretions, irrigate the canaliculus with penicillin G solution, 100,000 units/ml or iodine 1% solution (the patient is irrigated while in the upright position so the solution drains out of the nose and not into the nasopharynx).

If a fungus is found on smears and cultures, nystatin 1:20,000 drops tid + nystatin 1:20,000 solution irrigation several times per week may be effective.

If a herpes virus is found on smears, treat with trifluorothymidine 1% drops (e.g., Viroptic) 5 × /day for several weeks. Silicone intubation is sometimes required in viral cases, along with appropriate antiviral therapy.

3. Warm compresses to the punctal area qid.
4. More extensive surgical treatment is occasionally required.

Follow-up   This is generally not an urgent condition.

6.8   Dacryocystitis

(Inflammation of the Lacrimal Sac)

Symptoms   Pain, redness, and swelling over the innermost aspect of the lower eyelid (over the lacrimal sac), tearing, discharge, and fever. May be recurrent.

Critical Signs   Erythematous, tender swelling centered over the nasal aspect of the lower eyelid and extending around the periorbital area nasally. A mucoid or purulent discharge can be expressed from the punctum when pressure is applied over the lacrimal sac.

Other Signs   Fistula formation (often emerging from the skin beneath the medial canthal tendon), a lacrimal sac cyst, or a mucocele can occur in chronic cases. Rarely, orbital or facial cellulitis may develop as a complication.

Etiology   Nasolacrimal duct obstruction, diverticulum of the lacrimal sac, dacryolith, nasal or sinus surgery, trauma.

Differential Diagnosis   All of the following may produce inflammation of the periorbital area nasally.

- Facial cellulitis involving the medial canthus   (Discharge cannot be expressed from the punctum by placing pressure over the lacrimal sac. The lacrimal drainage system is patent on irrigation and special lacrimal drainage system radiographic studies.)
- Acute ethmoid sinusitis   (Pain, tenderness, and erythema over the nasal bone, just medial to the inner canthus. Frontal headache and nasal obstruction are common. Patients are often febrile.)
- Acute frontal sinusitis   (Inflammation predominantly involves the upper eyelid. The forehead is tender to palpation.)

Work-up

1. History: Previous episodes? Concomitant ear, nose, or throat infection?
2. External examination, including gentle compression of the lacrimal sac (nasal corner of the lower eyelid) with a cotton swab in an attempt to express discharge from the punctum. This should be performed bilaterally to uncover a subtle contralateral dacryocystitis.
3. Ocular examination, specifically checking extraocular motility and looking for proptosis (Hertel exophthalmometry).
4. Obtain a Gram's stain and blood agar culture (and chocolate agar culture in children) of any discharge expressed from the punctum.
5. Consider a CT scan (axial and coronal views) of the orbit and paranasal sinuses in atypical or severe cases or those which do not respond to, or get worse on, appropriate antibiotics.

NOTE   Do not attempt to probe the lacrimal system during the acute stage of the infection.

Treatment

1. Systemic antibiotic
   Children:
   a. Afebrile, systemically well, mild case, reliable parent: Amoxicillin/clavulanate (e.g., Augmentin) 20-40 mg/kg/day po in 3 divided doses. Alternative treatment: Cefaclor (e.g., Ceclor) 20-40 mg/kg/day po in 3 divided doses.
   b. Febrile or acutely ill or moderate-severe case or unreliable parent: Hospitalize and treat with cefuroxime 50-100 mg/kg/day iv in 3 divided doses.
   Adults:
   a. Afebrile, systemically well, mild case, reliable patient: Dicloxacillin 500 mg po q 6 hours.
   Alternative treatment: Cephalexin (e.g., Keflex) 500 mg po q 6 hours.
   b. Febrile or acutely ill: Hospitalize and treat with nafcillin 1 g iv q 4-6 hours.
   Alternative treatment: Cefazolin (e.g., Ancef) 500-1000 mg iv q 6-8 hours.
   The antibiotic regimen is adjusted according to the clinical response and the culture results. The IV antibiotics can be changed to comparable oral antibiotics depending on the rate of improvement, but systemic antibiotic therapy should be continued for a full 10 to 14-day course.
2. Topical antibiotic drops (e.g., sulfacetamide qid).
3. Warm compresses and gentle massage to the inner canthal region qid.
4. Pain medication (e.g., acetaminophen +/− codeine) prn.

5. Consider incision and drainage of a pointing abscess.
6. Consider surgical correction (e.g., dacryocystorhinostomy [DCR] with silicone intubation) once the acute episode has resolved, particularly with chronic dacryocystitis.

Follow-up Daily. If the condition of an outpatient worsens, hospitalization and intravenous antibiotics are recommended.

6.9 Acute Infectious Dacryoadenitis

(Infection of the Lacrimal Gland)

Symptoms Unilateral pain, redness, and swelling over the outer one-third of the upper eyelid, often with tearing or discharge. Typically occurs in children and young adults.

Critical Signs Erythema, swelling, and tenderness over the outer one-third of the upper eyelid; may be associated with hyperemia of the palpebral lobe of the lacrimal gland.

Other Signs Ipsilateral preauricular lymphadenopathy, ipsilateral conjunctival chemosis temporally, fever, elevated white blood cell count (WBC).

Etiology

• Bacterial (e.g., Staph. aureus, N. gonorrhea, streptococci)
• Viral (e.g., mumps, infectious mononucleosis, influenza, herpes zoster)

Differential Diagnosis

• Chalazion   (A palpable subcutaneous nodule or a blocked meibomian orifice may be present, afebrile, normal WBC.)
• Adenovirus conjunctivitis   (May produce eyelid swelling and erythema along with preauricular lymphadenopathy and a discharge. Typically produces inferior tarsal conjunctival follicles.)
• Preseptal cellulitis   (Erythema, edema, and warmth of the eyelid[s] and surrounding soft tissue. May have a periorbital skin laceration or site of infection.)

- Orbital cellulitis   (Proptosis and limitation of ocular motility often accompany eyelid erythema and swelling.)
- Inflammatory dacryoadenitis from orbital pseudotumor   (No preauricular lymphadenopathy. May have concomitant proptosis, downward displacement of the globe, or limitation of ocular motility. Typically afebrile with a normal WBC. Does not respond to antibiotics, but improves dramatically with systemic steroids.)
- Malignant lacrimal gland tumor   (Commonly produces displacement of the globe or proptosis, often palpable, evident on CT scan.)

Work-up   (The following is performed when an acute infectious etiology is suspected. When the disease does not respond to medical therapy or another etiology is being considered, see "Lacrimal-Gland Mass," Section 7.7.)

1. History: Acute or chronic? Fever? Discharge? Systemic infection or viral syndrome?
2. Palpate the eyelid and along the orbital rim for a mass.
3. Evaluate the resistance of each globe to retropulsion.
4. Look for proptosis (Hertel exophthalmometry).
5. Complete ocular examination, particularly extraocular motility assessment.
6. Smears and bacterial cultures of any discharge.
7. Examine the parotid glands (often, but not always, enlarged in mumps, sarcoidosis, tuberculosis, lymphoma, and syphilis.)
8. If the patient is febrile, a CBC with differential and, sometimes, blood cultures are obtained.
9. CT scan of the orbit and brain (axial and coronal views) when proptosis or a motility restriction is present or a mass is suspected.

Treatment

A. Bacterial or infectious (but unidentified) etiology

If mild-to-moderate: Amoxicillin/clavulanate (e.g., Augmentin)
  Adults: 250-500 mg po q 8 hours.
  Children: 20-40 mg/kg/day po in 3 divided doses.
 Alternative treatment: Cephalexin (e.g., Keflex)
  Adults: 250-500 mg po q 6 hours.
 Children: 25-50 mg/kg/day in 4 divided doses.

If moderate-to-severe, hospitalize and treat with: Ticarcillin/clavulanate (e.g., Timentin)
  Adults: 3.2 grams iv q 4-6 hours.
  Children: 200 mg/kg/day iv in 4 divided doses.

Alternative treatment: Cefazolin (e.g., Ancef)
Adults: 500-1000 mg iv q 6-8 hours.
Children: 50-100 mg/kg/day iv in 3-4 divided doses.

The antibiotic regimen should be adjusted according to the clinical response and culture and sensitivity results. IV antibiotics can be changed to comparable oral antibiotics depending on the rate of improvement, but systemic antibiotics should be continued for a full 7- to 14-day course.

If an abscess develops, incision and drainage are necessary.

B. Viral (e.g., mumps, infectious mononucleosis, etc.)
1. Cool compresses to the area of swelling and tenderness.
2. Analgesic prn (e.g., acetaminophen 650 mg po q 4 hours).

NOTE   Do not give aspirin to children with a viral syndrome because of the risk of Reye's syndrome.

Follow-up   Daily, watching for signs of orbital involvement (decreased motility or proptosis). Outpatients are admitted to the hospital for intravenous antibiotic therapy and an orbital CT scan if the condition worsens. Patients who fail to respond to medical therapy are managed as chronic dacryoadenitis (see "Lacrimal-Gland Mass," Section 7.7).

6.10   Preseptal Cellulitis

Symptoms   Tenderness and redness of the eyelid, mild fever, irritability.

Critical Signs   Eyelid erythema, edema, warmth, and tenderness. No proptosis, no restriction of extraocular motility, no pain with eye movement. The patient may not be able to open the eye due to the eyelid edema.

Other Signs   Conjunctival chemosis, tightness of the eyelid skin, fluctuant lymphedema of the eyelids.

NOTE   Preseptal cellulitis due to H. influenza generally occurs in children less than 5 years old and is characterized by the presence of an excessive amount of upper- and lower- eyelid edema which may extend into the cheeks. Typically, there is a distinctive red-purple discoloration of the involved area. The child may have malaise, ipsilateral otitis media, sinusitis, leukocytosis, or a bacteremia.

Etiology Puncture wound, laceration, retained foreign body from trauma, vascular extension, or extension from sinuses or another infectious site (e.g., dacryocystitis in children, chalazion). May be primarily infectious or inflammatory with secondary infectious potential.

Organisms Staph. aureus and streptococci most common, but H. influenza should be considered in children. Think of anaerobes if a foul-smelling discharge or necrosis is present or there is a history of an animal or human bite. Consider a viral cause if it is associated with a skin rash (e.g., herpes simplex or herpes zoster).

Differential Diagnosis

- Orbital cellulitis (Proptosis, pain with eye movement, restricted motility, decreased sensation along the first division of the trigeminal nerve, decreased vision, fever, or chemosis.)
- Other orbital disorders (Proptosis, globe displacement, or restricted ocular motility. See Section 7.1.)
- Chalazion (Focal eyelid inflammation, palpable mass, pointing meibomian gland.)
- Allergic eyelid swelling (Sudden onset, bright-red eyelid discoloration, prominent itching, absence of tenderness, history of allergies, or new eye or skin medication.)
- Viral conjunctivitis with eyelid swelling (Conjunctival follicles, palpable preauricular lymph node, itching, tearing, eyelid sticking, watery discharge.)
- Cavernous sinus thrombosis (Proptosis, paresis of the third, fourth, and sixth cranial nerves out of proportion of the eyelid swelling, decreased sensation of the first and second division of the trigeminal nerve, typically bilateral.)
- Erysipelas (Rapidly advancing streptococcus cellulitis, often with a clear demarcation line, high fever, and chills.)
- Others (e.g., insect bite, angioedema, trauma, maxillary osteomyelitis, others.)

Work-up

1. History: Pain with eye movements? Prior trauma or cancer?
2. Complete ocular examination, looking carefully for restriction of ocular motility or proptosis. An eyelid speculum or Desmarres eyelid retractor may facilitate the ocular examination if the eyelids are excessively swollen.
3. Check facial sensation in the distribution of first and second division of the trigeminal nerve.
4. Palpate the periorbital area and the head and neck lymph nodes for a mass.
5. Check vital signs.
6. Gram's stain and culture of any open wound or drainage.

7. If clinically suspect H. influenza then scrape the conjunctiva for Gram's stain and culture.
8. CT scan of the brain and orbits (axial and coronal views) if there is a history of significant trauma or a concern about the possibility of an orbital or intraocular foreign body, orbital cellulitis, a subperiosteal abscess, cavernous sinus thrombosis, or cancer.
9. Consider obtaining a CBC with differential and blood cultures in severe cases or when a fever is present.

Treatment

1. Antibiotic therapy
   A. Mild preseptal cellulitis and age >5 years:

     Amoxicillin/clavulanate (e.g., Augmentin)
      (20-40 mg/kg/day po in 3 divided doses in children)
      (250-500 mg po q 8 hours in adults)
     or cefaclor (e.g., Ceclor)
      (20-40 mg/kg/day po in 3 divided doses in children, maximum dose 1 g/day)
      (250-500 mg po q 8 hours in adults)

   If penicillin allergic, then:
   Trimethoprim/sulfamethoxazole (e.g., Bactrim)
    (8 mg/kg/day trimethoprim and 40 mg/kg/day sulfamethoxazole po in 2 divided doses in children)
    (160 mg trimethoprim and 800 mg sulfamethoxazole po bid in adults)

   If penicillin and sulfa allergic, then:
   Erythromycin
    (30-50 mg/kg/day po in 3-4 divided doses in children)
    (250-500 mg po q 6 hours in adults)

NOTE   Oral antibiotics are maintained for 10 days.

   B. Moderate-to-severe preseptal cellulitis or any one of the following:

- Patient appears toxic.
- Patient may be noncompliant with outpatient treatment and follow-up.
- Child ≤5 years old.
- Suspect H. influenza.
- No noticeable improvement or worsening after a few days of po antibiotics.

Admit to the hospital for IV antibiotics as follows:
Nafcillin or oxacillin
(150 mg/kg/day iv in 6 divided doses in children)
(1-2 g iv q 4 hours in adults)
and ceftazidime
(30-50 mg/kg iv q 8 h [maximum of 6 g/day] in children)
(1-2 g iv q 8 hours in adults)

NOTE   IV antibiotics can be changed to comparable oral antibiotics after significant improvement is observed. Systemic antibiotics are maintained for a total 10- to 14-day course.

2. Warm compresses to the inflamed area tid prn.
3. Polymyxin B/bacitracin ointment (e.g., Polysporin) to the eye qid if secondary conjunctivitis is present.
4. Tetanus toxoid if needed (see Appendix 11).
5. Exploration and debridement of the lesion if a fluctuant mass or abscess is present. Incise over the mass or reopen a healing laceration with a scalpel, fully explore the wound and Gram's stain and culture any drainage. Avoid the orbital septum if possible. A drain may need to be placed.

Follow-up   Daily until clear and consistent improvement is demonstrated, then every 2-7 days until the condition has totally resolved. If a preseptal cellulitis progresses despite antibiotic therapy, the patient is admitted to the hospital and a repeat (or initial) orbital CT scan is obtained. For patients on oral antibiotics, IV antibiotic treatment is started (see "Orbital Cellulitis," Section 7.4).

6.11   Malignant Tumors of the Eyelid

Symptoms   Asymptomatic or mildly irritating eyelid lump.

Signs   Skin ulceration and inflammation and distortion of the normal eyelid anatomy are common findings in malignant lesions.

Etiology

• Basal-cell carcinoma (most common malignant eyelid tumor)   Middle-aged to elderly patients. Two clinical presentations:

1. Nodular: Indurated, firm mass, commonly with telangiectasia over the tumor margins. Sometimes, the center of the lesion is ulcerated.
2. Morpheaform: Firm, flat, subcutaneous lesion with indistinct borders.

NOTE Basal-cell carcinoma does not metastasize, but it may be highly locally invasive, particularly when it is present in the medial canthal region.

- Squamous-cell carcinoma   Variable presentation, often appearing similar to a basal cell carcinoma. Metastasis may occur, but is uncommon. A premalignant lesion, an actinic keratosis, may appear as a scaly erythematous flat lesion or as a cutaneous horn.
- Sebaceous-gland carcinoma   Usually middle-aged to elderly patients. Most arise from the meibomian glands. Must be considered in the presence of a recurrent "chalazion" or intractable "blepharitis," as it may simulate each of these conditions. Loss of eyelashes and destruction of the meibomian gland orifices in the region of the tumor may occur. The tumor may be multifocal, involving both the upper and lower eyelids. Metastasis or orbital extension can occur.
- Others   (Malignant melanoma; lymphoma; sweat-gland carcinoma; metastasis, usually breast or lung).

Differential Diagnosis   (Benign eyelid masses)

- Seborrheic keratosis   (Middle-aged to elderly patients. Brown-black well-circumscribed crustlike lesion, usually elevated slightly and uninflamed. May be removed by shave biopsy if desired.)
- Hordeolum (Stye)   (Acute erythematous, tender, well-circumscribed lesion, often associated with blepharitis. See Section 6.1 for treatment.)
- Chalazion   (A chronic hordeolum which is no longer tender. See Section 6.1 for treatment.)
- Keratoacanthoma   (Appears similar to basal- and squamous-cell carcinomas, being elevated and possessing a central ulcer crater. These tumors, however, grow rapidly to a large size [1-2 cm] and then slowly shrink, often resolving spontaneously. Lesions which involve the eyelid or eyelash margin can be destructive and are surgically excised.)
- Cysts (e.g., epidermal inclusion, sudoriforous, sebaceous, etc.)   (Well-circumscribed white or yellow lesions on the eyelid margin or skin or underneath the skin. Ultrasound may help differentiate a cyst from a solid lesion. May be surgically excised.)
- Molluscum contagiosum   (Frequently multiple small papules with umbilicated centers. Viral in origin. May produce a chronic follicular conjuncti-

vitis. We usually surgically excise these lesions, but cryotherapy or other methods may be used.)

- Nevus   (Light to dark brown well-circumscribed lesion, sometimes with hair arising from the surface. It does not grow in size.)
- Xanthelasma   (Multiple, often bilateral, yellow plaques in the upper, and sometimes the lower, eyelids. Patients need to have a serum cholesterol and lipid profile evaluated to rule out a cholesterol or lipid disorder. Diabetes may also be present. Cosmetic surgery can be performed as desired.)
- Others   (Verrucae [viral warts], papilloma, benign tumors of hair follicles or sweat glands, inverted follicular keratosis, neurofibroma, neurilemoma, capillary hemangioma, cavernous hemangioma, pseudoepitheliomatis hyperplasia, necrobiotic xanthogranuloma nodules of multiple myeloma [yellow plaques or nodules often mistaken for xanthelasma].)

Work-up

1. History: How long has the lesion been present? Rapid or slow growth? Previous malignant skin lesion?
2. External examination: Check the skin for additional lesions, palpate the preauricular and submaxillary nodes for metastasis.
3. Slit-lamp examination: Look for telangiectasias on nodular tumors, evaluate for loss of eyelashes in the region of the tumor, and inspect the meibomian orifices, determining whether they have been destroyed.
4. Photograph and/or draw the lesion and its location for documentation.
5. Biopsy the lesion. An incisional biopsy is most commonly performed when a malignancy is suspected; although, an excisional biopsy with wide (10-mm) margins on all sides is preferable for malignant melanoma. Margins of potential malignant melanoma are sent for permanent section.
6. When a sebaceous-cell carcinoma is suspected, the pathologist needs to be alerted, and frozen or nonfixed tissue (for oil-red-O stain for fat) needs to be obtained. Patients confirmed to have this tumor are referred to a medical internist for a metastatic work-up (typically metastatic to the lymph nodes, lung, brain, liver, and bone).

Treatment

- Basal-cell carcinoma: Surgical excision with histologic evaluation of the tumor margins. Cryotherapy and radiation are used rarely. Patients are informed about the etiologic role of the sun and are advised to avoid sunlight when possible and to use protective sunscreens.
- Squamous-cell carcinoma: Same as for basal-cell carcinoma. Radiation therapy is the next best treatment after surgical excision. Warnings about the sun are given.

- Sebaceous-gland carcinoma: Surgical excision, taking wide margins of normal tissue on all sides. Frozen section evaluation of the margins is recommended.

Follow-up   After the initial follow-up period (e.g., every 1-4 weeks to ensure proper healing of the surgical site), patients are reevaluated every 6-12 months. Patients who have had one skin malignancy are at a greater risk for additional ones.

7
Orbit

7.1 Orbital Disease

This section helps distinguish a variety of orbital diseases. Specific work-ups and treatments are covered in sections on the individual disease entities.

Symptoms   Eyelid swelling, bulging eye(s), and double vision are common. Pain and decreased vision can occur.

Critical Signs   Proptosis and restriction of ocular motility, which can be confirmed by forced duction testing (see Appendix 6). There is often resistance on attempted retropulsion of the globe.

Other Signs   See the individual entities.

Etiology   One or more of the critical signs are usually present, but it is the specific characteristics listed below which help distinguish the individual entities.

- Thyroid eye disease   (Eyelid retraction and eyelid lag. Usually painless unless exposure keratopathy develops. Often bilateral. *CT scan:* Thickening of the extraocular muscles without involvement of the associated tendons.)
- Orbital inflammatory pseudotumor   (Often painful. Usually afebrile with a normal white blood cell count [WBC]. *CT scan:* Extraocular muscles are commonly thickened with involvement of the associated tendons. The sclera,

145

orbital fat, or lacrimal gland may be involved. Acute disease usually responds dramatically to systemic steroids.)

- Orbital cellulitis (Patients are usually febrile and often have an elevated WBC. *CT scan:* Sinusitis [especially ethmoid sinusitis] is usually present.)
- Orbital tumors (A palpable mass may be present. The globe may be displaced away from the location of the tumor. *CT scan:* A mass lesion is evident.)
- Lacrimal-gland tumors (A form of orbital tumor located in the outer one-third of the upper eyelid. The globe is usually displaced inferiorly and medially with ptosis of the involved eyelid. *CT scan:* A mass lesion is present in the lacrimal gland.)
- Trauma (e.g., retrobulbar hemorrhage, intraorbital foreign body) (Both occur at the time of trauma, however, an intraorbital foreign body may not produce orbital signs for a long period of time. CT scan +/− orbital ultrasound are diagnostic.)
- Orbital vasculitis (e.g., Wegener's granulomatosis, polyarteritis nodosa, others) (Systemic signs and symptoms [especially sinus, renal, pulmonary, and skin disease], fever, markedly elevated ESR.)
- Mucormycosis (Orbital, nasal, and sinus disease in a diabetic, immuno-compromised, or debilitated patient. Life-threatening. See "Cavernous Sinus/ Superior Orbital Fissure Syndrome," Section 11.8.)
- Varix (A large dilated vein within the orbit which produces proptosis when it fills and dilates [e.g., during a Valsalva maneuver or while placing the head in the dependent position]. When the vein is not engorged, the proptosis is not present. *CT scan:* Demonstrates the dilated vein if an enhanced scan is performed during a Valsalva maneuver. Venography may need to be performed if the CT scan is negative and a varix is still suspected.)

Differential Diagnosis

- Arteriovenous fistula (e.g., carotid-cavernous fistula) (May mimic orbital disease. It follows trauma or can occur spontaneously. A bruit is often heard by the patient and may be heard by the examiner if ocular auscultation is performed. *CT scan:* Enlarged superior ophthalmic vein, sometimes accompanied by enlarged extraocular muscles.)
- Cavernous sinus thrombosis (Orbital cellulitis signs plus decreased sensation of the fifth cranial nerve, dilated and sluggish pupil, paresis of the third, fourth, and sixth cranial nerves out of proportion to the degree of orbital edema, decreasing level of consciousness, nausea, vomiting, usually bilateral.)
- Cranial-nerve palsy (May produce mild proptosis with limitation of eye movement in specific directions. No resistance to retropulsion or on forced duction testing. Orbital CT scan is normal.)

- Enlarged globe (e.g., myopia)   (May produce pseudoproptosis. Large myopic eyes frequently have tilted discs and peripapillary crescents, and ultrasound reveals a large axial length.)
- Enophthalmos of the fellow eye (e.g., after an orbital floor fracture)   (May produce pseudoproptosis.)

Work-up

1. History: Rapid or slow onset? Pain? Ocular bruit? Fever, chills, systemic symptoms? History of cancer, diabetes, pulmonary, or renal disease? Skin rash? Trauma?
2. External examination:
   a. Look from over the patient's forehead to examine for proptosis (measure the amount with a Hertel exophthalmometer.[1])
   b. Look for displacement of the globe (measure from the bridge of the nose with a ruler.)
   c. Test for resistance to retropulsion (have the patient close his eyes while you gently push each globe back into the orbit with your thumb. Assess the resistance of each eye.)
   d. Feel along the orbital rim for a mass.
   e. Measure the ocular misalignment with prisms (see Appendix 2).
3. Ocular examination, specifically checking the pupils, visual fields, color vision (by color plates), intraocular pressure, optic nerve, and peripheral retina.
4. Orbital CT scan (axial and coronal views).
5. Occasionally an MRI or orbital ultrasound is obtained in addition when the diagnosis is uncertain or the extent of the lesion needs to be better defined.
6. Vital signs, particularly temperature.
7. Lab work when appropriate: T3, T4, TSH, CBC, ESR, ANA, BUN, creatinine, fasting blood sugar, blood cultures, others.
8. Consider a forced duction test (see Appendix 3 for the technique.)
9. Consider an excisional, incisional, or fine-needle biopsy as dictated by the working diagnosis.

Additional work-up, treatment, and follow-up vary according to the suspected diagnosis. See the individual sections.

---

[1]Normal upper limits for proptosis are approximately 22 mm in whites and 24 mm in blacks. There should be no more than a 2-mm difference between the two eyes.

7.2 Thyroid Eye Disease (Graves' Ophthalmopathy)

Ocular Symptoms   Prominent eyes, eyelid swelling, double vision, foreign-body sensation, pain, photophobia, decreased vision in one or both eyes.

Critical Ocular Signs   Retraction of the upper eyelid, eyelid lag on downward gaze, and often unilateral or bilateral proptosis. When extraocular muscles are involved, limitation of elevation and outward movement are most common. There is resistance on forced duction testing. Orbital CT scan shows thickening of the involved extraocular muscles with sparing of the tendon which attaches the muscle to the globe.

NOTE   Optic-nerve compression secondary to thickened extraocular muscles at the orbital apex can produce an afferent pupillary defect, reduced color vision, and visual field and visual acuity loss. The optic disc may be swollen. Optic-nerve compression can develop in the presence of minimal exophthalmos. Involvement of more than one muscle with restriction of both elevation and horizontal eye movements is an indication that the patient is at risk for this complication.

Other Ocular Signs   Reduced frequency of blinking (stare), injection of the blood vessels over the insertion sites of involved extraocular muscles, resistance to retropulsion, eyelid edema, corneal superficial punctate keratitis or ulceration from exposure keratopathy.

Systemic Signs   Hyperthyroidism most commonly (rapid pulse, hot and dry skin, diffusely enlarged thyroid gland [goiter], weight loss, muscle wasting with proximal muscle weakness, hand tremor, pretibial dermopathy or myxedema, and sometimes cardiac arrhythmias). Some patients are euthyroid. Myasthenia gravis (fluctuating double vision and ptosis) is often present.

Differential Diagnosis   (See "Orbital Disease," Section 7.1, for conditions which produce proptosis.)   Two rare conditions which may produce eyelid retraction or eyelid lag are:

- Third-nerve palsy with aberrant regeneration   (The upper eyelid may elevate with downward gaze, simulating eyelid lag. Ocular motility may be limited, but forced duction testing and the orbital CT scan are normal.)
- Parinaud's syndrome   (Eyelid retraction and limitation of up-gaze may accompany mildly dilated pupils which react poorly to light, but normally to convergence.)

Work-up   (See "Orbital Disease," Section 7.1, for a general work-up of proptosis with an unknown etiology.)

1. History: Duration of symptoms? Pain? Known thyroid disease or cancer?
2. Complete ocular examination to establish the diagnosis and to determine whether the patient is developing exposure keratopathy (slit-lamp examination with fluorescein staining) or optic-nerve compression (pupillary assessment and evaluation of color vision with color plates). Limitation of motility is measured with prisms (see Appendix 2) and proptosis is measured with a Hertel exophthalmometer.
3. CT scan of the orbit (axial and coronal views) is performed when the diagnosis is uncertain (e.g., proptosis is present without other signs of thyroid disease) or surgery is planned.
4. Forced duction testing as needed to establish the diagnosis (see Appendix 6).
5. Formalized visual field examination when the vision is reduced (e.g., Humphrey, Octopus, or Goldmann).
6. Thyroid function tests (T3, T4, TSH).
7. Edrophonium chloride (e.g., Tensilon) test for suspected myasthenia gravis (see Section 11.9).

Treatment

1. Referral to a medical internist or endocrinologist for management of systemic thyroid disease if present.
2. Treat exposure keratopathy with artificial tears and lubricating ointment (e.g., Refresh drops q 1-6 hours and/or Refresh PM ointment qhs-tid). (See Section 4.4.)
3. Elevate the head of the bed at night if the patient is developing eyelid edema.
4. Orbital disease may need to be treated more aggressively when exposure keratopathy is worsening despite treatment (or is already severe), bothersome diplopia is present (particularly when looking straight ahead or reading), or optic-nerve compression is developing.
   The following recommendations may be controversial:
   a. Proptosis with corneal ulceration: Prednisone 100 mg po q day for 1-2 days maximum followed by orbital decompression surgery.
   b. Acute disturbing double vision with an inflamed eye: Prednisone 60-100 mg po q day, which may be tapered slowly as the condition improves. If no improvement occurs within 10 days then taper the patient off of the steroids quickly. When the thyroid disease is no longer active, extraocular muscle surgery may be performed as needed.
   c. Visual loss from optic neuropathy: Treat immediately. Options include prednisone 100 mg po q day, radiation therapy, and posterior orbital

decompression surgery. Often prednisone is started immediately in preparation for radiation or surgical therapy. If the vision does not improve or continues to deteriorate after 2-7 days of systemic steroids, one of the other modalities is employed. We prefer posterior orbital decompression surgery if it can be performed by a surgeon very familiar with the technique.

NOTE   See Appendix 5 for a systemic steroid work-up.

Follow-up   Optic-nerve compression is the most urgent ocular complication of thyroid eye disease, requiring immediate attention. Patients with advanced exposure keratopathy and severe proptosis also require prompt attention. Patients with minimal-to-no exposure problems and mild-to-moderate proptosis are reevaluated every 3-6 months. Patients who develop fluctuating diplopia and/or ptosis should receive an edrophonium chloride (e.g., Tensilon) test to rule out myasthenia gravis.

7.3   Orbital Inflammatory Pseudotumor

(Nonspecific Orbital Inflammatory Disease)

Symptoms   May be acute, recurrent, or chronic. Pain, prominent red eye, double vision, or decreased vision are common in acute disease. Children may have concomitant constitutional symptoms (including fever), which are not typical in adults. Asymptomatic proptosis may develop in chronic disease.

Critical Signs   Proptosis and/or restriction of ocular motility, usually unilateral. Orbital CT scan shows a thickened posterior sclera (or a ring of scleral thickening 360 degrees around the globe), orbital-fat or lacrimal-gland involvement, or thickening of extraocular muscles (including the tendons attaching the involved muscles to the globe). Bone destruction is very rare.

Other Signs   Eyelid erythema and edema, lacrimal-gland enlargement or a palpable orbital mass, decreased vision, uveitis, elevated intraocular pressure (IOP), hyperopic shift, optic-nerve swelling or atrophy, decreased sensitivity of the first division of the trigeminal nerve, conjunctival chemosis and injection.

NOTE   Bilateral pseudotumor in adults can occur, but should prompt a careful evaluation to rule out a systemic vasculitis (e.g., Wegener's granulomatosis or polyarteritis nodosa) and lymphoma. Bilateral pseudotumor in children is more common than in adults.

Etiology   Idiopathic.

Differential Diagnosis   See ''Orbital Disease,'' Section 7.1.

Work-up   (See Section 7.1, for a general orbital work-up.)

1. History: Previous episodes? Any other systemic symptoms or diseases? History of cancer?
2. Complete ocular examination (including ocular motility, exophthalmo-metry, IOP and optic-nerve evaluation).
3. Vital signs, particularly temperature.
4. Orbital CT scan (axial and coronal views).
5. Blood tests as needed (e.g., bilateral or atypical cases): ESR, CBC with differential, ANA, BUN and creatinine (rule out vasculitis), and fasting blood sugar (need to rule out mucormycosis in diabetics and immunocom-promised hosts).
6. Orbital biopsy (fine-needle aspiration or incisional biopsy) when the di-agnosis is uncertain, the case is atypical, the patient has a history of cancer, or an acute case does not respond to systemic steroids within a few days.

Treatment   Prednisone 80-100 mg po q day plus an antiulcer medication (e.g., ranitidine 150 mg po bid). Low-dose radiation therapy may be used when the patient does not respond to the systemic steroids or when the steroids pose a significant risk to the patient (see Appendix 5).

Follow-up   Reevaluate in 3-5 days. Patients who respond to the systemic ste-roids are maintained on them at the initial dose for 1-2 weeks and then tapered off of them slowly, usually over several months. Patients who do not respond to the steroids usually undergo biopsy (unless the diagnosis is known for certain, in which case radiation therapy is attempted). The IOP must be fol-lowed in patients being treated with steroids.

7.4   Orbital Cellulitis

Symptoms   Swollen eyelids, red eye, pain, blurred vision, fever, headache, double vision.

Critical Signs Eyelid edema, erythema, warmth, and tenderness. Conjunctival chemosis and injection, proptosis, and restricted ocular motility with pain on attempted eye movement are usually present.

Other Signs Decreased sensation of the first division of the fifth cranial nerve, typically with sparing of the second division, decreased vision, retinal venous congestion, optic-disc edema, purulent discharge, and fever. CT scan usually shows a sinusitis (typically an ethmoid sinusitis).

Etiology

- Direct extension from a sinus infection (especially ethmoiditis), focal orbital infection (e.g., dacryoadenitis, dacryocystitis, panophthalmitis), orbital fracture, or dental infection.
- Status post orbital trauma (NOTE When a foreign body is retained, the cellulitis may develop months after the injury.)
- Status post eye surgery (especially orbital surgery).
- Vascular extension (from a bacteremia).

Organisms Staphylococcus, streptococcus, H. influenzae (especially in children), bacteroides, gram negative rods (especially after trauma).

Differential Diagnosis See "Orbital Disease," Section 7.1.

Work-up (See Section 7.1 for a nonspecific orbital work-up.)

1. History: Trauma? Ear, nose, throat, or systemic infection? Stiff neck or mental status changes? Diabetes or an immunosuppressive illness?
2. Complete ophthalmic examination (especially looking for an afferent pupillary defect, limitation of or pain with eye movements, proptosis, decreased skin sensation, or an optic-nerve or fundus abnormality).
3. Check vital signs, mental status, and neck flexibility.
4. CT scan of the orbits and sinuses (axial and coronal views, with and without contrast if possible) to confirm the diagnosis and to rule out a foreign body and orbital or subperiosteal abscess.
5. CBC with differential.
6. Blood cultures.
7. Explore and debride any wound and obtain a Gram's stain and culture of any drainage (blood and chocolate agars, Sabouraud's medium, thioglycolate broth).
8. Obtain a lumbar puncture for suspected meningitis. Consider a neurology consult.

NOTE   Mucormycosis, a life-threatening disease, must be considered in all
diabetics and immunocompromised patients with orbital cellulitis. Immediate
action may need to be taken. (See "Cavernous Sinus/Superior Orbital Fissure
Syndrome," Section 11.8.)

Treatment

1. Admit to the hospital.
2. IV antibiotics for at least 1 week or until the condition improves significantly. We prefer the following (or equivalent) drugs:

CHILDREN

	nafcillin	(150 mg/kg/day iv in 6 divided doses)
or	vancomycin	(40 mg/kg/day iv in 2-3 divided doses)
plus	ceftazidime	(30-50 mg/kg iv q 8 hours [maximum of 6 g/day])

ADULTS

	ceftazidime	(1-2 g iv q 8 hours)
or	gentamicin	(1.75 mg/kg iv loading dose, then 1 mg/kg q 8 hours)
plus	nafcillin	(1-2 g iv q 4 hours)

Consider adding clindamycin (300 mg iv q 6 hours) for adults with chronic
orbital cellulitis or when an anaerobic infection is suspected.

If penicillin/cephalosporin allergic:

	vancomycin	(1 g iv q 12 hours)
or	clindamycin	(300 mg iv q 6 hours)
plus	gentamicin	(1.75 mg/kg iv loading dose, then 1 mg/kg q 8 hours)

NOTE   Antibiotic dosages may need to be reduced in the presence of renal
insufficiency or failure. Peak and trough levels of vancomycin and gentamicin are usually drawn ½ hour before and after the fifth dose, and
dosages are adjusted as needed. BUN and creatinine levels are followed
closely.

3. ENT consult for surgical drainage of the sinuses as needed, usually after
the initial episode is treated.
4. Nasal decongestant spray (e.g., Afrin bid) as needed.
5. Erythromycin ointment to the eye qid for corneal exposure if there is severe
proptosis.

Follow-up   Need to reevaluate every day in the hospital.

1. Progress may be monitored by:
   a. Temperature and white blood cell count.
   b. Vision.
   c. Ocular motility.
   d. Degree of proptosis and any displacement of the globe (significant displacement may indicate an abscess).

If any of the above are worsening then a CT scan of the orbit and brain needs to be repeated looking for an abscess. If an abscess is found, then surgical drainage may be required. Other conditions which need to be considered when the patient is not improving are cavernous sinus thrombosis and meningitis.

2. Evaluate the cornea for signs of exposure.
3. Check the intraocular pressure.
4. Examine the retina and optic nerve for signs of posterior compression (e.g., choroidal folds), inflammation, or an exudative retinal detachment.

When the orbital cellulitis is clearly and consistently improving, then the regimen can be changed to oral antibiotics (depending on the culture and sensitivity results) to complete a total 14-day course. We often use:

amoxicillin/clavulanate (e.g., Augmentin) (20-40 mg/kg/day in 3 divided doses in children; 250-500 mg tid in adults)

or

cefaclor (e.g., Ceclor) (20-40 mg/kg/day in 3 divided doses in children; 250-500 mg tid in adults)

The patient is followed every few days as an outpatient until the condition resolves.

7.5   Orbital Tumors in Children

Presentation   Proptosis and/or globe displacement. See the specific etiologies below for additional presenting signs.

Etiology

• Dermoid and epidermoid cysts   (Birth to young adulthood. Progresses slowly, unless the cyst ruptures. May develop in the orbit superiorly (especially superotemporally) or outside of the orbit in the temporal upper eyelid or brow. When external to the orbit, it is usually a smooth, round, and nontender

mass. *CT scan:* Well-defined lesion that may mold the bone of the orbital walls. *Ultrasound [B-scan]:* Cystic lesion with good transmission of echoes.)
- Capillary hemangioma (Birth to early infancy, slow progression, usually in the superonasal orbit. It may be observed through the eyelid as a bluish mass or be accompanied by a red hemangioma of the skin) a ("strawberry nevus," which blanches with pressure. Proptosis may be exacerbated by crying. It can enlarge over the first year, but spontaneously regresses over the following several years. *CT scan:* Irregular, contrast-enhancing, and usually extraconal lesion.)
- Rhabdomyosarcoma (Usually presents around 7 years of age, but may occur from infancy to adulthood. Malignant and may metastasize. Rather rapid onset and progression. May have edema of the eyelids, a palpable superonasal eyelid or subconjunctival mass, or a history of nosebleeds. Needs to be managed by urgent biopsy. *CT scan:* Bone destruction is typical. The mass may be well circumscribed, commonly in the superior orbit, especially nasally.)
- Lymphangioma (Usually presents in the first decade of life with a slowly progressive course, but may abruptly worsen if the tumor bleeds. Proptosis may be intermittent and exacerbated by upper respiratory infections. Concomitant conjunctival, eyelid, or oropharyngeal lymphangiomas may be noted [a conjunctival lesion appears as a multicystic mass]. *CT scan:* Nonencapsulated, irregular mass. *Ultrasound [B-scan]:* Cystic spaces are often seen.)
- Optic-nerve glioma (juvenile pilocytic astrocytoma) (Usually presents at age 2-6 years and is slowly progressive. Decreased visual acuity and a relative afferent pupillary defect usually develop. Optic atrophy or optic-nerve swelling may be present. May be associated with neurofibromatosis [in which case it may be bilateral]. *CT scan:* Fusiform enlargement of the optic nerve. The optic canal or chiasm may be involved.)
- Leukemia (granulocytic sarcoma) (Presents in the first decade of life with rapidly evolving unilateral or bilateral proptosis and occasionally swelling of the temporal fossa area due to a mass. Typically these lesions precede blood or bone marrow signs of leukemia, usually acute myelogenous leukemia, by several months. *CT scan:* Irregular mass sometimes with bony erosion. There may also be extension of the mass into the temporal fossa.) NOTE: Acute lymphoblastic leukemia can also produce unilateral or bilateral proptosis.
- Metastatic neuroblastoma (First few years of life. Abrupt presentation with unilateral or bilateral proptosis, eyelid ecchymosis, and globe displacement. The child is usually systemically ill, with the vast majority of patients having already been diagnosed with the abdominal cancer. *CT scan:* Poorly defined mass with bony destruction—especially of the lateral orbital wall.)
- Plexiform neurofibroma (Presents in the first decade of life and is pathognomonic of neurofibromatosis. Ptosis, eyelid hypertrophy, an S-shaped

deformity of the upper eyelid, or pulsating proptosis may be present. Facial asymmetry and a palpable anterior orbital mass may also be evident. *CT scan:* Diffuse, irregular soft tissue mass. A defect in the orbital roof may be seen. See Section 14.11.)
- Teratoma   (Presents at birth with severe unilateral proptosis that may progress. Vision is often lost from increased intraocular pressure [IOP], optic-nerve atrophy, and corneal exposure. The mass transilluminates. *CT scan:* Multiloculated soft tissue mass, enlarged orbit, intracranial extension is possible.)

Differential Diagnosis   See Section 7.1.

Work-up

1. History: Determine the age of onset and the rate of progression. Does the proptosis vary in degree (e.g., with crying)? Nosebleeds? Systemic illness?
2. External examination: Look for an anterior orbital mass, a skin hemangioma, or a temporal fossa lesion. Measure any proptosis (Hertel exophthalmometer) or globe displacement (measure from the bridge of the nose with a ruler). Abdominal examination is needed.
3. Complete ocular examination, including vision, pupillary assessment, color vision if possible, IOP, refraction, and an optic-nerve evaluation.
4. CT scan (axial and coronal views) of the orbit and brain.
5. Orbital ultrasound or MRI of the orbit as needed to further define the lesion.
6. In cases of acute onset and rapid progression, an emergent incisional biopsy for frozen, permanent, and electron microscopic evaluation may be advisable to rule out an aggressive malignancy (e.g., rhabdomyosarcoma).
7. Other tests as determined by the working diagnosis (usually performed by a pediatric oncologist):

   Rhabdomyosarcoma   Physical examination (looking especially for enlarged lymph nodes), chest and bone x-rays, bone marrow aspiration, lumbar puncture, liver function studies.
   Leukemia   CBC with differential, bone marrow studies, others.
   Neuroblastoma   Abdominal CT scan, urine for vanilyllmandelic acid (VMA).

Treatment

- Dermoid and epidermoid cysts: Complete surgical excision with the capsule intact. If the cyst ruptures, the contents can incite an acute inflammatory response.
- Capillary hemangioma: Observe if mild. A local steroid injection (e.g., betamethasone 6 mg and triamcinolone 40 mg) may be given to shrink the

lesion if necessary. Treatment is often indicated if strabismus, anisometropia, or amblyopia develop (see ''Amblyopia,'' Section 9.5).

- Rhabdomyosarcoma (managed by a pediatric oncologist in most cases): Local radiation therapy plus systemic chemotherapy is given once the diagnosis is confirmed by biopsy.
- Lymphangioma: Surgical excision is performed for a significant cosmetic deformity, ocular dysfunction (e.g., strabismus and amblyopia), or compressive optic neuropathy from acute orbital hemorrhage. Recurrences may occur after surgical excision.
- Optic-nerve glioma: Controversial. Observation, surgery, or radiation is used.
- Leukemia (managed by a pediatric oncologist in most cases): Systemic chemotherapy for the leukemia. Some physicians administer orbital radiation therapy alone when systemic leukemia cannot be confirmed on bone marrow studies.
- Metastatic neuroblastoma (managed by a pediatric oncologist in most cases): Local radiation plus systemic chemotherapy.
- Plexiform neurofibroma: Surgical excision is reserved for significant symptoms or disfigurement.
- Teratoma: Surgical excision (sometimes with the help of a neurosurgeon). Aspiration of the cyst may facilitate complete removal of large lesions. Preservation of ocular function may be possible.

Follow-up Tumors with a rapid onset and progression require urgent attention to rule out malignancy. Tumors which present more slowly may be managed less urgently.

7.6 Orbital Tumors in Adults

Symptoms Prominent eye, double vision. Pain or decreased vision may be experienced. May be asymptomatic.

Critical Signs Proptosis, displacement of the globe away from the location of the tumor, orbital mass on CT scan.

Other Signs A palpable mass, optic disc edema, or choroidal folds may be present. See the individual tumors below for more specific findings.

Etiology

- Metastatic (Usually middle-aged to elderly with a rapid onset of orbital signs. Common primary sources include the breast (most common), lung, genitourinary tract (especially prostate), and gastrointestinal tract. Enophthalmos (not proptosis) may be seen with scirrhous breast carcinoma. *CT scan:* Poorly defined, diffuse tumor which may conform to the shape of the adjacent orbital structures. Bone destruction may be seen.)

- Cavernous hemangioma (Typically young adulthood to middle age with a slow onset of orbital signs. *CT scan:* Well-defined mass, usually within the muscle cone. *Ultrasound [A-scan]:* High amplitude internal echoes.)

- Mucocele (Often have a frontal headache and a history of chronic sinusitis. Usually nasally or superonasally located. *CT scan:* A frontal or ethmoid sinus cyst can usually be noted to extend through eroded bone into the orbit. Affected sinuses may be opacified.)

- Lymphoid tumors (Usually middle-aged adults. Slow onset and progression. Typically develop superiorly in the anterior aspect of the orbit. May be accompanied by a subconjunctival "salmon-colored" lesion. *CT scan:* Irregular mass conforming to the shape of the orbital bones or globe. No bony erosion. Less responsive to systemic steroids than orbital pseudotumor. Can occur without evidence of systemic lymphoma.)

- Optic-nerve-sheath meningioma (Typically middle-aged females with painless, slowly progressive visual loss, often with mild proptosis. An afferent pupillary defect develops with visual loss. Ophthalmoscopy can reveal optic-nerve swelling, optic atrophy, or abnormal collateral vessels around the disc [optociliary shunt vessels]. Meningiomas arising intracranially can produce a temporal fossa mass. *CT scan:* Tubular enlargement of the optic nerve, sometimes with a "railroad tract" appearance [a linear shadow is seen within the lesion].)

- Localized neurofibroma (Young to middle-aged adult with slow development of orbital signs. Some have neurofibromatosis, but most do not. *CT scan:* Well-defined mass in the superior orbit [rarely inferiorly].)

- Neurilemoma (benign schwannoma) (Progressive painless proptosis. Mass usually located in the superior orbit. Rarely associated with neurofibromatosis. *CT scan:* Well-circumscribed fusiform or ovoid mass.)

- Fibrous histiocytoma (Any age. *CT scan:* Well-circumscribed mass anywhere in the orbit. Cannot be distinguished from a hemangiopericytoma before biopsy. See below.)

- Hemangiopericytoma (Any age. Relatively slow development of signs. Usually superiorly located. *CT scan:* May appear well defined and indistinguishable from a cavernous hemangioma or fibrous histiocytoma. Sometimes extends through the orbital bones into the temporal fossa and cranial cavity. *Ultrasound [A-scan]:* Low-to-medium internal reflectivity.)

- Others (Dermoid cyst, osteoma, hematocele, lymphangioma, extension of an ocular or periocular tumor, etc.)

Differential Diagnosis   See Sections 7.1 and 7.7.

Work-up

1. History: Determine the age of onset and the rate of progression. Headache or chronic sinusitis? History of cancer? Trauma (hematocele, orbital foreign body)?
2. Complete ocular examination, particularly vision, pupillary response, ocular motility, color vision and visual field of each eye, measurement of globe displacement (from the bridge of the nose with a ruler) and proptosis (Hertel exophthalmometer), intraocular pressure, and optic-nerve evaluation.
3. CT scan (axial and coronal views) of the orbit and brain.
4. Orbital ultrasound or MRI as needed to further define the lesion.
5. When a metastasis is suspected, the following should be performed:
    a. Fine-needle aspiration biopsy or incisional biopsy to confirm the diagnosis, with estrogen receptor assay if breast carcinoma is suspected.
    b. Breast examination and palpation of axillary lymph nodes.
    c. Medical work-up as directed by the biopsy result (e.g., chest x-ray, mammogram, etc.).
6. When a lymphoma is suspected, a medical consult is obtained and a systemic work-up is instituted (e.g., CBC with differential, serum protein electrophoresis, bone marrow biopsy, and CT scan of the abdomen and brain). If the work-up is negative, an incisional biopsy is performed (often need nonfixed tissue). If the work-up is positive, the systemic lymphoma is treated and the orbital lesion is observed for its response to treatment. Occasionally, a fine-needle biopsy is performed to confirm the orbital diagnosis.

Treatment

METASTATIC DISEASE

Systemic chemotherapy (or hormonal therapy) as required for the primary malignancy. Radiotherapy is often used for the orbital mass. Carcinoid tumors are occasionally resected.

CAVERNOUS HEMANGIOMA

Complete surgical excision is performed for compromised visual function or cosmetic purposes. If the patient is asymptomatic, they can be followed every 6-12 months.

MUCOCELE

1. Systemic antibiotics (e.g., nafcillin 1 g iv q 4 hours + ceftazidime 1 g iv q 8 hours) pre- and postoperatively.
2. Surgical drainage of the mucocele and exenteration of the involved sinus.

LYMPHOID TUMORS

Lymphoid hyperplasia and orbital lymphoma without systemic involvement are treated with local radiation therapy. Systemic lymphoma is treated with chemotherapy.

OPTIC-NERVE-SHEATH MENINGIOMA

Surgery is usually indicated when the tumor is growing and producing visual loss. Otherwise, the patient may be followed every 3-6 months.

LOCALIZED NEUROFIBROMA

Surgical removal is performed for enlarging tumors producing symptoms.

NEURILEMOMA

Same as cavernous hemangioma, see above.

FIBROUS HISTIOCYTOMA

Complete surgical removal. Recurrences are generally more aggressive and more malignant, sometimes necessitating orbital exenteration.

HEMANGIOPERICYTOMA

Complete surgical excision (as there is a potential for malignant transformation and metastasis).

Follow-up   Variable. Referral for treatment is not emergent, except when optic-nerve compromise is present. Metastatic disease should be worked-up without much delay.

NOTE   Also see "Lacrimal-Gland Mass," Section 7.7, especially if the mass is in the outer one-third of the upper eyelid, and "Orbital Tumors in Children," Section 7.5.

7.7   Lacrimal-Gland Mass / Chronic Dacryoadenitis

Symptoms   Persistent or progressive swelling of the outer one-third of the upper eyelid. Pain and/or double vision may or may not be present.

Critical Signs   Chronic eyelid swelling and erythema, predominantly in the outer one-third of the upper eyelid, with or without proptosis and displacement of the globe inferiorly and medially.

Other Signs   A palpable mass may be present in the upper outer one-third of the eyelid, extraocular motility may be restricted.

Etiology

- Sarcoidosis   (May have concomitant lung, skin, or ocular disease. Lymphadenopathy, parotid-gland enlargement, or a seventh-nerve palsy may be present. More common in blacks. Angiotensin-converting enzyme [ACE] level may be elevated.)
- Orbital inflammatory pseudotumor   (Commonly, pain and swelling develop acutely with or without limitation of ocular motility, displacement of the globe, or proptosis. A rapid response to systemic steroids is typical in acute cases.)
- Benign mixed epithelial tumor (pleomorphic adenoma)   (Slowly progressive, painless proptosis or displacement of the globe in middle-aged adults. CT scan may show a well-circumscribed mass with pressure-induced remodeling and enlargement of the lacrimal-gland fossa. No bony erosion occurs.)
- Dermoid   (Typically a painless, subcutaneous mass in a child that enlarges slowly. Well-defined, extraconal mass noted on CT scan.)
- Lymphoid tumor   (Slowly progressive proptosis and globe displacement in a middle-aged patient. May have a pink-white [''salmon-patch''] subconjunctival extension. CT scan shows an irregularly shaped lesion, conforming to the globe and lacrimal fossa. Bony erosion is not usually found.)
- Adenoid cystic carcinoma   (Acute onset of pain and proptosis progressing rapidly. Globe displacement, ptosis, and a motility disturbance are common. CT scan often shows an irregular mass, often with bony erosion.)
- Malignant mixed epithelial tumor (pleomorphic adenocarcinoma)   (Occurs primarily in older patients, acutely producing pain and progressing rapidly. Usually develops within a long-standing benign mixed epithelial tumor, or secondarily as a recurrence of a previously resected benign mixed tumor. CT scan findings are similar to adenoid cystic carcinoma.)
- Lacrimal gland cyst (dacryops)   (Usually an asymptomatic mass which may fluctuate in size. Typically a young adult or middle-aged patient.)
- Others   (Tuberculosis, syphilis, leukemia, mumps, mucoepidermoid carcinoma, plasmacytoma, etc.)

NOTE   Primary neoplasms (except lymphoma) are almost always unilateral; inflammatory disease may be bilateral. Lymphoma is more commonly unilateral, but may be bilateral.

Work-up

1. History: Determine the duration of the abnormality and the rate of progression. Associated pain, tenderness, double vision? Weakness, weight loss, fever, or other signs of systemic malignancy? Breathing difficulty, skin rash, or prior history of uveitis (sarcoidosis)? Any known medical problems? Prior lacrimal-gland biopsy or surgery?
2. Complete ocular examination, specifically looking for keratic precipitates on the posterior corneal surface, iris nodules, posterior synechiae, or old retinal periphlebitis from sarcoidosis.
3. Orbital CT scan—axial and coronal views (MRI is rarely required).
4. Consider a chest x-ray (may diagnose sarcoidosis and rarely tuberculosis).
5. Consider a CBC with differential, ACE, RPR, FTA-ABS, and PPD with anergy panel.
6. Systemic work-up by an internist or hematologist/oncologist when a lymphoma is suspected (e.g., abdominal and head CT scan, bone marrow biopsy, etc.).
7. Lacrimal-gland biopsy is indicated when:
   a. A malignant tumor is suspected (This may be unnecessary when a lymphoma is suspected clinically and is found on systemic work-up.)
   or
   b. The diagnosis is uncertain, but a malignancy or inflammatory etiology is suspected.

NOTE   Do not biopsy lesions thought to be benign mixed tumors or dermoids. Incomplete excision of a benign mixed tumor may lead to a recurrence with or without malignant transformation. Rupture of a dermoid cyst may lead to a severe inflammatory reaction. These two lesions need to be completely excised without rupturing the capsule or pseudocapsule.

Treatment

- Sarcoidosis: Systemic steroids (see Section 13.4)
- Orbital inflammatory pseudotumor: Systemic steroids (see Section 7.3).
- Benign mixed epithelial tumor: Complete surgical removal.
- Dermoid cyst: Complete surgical removal.
- Lymphoid tumor:
  a. Confined to the orbit: Orbital irradiation.

    b. Systemic involvement: Chemotherapy (orbital irradiation is usually with-
       held until the response of the orbital lesion to chemotherapy can be
       evaluated).
- Adenoid cystic carcinoma: Consider orbital exenteration +/− irradiation.
  (Chemotherapy is used rarely.)
- Malignant mixed epithelial tumor: Same as adenoid cystic carcinoma.
- Lacrimal-gland cyst: Excise if symptomatic.

Follow-up   Depends on the specific cause.

8

Ocular Tumors

8.1 Conjunctival Tumors

Below are listed the most common and important conjunctival tumors. Pterygium/pingueculum and phlyctenulosis are discussed elsewhere in this book.

Amelanotic Lesions

LIMBAL DERMOID

Congenital benign tumor, usually located at the temporal limbus; it may involve the cornea. Lesions are white, solid, fairly well circumscribed, elevated, and may have hair arising from their surface. They may be associated with eyelid colobomas, preauricular skin tags, and vertebral abnormalities (Goldenhar's syndrome). Surgical removal may be performed for cosmetic purposes, although a white corneal scar may persist postoperatively.

NOTE   The cornea or sclera underlying a dermoid may be very thin or even absent, and penetration of the eye can occur with surgical resection.

DERMOLIPOMA

Congenital benign tumor, usually occurring under the bulbar conjunctiva in the temporal-most aspect of the eye. It appears as a yellow-white solid tumor, often with hair arising from its surface. Surgical removal is usually avoided if possible because of the frequent extension of this tumor into the orbit, involving some of the orbital structures.

PYOGENIC GRANULOMA

Benign, deep-red pedunculated mass. It typically develops at a site of prior surgery, trauma, or chalazion. It may respond to topical steroids (we usually give a topical steroid-antibiotic combination, as infection may be present, e.g., prednisolone acetate-gentamicin qid for 1-2 weeks), but it often needs to be excised if it persists.

LYMPHANGIOMA

Probably congenital, but often not detected until years after birth. The lesion is benign, yet slowly progressive and appears as a diffuse, multiloculated, cystic mass. Hemorrhage into the cystic spaces may produce a "chocolate cyst." Concomitant eyelid, orbital, facial, nasal, or oropharyngeal lymphangiomas may be present. Surgical excision may be performed for cosmetic or functional purposes (it often needs to be repeated, as it is difficult to remove the entire tumor with one surgical procedure). Lesions often stabilize in early adulthood.

GRANULOMA

Any age. Predominantly occurs on the tarsal conjunctiva. No distinct clinical appearance, but patients may have an associated embedded foreign body, sarcoidosis, tuberculosis, or another granulomatous disease. Management often includes an incisional or excisional biopsy.

PAPILLOMA

Two types:

A. *Viral* Frequently multiple pedunculated or sessile lesions in children and young adults. These lesions are benign and are generally left untreated because of their high recurrence rate (which is often multiple) and their tendency for spontaneous resolution.
B. *Nonviral* Typically a single sessile or pedunculated lesion found in older patients. These may represent precancerous lesions with malignant potential. Complete excisional biopsy, flush with the surface, is the preferred treatment. Supplemental cryotherapy may be applied.

NOTE In dark-skinned individuals, papillomas may appear pigmented and may be mistaken for malignant melanoma.

KAPOSI'S SARCOMA

Malignant, subconjunctival nodule, usually red or purple in color. Patients need to be evaluated for AIDS (see Section 14.1).

CONJUNCTIVAL INTRAEPITHELIAL NEOPLASIA (DYSPLASIA AND CARCINOMA-IN-SITU)

Typically, middle-aged to elderly patients with a leukoplakic or gray-white gelatinous lesion, which usually begins at the limbus. Occasionally a papillomatous, cauliflowerlike appearance develops. The lesions are usually unilateral and unifocal. Lesions may evolve into invasive squamous-cell carcinoma if not treated early and successfully. They can spread over the cornea or, less commonly, invade the eye or metastasize. A complete excisional biopsy followed by supplemental cryotherapy to the remaining adjacent conjunctiva is the preferred treatment. (Excision may require lamellar dissection into the corneal stroma and sclera.) Periodic follow-up examinations are required to detect recurrences.

LYMPHOID TUMORS (RANGE FROM BENIGN REACTIVE LYMPHOID HYPERPLASIA TO LYMPHOMA)

Young to middle-aged adults. Usually appears as a light pink, "salmon-colored" lesion. It may appear in the bulbar conjunctiva, where it is typically oval in shape, or in the fornix, where it is usually horizontal in shape, conforming to the contour of the fornix. Excisional or incisional biopsy is performed for immuno-histochemical studies (may require nonfixed tissue). Symptomatic benign reactive lymphoid hyperplasia may be treated by excisional biopsy, low-dose radiation, or topical steroid drops. Lymphomas should be completely excised. Patients with the latter tumor are referred to an internist for systemic evaluation. Systemic lymphoma may or may not develop if it is not already present.

EPIBULBAR OSSEOUS CHORISTOMA

Congenital, benign, hard bony mass, usually on the superotemporal bulbar conjunctiva. Surgical removal may be performed for cosmetic purposes.

Melanotic Lesions

OCULAR OR OCULODERMAL MELANOCYTOSIS

Congenital. Not a conjunctival lesion, but an episcleral lesion, as demonstrated (after topical anesthesia) by moving the conjunctiva back and forth over the area of pigmentation with a sterile cotton swab. (Conjunctival pigmentation will move with the conjunctiva.) Typically it is unilateral and blue-gray in appearance often accompanied by a darker-colored ipsilateral iris and choroid.

In oculodermal disease, the periocular skin is also pigmented. Both conditions predispose to malignant melanoma of the uveal tract, orbit, and brain (most commonly in whites).

PRIMARY ACQUIRED MELANOSIS

Appears in middle-aged adults as flat brown patches of pigmentation without small cysts within the conjunctiva. It predisposes to malignant melanoma of the conjunctiva, which should be suspected when an elevation in one of these areas develops. Management options include incisional or excisional biopsy followed by cryotherapy.

NEVUS

Commonly develops during puberty, most often within the palpebral fissure on the bulbar conjunctiva. It is usually well demarcated and may or may not be pigmented (the degree of pigmentation may also change with time). A key sign in the diagnosis is the presence of small cysts within the lesion. Benign nevi may enlarge; however, malignant melanoma may occasionally develop from a nevus and enlargement may be an early sign of malignant transformation. Nevi of the palpebral conjunctiva are rare; primary acquired melanosis and malignant melanoma must be considered in such lesions. A baseline photograph of the nevus should be taken and the patient should be observed every 6-12 months. Surgical excision is elective.

MALIGNANT MELANOMA

Typically middle-aged to elderly patients with a nodular brown mass. The tumor is well vascularized, and a large conjunctival vessel can often be seen to be feeding the tumor. It may develop from a nevus or primary acquired melanosis, but it may also develop de novo. An underlying ciliary body melanoma must be checked for (dilated fundus examination, transillumination, and B-scan ultrasound). Intraocular and orbital extension may occur. Excisional biopsy (often with supplemental cryotherapy) is performed unless intraocular or orbital involvement is present (in which case an incisional biopsy may be performed if the diagnosis is uncertain, followed by enucleation or exenteration).

8.2 Malignant Melanoma of the Iris

Malignant melanoma (MM) of the iris may occur as a localized or diffuse pigmented (melanotic) or nonpigmented (amelanotic) lesion.

Critical Signs Unilateral brown or translucent iris mass lesion exhibiting slow growth. It is more common in the inferior half of the iris and in light-skinned individuals. It is rare in blacks.

Other Signs

A *localized* MM is generally greater than 3 mm in diameter at the base and greater than 1 mm in depth and often has prominent feeder vessels which ramify throughout the mass. It may produce secondary glaucoma. Although nonspecific, it may cause a sector cortical cataract, ectropion iridis, spontaneous hyphema, seeding of tumor cells into the anterior chamber, or direct invasion of tumor into the trabecular meshwork.

A *diffuse* MM causes progressive darkening of the involved iris, loss of iris crypts, and increased intraocular pressure (IOP). Focal iris nodules may be present.

Differential Diagnosis

A. Melanotic masses
  • Nevi (Typically become clinically apparent at the time of puberty, usually flat or minimally elevated (i.e., less than 1 mm) and uncommonly exceed 3 mm in diameter. Can cause ectropion iridis, sector cortical cataract, or secondary glaucoma. Generally *not* vascular. More common in the inferior half of the iris. *Nevi do not usually grow.*)
  • Tumors of the iris pigment epithelium (Usually black, in contrast to melanomas which are often dark brown or amelanotic.)
B. Amelanotic masses
  • Metastasis (Grows rapidly. More likely to be multiple or bilateral than MM. Frequently liberates cells and produces a pseudohypopyon. Involves the superior and inferior halves of the iris equally.)
  • Leiomyoma (Transparent and vascular. May be difficult to distinguish from a melanoma.)
  • Iris cyst (Unlike MM, most transmit light with transillumination.)
  • Inflammatory granuloma (e.g., sarcoidosis or tuberculosis) (Often have other signs of inflammation such as keratic precipitates, synechiae, and posterior subcapsular cataracts. A history of iritis or a systemic inflammatory disease may be elicited.)
C. Diffuse lesions
  • Congenital iris heterochromia (The darker iris is present at birth or in early childhood. It is nonprogressive and usually not associated with glaucoma. The iris has a smooth appearance.)
  • Fuchs' heterochromic iridocyclitis (Asymmetry of iris color, mild iritis in the eye with the lighter-colored iris, usually unilateral. Often associated with a cataract and/or glaucoma.)

- Iris nevus syndrome   (Corneal edema, peripheral anterior synechiae, iris atrophy, or an irregular pupil may be present along with multiple iris nodules and glaucoma.)
- Pigment dispersion   (Usually bilateral, the iris is rarely heavily pigmented [although the trabecular meshwork may be], and iris transillumination defects are often present.)
- Hemosiderosis   (A dark iris may result after iron breakdown products from old blood deposit on the iris surface. Patients have a history of a traumatic hyphema or vitreous hemorrhage.)

Work-up

1. History: Previous cancer, ocular surgery or trauma? Weight loss? Anorexia?
2. Slit-lamp examination: Carefully evaluate the irides. Check the IOP.
3. Gonioscopy of the anterior-chamber angle.
4. Dilated fundus examination using indirect ophthalmoscopy.
5. Transillumination (used to differentiate epithelial cysts which transmit light from pigmented lesions which do not).
6. Photograph the lesion and accurately draw it in the chart, including dimensions.

Treatment/Follow-up

1. Observe with periodic examinations and photographs every 3-12 months, depending on your suspicion of malignancy.
2. Surgical resection is indicated if growth is documented, the tumor interferes with vision, or it produces intractable glaucoma.
3. Diffuse iris MM with secondary glaucoma may require enucleation.

8.3   Malignant Melanoma of the Choroid

Symptoms   Patients may be asymptomatic or complain of decreased vision, a visual field defect, floaters, light flashes, or pain.

Critical Signs   Gray-green or brown (melanotic) or yellow (amelanotic) choroidal mass which exhibits one or more of the following:

1. Growth.
2. A large amount of subretinal fluid (i.e., retinal detachment).

3. A height greater than 2 mm, especially with an abrupt elevation from the choroid.
4. Ill-defined, large areas of orange pigment over the lesion.
5. A mushroom shape with congested blood vessels in the dome of the tumor.

NOTE   A diffuse choroidal malignant melanoma can appear as a thickened choroid, without a distinct mass.

Other Signs   Overlying cystoid retinal degeneration, vitreous hemorrhage or vitreous pigment cells, drusen on the tumor surface, a choroidal neovascular membrane, or proptosis (from orbital invasion). Choroidal malignant melanoma (MM) rarely occurs in blacks and more commonly occurs in light-skinned individuals.

Differential Diagnosis

A. Pigmented lesions
   - Nevi   (Melanotic or amelanotic choroidal lesions which rarely exhibit significant growth, are not mushroom-shaped, are generally less than 2 mm in thickness and show gradual elevation from the choroid. They may have an associated shallow retinal detachment or well-defined small areas of orange pigment on their surface, but surface drusen are more typical.)
   - Congenital hypertrophy of the retinal pigment epithelium (RPE)   (Flat lesions which are often black in color, but may appear gray-green. The margins are often well delineated with a surrounding depigmented halo. Depigmented areas frequently appear on the surface of the lesion.)
   - Reactive hyperplasia of the RPE   (Related to previous trauma or inflammation. Lesions are dark black in color, flat, have irregular margins, and may have associated white gliosis. Often multifocal.)
   - Age-related disciform macular degeneration   (Subretinal blood can simulate a melanoma. This disease is typically bilateral in the posterior pole and associated with extensive exudate. Fluorescein angiography [FA] easily differentiates.)
   - Peripheral disciform degeneration   (Peripheral elevated yellow-to-red mass with extensive exudation and hemorrhage. It may extend into the vitreous. The opposite eye often shows peripheral RPE changes.)
   - Melanocytoma of the optic nerve   (A dark-black optic nerve lesion with fibrillated margins. It may grow slowly. FA may differentiate.)
   - Choroidal detachment   (Follows ocular surgery, trauma, or hypotony of another etiology. Dark peripheral multilobular fundus mass. The ora serrata is often visible without scleral depression. It transilluminates [unless it is a hemorrhagic choroidal detachment], unlike a pigmented melanoma. Ultrasound may be required to differentiate the two.)

B. Nonpigmented lesions
  - Choroidal hemangioma   (Red-orange in color, may be elevated, but never mushroom-shaped.)
  - Metastatic carcinoma   (Creamy or light-brown color, flat or slightly elevated, extensive subretinal fluid, may be multifocal or bilateral. May have history of cancer [especially breast or lung cancer].)
  - Choroidal osteoma   (Yellow-orange in color, generally close to the optic disc, pseudopodium-like projections of the margin, often bilateral, typically in young women [teens or twenties]. Ultrasound may show a calcified mass.)
  - Posterior scleritis   (May have choroidal folds, pain, proptosis, uveitis, or anterior scleritis associated with an amelanotic mass.)

Work-up

1. History: Ocular surgery or trauma, cancer, anorexia, weight loss, or systemic illness?
2. Dilated fundus examination using indirect ophthalmoscopy.
3. Fluorescein angiography.
4. Ultrasound (A and B scans) (Documents thickness and confirms clinical impression).
5. Consider a phosphorus 32 test, CT scan or MRI of the orbit and brain, or fine-needle aspiration biopsy in selected cases.
6. If MM is confirmed:
   a. Blood work: LDH, GGT (gamma glutamyl transpeptidase), SGOT, SGPT, and alkaline phosphatase. Consider a liver scan if liver enzymes are elevated to rule out a liver metastasis.
   b. Chest x-ray.
   c. Complete physical examination by a medical internist.
7. Consider a CEA if a choroidal metastasis is suspected.

Treatment   Depending on the results of the metastatic work-up, the tumor characteristics, the status of the opposite eye, and the age and general health of the patient, malignant melanoma of the choroid may be managed by observation, photocoagulation, radiotherapy, local resection, or enucleation.

9
Pediatrics

9.1 Leukocoria

Definition   A white pupillary reflex.

Etiology

- Retinoblastoma   (A malignant tumor appearing as a flat or elevated white lesion in the inner retina which may be accompanied by indistinct white vitreous particles or a retinal detachment. Iris neovascularization is common and a pseudohypopyon may occur. There is almost never a cataract nor an abnormally-sized eye. It may be bilateral and/or multifocal and is usually diagnosed between ages 12 and 18 months. A positive family history may be elicited.)
- Toxocariasis   (A nematode infection producing a white, dome-shaped retinal granuloma, vitreous cells and haze, vitreous traction bands which can drag the macula or disc, and/or a traction retinal detachment. Anterior-chamber cells and flare may additionally be present. Rarely bilateral or multifocal, usually diagnosed between 7 and 8 years of age, often a history of contact with puppies or eating dirt, and no family history. A paracentesis of the anterior chamber may reveal eosinophils, and a serum ELISA test for Toxocara will be positive.)
- Coats' disease   (A retinal vascular abnormality resulting in small multifocal outpouchings of the retinal vessels associated with yellow intraretinal and subretinal exudate. An exudative retinal detachment may account for the

leukocoria. It usually develops in males during the first two decades of life, more severe cases occurring in the first decade of life. Rarely bilateral, no family history.)

- Persistent hyperplastic primary vitreous (PHPV)   (A developmental ocular anomaly producing a small eye, a shallow anterior chamber, a cataract, a fibrovascular membrane behind the lens, elongated ciliary processes, and large iris blood vessels. Angle-closure glaucoma can develop from lens swelling. The condition is congenital, but may not be detected until later in childhood. Rarely bilateral, no family history.)
- Congenital cataract   (Opacity of the lens present at birth, unilateral or bilateral. There may be a positive family history or an associated systemic disorder.)
- Retinal astrocytoma   (A white retinal lesion often, but not always, associated with tuberous sclerosis or, less commonly, neurofibromatosis.)
- Retinopathy of prematurity   (Predominantly in premature children; may have received supplemental oxygen therapy. Leukocoria is usually due to a retinal detachment. See "Retinopathy of Prematurity," Section 9.2.)
- Others (Retinochoroidal coloboma, retinal detachment, familial exudative vitreoretinopathy, myelinated nerve fibers, others)

Work-up

1. History: Age at onset? Family history of one of the conditions mentioned above? Prematurity or supplemental oxygen therapy? Contact with puppies or habit of eating dirt?
2. Complete ocular examination, including a measurement of corneal diameters (look for a small eye), an examination of the iris (look for neovascularization or abnormally dilated blood vessels), and an inspection of the lens (looking for a cataract). (A hand-held slit lamp is often most helpful.) A dilated fundus examination and anterior vitreous examination are essential.
3. Any or all of the following may be helpful in diagnosis and planning treatment:
   a. B-scan ultrasound (retinoblastoma, PHPV, cataract).
   b. IV fluorescein angiogram (Coats' disease, retinopathy of prematurity, retinoblastoma).
   c. CT scan or MRI of the orbit and brain (retinoblastoma), particularly for bilateral cases or those with a positive family history.
   d. Serum ELISA test for toxocara (Positive at 1:8 in the vast majority of infected patients.)
   e. Systemic examination (retinal astrocytoma, retinoblastoma).
   f. Anterior chamber paracentesis (toxocariasis).

NOTE   A paracentesis in a patient with a retinoblastoma can lead to tumor cell dissemination.

4. Consider an examination under anesthesia (EUA) in young or uncooperative children, particularly when retinoblastoma, toxocariasis, Coats' disease, or retinopathy of prematurity is being considered.

See "Congenital Cataract," Section 9.6, for a more specific cataract work-up.

Treatment

- Retinoblastoma: Enucleation, irradiation, photocoagulation, cryotherapy, or occasionally other therapeutic modalities. Systemic chemotherapy is used in metastatic disease.
- Toxocariasis:
  1. Steroids   (The route and dosage depend on the degree of inflammation and physician preference. In moderate-to-severe cases, a periocular depot steroid may be given at the time of an EUA, and topical steroids may be given in the presence of anterior-segment inflammation. Systemic steroids may also be used.)
  2. Consider a surgical vitrectomy when vitreoretinal traction bands form or when the condition does not improve or worsens with medical therapy.
- Coats' disease: Laser photocoagulation and/or cryotherapy to leaking vessels; surgery may be required for a retinal detachment.
- Persistent hyperplastic primary vitreous:
  1. Cataract extraction.
  2. Possible vitreal membrane excision.
  3. Treat any amblyopia.
- Congenital cataract: See Section 9.6.
- Retinal astrocytoma: Observation.
- Retinopathy of prematurity: See Section 9.2.

Follow-up   Variable, depending on the diagnosis.

9.2   Retinopathy of Prematurity (ROP)

Risk Factors

- Prematurity (especially <36 weeks gestation).
- Birthweight <2000 grams (4 lbs 6 oz), especially <1250 grams (2 lbs 12 oz).
- Supplemental oxygen therapy.

Critical Signs   An avascular peripheral retina with a distinct border, can have dragging of the posterior pole.

Other Signs   Usually bilateral, decreased visual acuity, leukocoria, retinal neovascularization, retinal detachment.

Differential Diagnosis

- Familial exudative vitreoretinopathy (FEV)   (Same as ROP except autosomal dominant, although family members may be asymptomatic, and no history of prematurity or oxygen therapy.)
- See "Leukocoria," Section 9.1 for further differential diagnosis.

Work-up

A. *Infants <1250 grams*   Dilated, depressed retinal examination at age 4-6 weeks, ideally prior to discharge from the hospital, with accurate staging of the disease. Can dilate with phenylephrine 2.5%, tropicamide 0.5-1% and homatropine 2%.

B. *Other premature or low-birth-weight infants*   Examination at age 6-10 weeks or prior to discharge from the hospital as above.

Classification

LOCATION

Zone 1   Posterior pole: 2 × disc-fovea distance (8 mm) centered around the disc.

Zone 2   From Zone 1 to the nasal periphery and equidistant temporally from the disc.

Zone 3   The remaining temporal periphery.

EXTENT

Number of clock hours involved.

SEVERITY

Stage 1   A flat demarcation line separating the vascular posterior retina from the avascular peripheral retina.

Stage 2   A ridged demarcation line.

Stage 3   A ridge with orange extraretinal neovascularization.

Stage 4   A retinal detachment.

"PLUS" DISEASE

Engorged veins and tortuous arteries in the posterior pole (a poor prognostic sign).

Treatment (based on severity)

Stage 1 Usually not treated. See indications for stage 2.

Stage 2 Cryotherapy may be indicated when vascularization does not extend beyond zone 1 and there is marked "plus" disease.

Stage 3 Cryotherapy is employed if zones 1 or 2 are involved with at least five confluent clock hours or eight total clock hours of extraretinal neovascularization and "plus" disease. Treatment should be instituted within 72 hours once this degree of involvement is reached.

Stage 4 Surgical repair of retinal detachment (regardless of zone).

Follow-up

A. *Infants <1250 grams* Repeat the examination every 2 weeks until age 14 weeks, then follow every 1-2 months at first and later every 6-12 months, as these children have a higher incidence of retinal detachment, dragged macula, cataracts, glaucoma, and amblyopia. If any stage of ROP is found in zone 1, if a ridge with "plus" disease is found in zone 2, or if any degree of extraretinal neovascularization is found in zone 2, then repeat examinations need to be performed weekly.

B. *Other premature or low birth weight infants* If signs of ROP are found on initial examination, follow as outlined for infants <1250 grams. If no signs of ROP are present initially, a repeat examination at 12-14 weeks of age may be considered, although the likelihood of ROP is minimal.

REFERENCES

COMMITTEE FOR THE CLASSIFICATION OF RETINOPATHY OF PREMATURITY. The international classification of retinopathy of prematurity. *Arch Ophthalmol* 102:1130, 1984.

CRYOTHERAPY FOR RETINOPATHY OF PREMATURITY COOPERATIVE GROUP. Multicenter trial of cryotherapy for retinopathy of prematurity. *Arch Ophthalmol* 106:471, 1988.

9.3 Esodeviations in Children

Critical Signs Either eye is turned inward ("cross-eyed"). On the cover-uncover test, when the fixating eye is covered, the nonfixating eye turns outward to fixate. See Appendix 2.

Other Signs   Amblyopia, overaction of the superior or inferior oblique muscles (producing an "A" or "V" pattern), latent nystagmus, vertical deviation.

Types

A. Comitant esodeviations   (The amount of esodeviation is constant in all fields of gaze at distance fixation. This is determined by prisms. See Appendix 2.)

- Congenital (infantile) esotropia   (Present by age 6 months, the angle of deviation is large [usually >30-40 prism diopters], and distance and near deviations are about equal.)
- Accommodative esotropia   (Onset is usually from 6 months to 7 years of age, moderate-to-severe hyperopia [farsightedness] is common, and the correction of the hyperopia eliminates the esotropia at distance. The deviation may progress from an intermittent to a constant esotropia.)
  Types:
  Normal AC/A (accommodative convergence to accommodation) ratio: Approximately equal deviation at near and distance fixation.
  High AC/A ratio: Greater esotropia at near than at distance fixation (these patients are not necessarily hyperopic).
- Nonaccommodative esotropia   (An esodeviation which cannot be fully straightened for distance by the full hyperopic correction. There is no history of a successfully treated accommodative esotropia.)
- Decompensated accommodative esotropia   (An accommodative esotropia with a new nonaccommodative component. That is, the accommodative esotropia was straight at distance in the past with correction, but now there is residual esotropia at distance when wearing the full hyperopic correction.)
- Sensory deprivation esotropia   (Esotropia secondary to a monocular or asymmetric organic lesion such as anisometropia, a cataract, a corneal opacity, a retinal scar, a retinoblastoma, an optic neuropathy, etc.)
- Divergence insufficiency/paralysis   (Esotropia is greater at distance than at near.)

B. Incomitant esodeviations   (The amount of deviation varies with the direction of gaze. One eye is usually limited in abduction. See "Isolated Sixth-Nerve Palsy," Section 11.7, and its differential diagnosis.)

Differential Diagnosis

- Pseudoesotropia   (The eyes appear esotropic; however, there is no movement on the cover-uncover test despite good vision in each eye. Typically it is seen in infants with a wide, flat nasal bridge, prominent epicanthal folds, or a small interpupillary distance. No treatment is needed.)

Work-up

1. History: When were the eyes first noted to be "crossed"? Any old photographs? Constant or intermittent? Straightened by glasses? Trauma?
2. Visual acuity of each eye separately with correction and pinhole to evaluate for amblyopia.
3. Ocular motility examination, observing for restricted movements.
4. Measure the distance deviation in all fields of gaze and the near deviation in the primary position (straight ahead) using prisms. See Appendix 2.
5. Manifest and cycloplegic refractions.
6. Pupillary, slit-lamp, and fundus examinations, looking for causes of sensory deprivation.
7. If divergence insufficiency/paralysis is present, the patient needs a head CT scan (axial and coronal views) or an MRI and a neurological evaluation to rule out an intracranial mass lesion.
8. If abduction is limited and the esodeviation is incomitant, see "Isolated Sixth-Nerve Palsy," Section 11.7, for the appropriate work-up.

Treatment In *all* cases correct refractive errors of $> +2.00$ to $+3.00$ diopters and treat any amblyopia by patching the better seeing eye (see "Amblyopia," Section 9.5).

- Congenital esotropia: When equal vision is obtained in the two eyes, corrective muscle surgery is usually performed.
- Accommodative esotropia:
  1. If the patient is <5-6 years old, correct the hyperopia with the full cycloplegic refraction.
  2. If over age 5-6 years, push plus lenses during the manifest (noncycloplegic) refraction until distance vision blurs, and give the most plus without blurring distance vision.
  3. If the patient is straight at distance with his full correction, but still esotropic at near (high AC/A ratio), then consider bifocals to straighten the eyes at near. (An "Executive" Style Bifocal with a $+2.50$ to $+3.00$ diopter add, the top of the bifocal segment crossing the lower pupillary border, is usually used.)

NOTE Glasses for accommodative esotropia need to be worn full-time.

- Nonaccommodative esotropia and decompensated accommodative esotropia: Muscle surgery is usually performed to correct any significant esotropia remaining with the glasses on.
- Sensory-deprivation esotropia:
  1. Attempt to correct the cause of poor vision.

2. Give the full plus correction to the fixating eye.
3. Muscle surgery to correct the esotropia is usually cosmetic.
4. All patients with very poor vision in one eye need to wear protective glasses (e.g., polycarbonate lenses) at all times.

NOTE   In children less than 9-11 years of age, a trial of patching to correct any superimposed amblyopia is usually attempted.

Follow-up   At each visit, evaluate for amblyopia and measure the degree of deviation with prisms (with glasses on if the patient has a pair).

• If amblyopia is present, see Section 9.5 for management and follow-up guidelines.
• If amblyopia is not present, the child is reevaluated 3-6 weeks after a new prescription is given or in 1-6 months if no changes are made and the eyes are straight.
• When a residual esotropia is present while the patient wears glasses, an attempt is made to add more plus power to the current prescription. Children less than 6 years old should receive a new cycloplegic refraction; plus lenses are pushed without cycloplegia in older children. The maximum additional plus lens which does not blur distance vision is prescribed. If the eyes cannot be straightened with more plus power, then a decompensated accommodative esotropia has developed (see above).
• Hyperopia (farsightedness) often decreases slowly after 5-7 years of age and the strength of the glasses may need to be reduced so as not to blur distance vision (on manifest refraction). If the strength of the glasses must be reduced to improve visual acuity and the esotropia returns, then this is a decompensated accommodative esotropia, see above.

9.4   Exodeviations in Children

Critical Signs   Either eye is turned outward (''wall-eyed'') either constantly or intermittently. On the cover-uncover test, when the fixating eye is covered, the uncovered eye turns inward to fixate. See Appendix 2.

Other Signs   Amblyopia, overaction of the superior or inferior oblique muscles (producing an ''A'' or a ''V'' pattern), vertical deviation.

Types

- Intermittent exotropia   (The most common type of exodeviation in children. Onset is usually from infancy to age 4 years and it is often, but not always, progressive in frequency.)

  Phases:
  Phase 1
     One eye turns out at distance fixation spontaneously or when it is covered.
     Primarily occurs when the patient is fatigued, sick, or not concentrating.
     The eyes become straight within 1-2 blinks of the cover being removed.
     The eyes are straight at near fixation.
  Phase 2
     Increasing frequency of exotropia at distance fixation.
     The exotropia begins to occur at near fixation.
  Phase 3
     There is a constant exotropia at distance and near fixations.

- Sensory deprivation exotropia   (An eye that does not see well, for any reason, turns outward.)
- Duane's syndrome—Type 2   (Limitation of adduction of one eye, with globe retraction and narrowing of the palpebral fissure on attempted adduction. Rarely bilateral.)
- Third-nerve palsy   (Limitation of eye movement superiorly, medially, and inferiorly, usually with ptosis.)
- Orbital disease (e.g., tumor, orbital pseudotumor, etc.)   (Proptosis and restriction of ocular motility are usually evident.)
- Myasthenia gravis   (Ptosis and limitation of eye movement can vary throughout the day, positive edrophonium chloride [e.g., Tensilon] test.)
- Convergence paralysis   (Blurred near vision, difficulty reading. Exodeviation at near fixation, but straight at distance fixation. A CT scan or MRI of the brain is often obtained.)

Differential Diagnosis

- Pseudoexotropia   (The patient appears to have an exodeviation, but no movement is noted on cover-uncover testing despite good vision in each eye. A wide interpupillary distance or temporal dragging of the macula from retinopathy of prematurity, toxocariasis, or other retinal disorders may be responsible.)

Work-up

1. Visual acuity of each eye with correction and pinhole to evaluate for amblyopia.

2. Motility examination, observing for restricted eye movements or signs of Duane's syndrome.
3. Measure the exodeviation in all fields of gaze at distance and in primary position (straight ahead) at near, using prisms. (See Appendix 2.)
4. Check for proptosis (Hertel exophthalmometry).
5. Pupillary, slit lamp, and fundus examinations, checking for causes of sensory deprivation.
6. Manifest and cycloplegic refractions.
7. Consider an edrophonium chloride (e.g., Tensilon) test when myasthenia gravis is suspected.
8. Consider a CT scan (axial and coronal views) and/or an MRI of the orbit and the brain as needed.

Treatment In *all* cases correct significant refractive errors and treat amblyopia, see Section 9.5.

- Intermittent exotropia:
    Phase 1: Follow closely.
    Phase 2: Muscle surgery may be indicated to maintain normal binocular vision.
    Phase 3: Muscle surgery is often cosmetic at this point; however, bifixation and peripheral fusion can occasionally be attained.

- Sensory-deprivation exotropia:
    1. Correct the underlying cause, if possible.
    2. Muscle surgery may be performed for cosmetic purposes.
    3. When one eye has very poor vision, protective glasses (e.g., polycarbonate lenses) should be worn at all times to protect the good eye.

- Duane's syndrome: Consider muscle surgery if an abnormal head position is present.
- Third-nerve palsy: See Section 11.5.

Follow-up

- If amblyopia is being treated see Section 9.5.
- If no amblyopia is present then reexamine every 4-6 months. The parents and patient are told to return sooner if the deviation increases or becomes more frequent.

9.5 Amblyopia

Symptoms Decreased vision in one eye.[1] A history of patching, strabismus, and/or muscle surgery as a child may be elicited.

Critical Sign Poorer vision in one eye, not improved with refraction and not entirely explained by an organic lesion. The decrease in vision develops during the first decade of life and does not deteriorate after that.

Other Signs Crowding phenomenon (individual letters can be read better than a whole line), occasionally a trace afferent pupillary defect is present. A neutral density filter significantly reduces vision in organic disease, but generally does not in pure amblyopia.

Etiology

- Anisometropia   (A difference in refractive error between the two eyes.)
- Strabismus   (The eyes are not straight. Vision is worse in the nonfixating eye. Strabismus can lead to, or be the result of, amblyopia.)
- Occlusion   (Ptosis [congenital or secondary, e.g., eyelid hemangioma], or iatrogenic [e.g., patching].)
- Organic   (Media opacity such as a cataract, corneal scar, persistent hyperplastic primary vitreous, retinal/macular lesion, etc.)

Work-up

1. History: Eye problem in childhood, particularly misaligned eyes? Patching or muscle surgery as a child?
2. Complete ocular examination to rule out an organic cause for the reduced vision. Carefully check the pupils, optic disc, and macula.
3. Cover-uncover test to evaluate eye alignment, see Appendix 2.
4. Cycloplegic refraction.

Treatment/Follow-up

A. Age <9-11 years:
   1. Spectacle correction if significant anisometropia is present.

---

[1]Amblyopia occasionally occurs bilaterally due to bilateral visual deprivation (e.g., congenital cataracts or high refractive errors).

2. Full-time patching (e.g., Coverlet or Opticlude eye patch) over the preferred eye, one week per year of age (e.g., 3 weeks for a 3-year-old), followed by a repeat eye examination.
3. Continue patching as above until the vision is equalized, or until vision is not improving after three compliant cycles of patching. If a recurrence of amblyopia is likely then part-time patching (e.g., 2-6 hours/day) is used until the child reaches 9-11 years of age.
4. In noncompliant patients consider placing atropine 1% tid into the better eye to reduce its vision. This may only succeed if the vision of the better eye is reduced below that of the poorer seeing eye.
5. If occlusion amblyopia (i.e., worsened vision in the patched eye) develops, patch the eye with the poorer vision for a short period of time (e.g., 1 *day* per year of age), and repeat the examination.
6. In strabismic amblyopia, delay strabismus surgery until the vision in the two eyes is equal or maximum vision has been obtained in the amblyopic eye.

B. Age >11 years:

No treatment is useful. Protective glasses (e.g., polycarbonate lenses) should be worn at all times if only one eye has good vision.

NOTE

1. "Pirate" patches and patches worn over glasses are less effective than patches that are placed directly over the eye and adhere to the skin.
2. When a patch causes periorbital erythema and irritation, have the parent apply tincture of benzoin to the skin before applying the patch. The patch can often be removed with less irritation if a warm-water compress is placed on the patch for several minutes before removal.

9.6 Congenital Cataract

Presentation A white fundus reflex (leukocoria) or abnormal eye movements (nystagmus) in one or both eyes. Infants with bilateral cataracts may be noted to be visually inattentive.

Critical Sign Opacity of the lens (see types below).

Other Signs Eye misalignment (strabismus), nystagmus, or a blunted red reflex may be present. In cases of a monocular cataract, the involved eye is often smaller. A cataract alone does not cause a relative afferent pupillary defect.

Types of Cataracts

A. Polar   (Opacity of the lens capsule and adjacent cortex. May be anterior or posterior.)

B. Zonular (lamellar)   (Small white opacities, usually in a concentric zone around the nucleus. Bilateral.)

C. Lenticular   (Opacity involves the lens nucleus or a zonular band outside of it.)

D. Sutural   (Y-shaped or inverted Y-shaped cataracts in the central area of the lens. These rarely affect vision.)

E. Capsular   (Opacification of the most anterior portion of the lens, the lens capsule. Generally does not affect vision.)

Etiology

- Idiopathic
- Galactosemia   (Cataract may be the sole manifestation when galactokinase deficiency is responsible. A deficiency of galactose-1-phosphate uridyl transferase may produce mental retardation and symptomatic cirrhosis along with cataracts. The typical "oil droplet" opacity may or may not be seen.)
- Persistent hyperplastic primary vitreous (PHPV)   (Unilateral. The involved eye is smaller than the normal fellow eye. Examination after pupil dilatation may reveal a plaque of fibrovascular tissue behind the lens with elongated ciliary processes extending to it. Progression of the lens opacity often leads to angle-closure glaucoma.)
- Rubella   (Nuclear cataract, "salt and pepper" chorioretinitis, iritis, a smaller involved eye than the normal fellow eye, and sometimes glaucoma. Hearing defects and heart abnormalities are common.)
- Lowe's syndrome (oculocerebrorenal syndrome)   (Opaque lens +/− posterior lenticonus, congenital glaucoma, renal disease, and mental retardation. X-linked recessive. Patient's mothers may have small white opacities within their lens cortex.)
- Others   (Hereditary, chromosomal disorders, systemic syndromes, other intrauterine infections, trauma, drugs, other metabolic abnormalities)

Differential Diagnosis   See "Leukocoria," Section 9.1.

Work-up

1. History: Maternal illness or drug ingestion during pregnancy? Systemic or ocular disease in the infant or child? Radiation exposure or trauma? Family history of congenital cataracts?
2. Visual assessment of each eye alone if possible (illiterate E's, pictures, or following small toys or a light).

3. Ocular examination, attempting to determine the visual significance of the cataract: Evaluate the size and location of the cataract and whether you can see the retina with a direct ophthalmoscope when looking through an undilated pupil. A portable slit lamp is helpful when available, as is a retinoscope (a blunted retinoscopic reflex suggests the cataract is visually significant). Check for signs of associated glaucoma (large corneal diameter, corneal edema, breaks in Descemet's membrane, etc.) and examine the retina for pathology, if possible.

NOTE   Cataracts 3 mm in diameter or larger usually affect vision.

4. Cycloplegic refraction.
5. B-scan ultrasonography is necessary when the fundus view is obscured.
6. Medical examination by a pediatrician looking for associated abnormalities.
7. Red blood cell (RBC) galactokinase activity (galactokinase levels) +/− RBC galactose-1-phosphate-uridyltransferase activity (rule out galactosemia).
8. Other tests as suggested by the systemic or ocular examination:
   a. Blood: Calcium and phosphorus levels (hypocalcemia, hypoparathyroidism), glucose levels (hypoglycemia, diabetes mellitus).
   b. Urine: Sodium nitroprusside test (homocystinuria), blood and protein quantitation (Alport's syndrome), amino acid content (Lowe's syndrome), copper level (Wilson's disease).
   c. Antibody titers (rubella, other infectious agents).

NOTE   The chance that one of these conditions is present in a healthy child is small.

Treatment

1. Referral to a pediatrician to correct any underlying disorder (e.g., galactosemia requires dietary restriction of milk and other galactose-containing products).
2. Treat associated ocular diseases (e.g., glaucoma, see "Congenital Glaucoma," Section 9.9).
3. Treat amblyopia in children under 9-11 years of age (see "Amblyopia," Section 9.5).
4. Cataract extraction, usually within days to weeks of discovery, is performed when:
   a. Vision is obstructed and the eye's visual development is at risk.
   b. The lens is responsible for intraocular disease (e.g., lens-related glaucoma or uveitis).
   c. Cataract progression threatens the health of the eye (e.g., in PHPV).

NOTE   Unlike adult cataracts, significant delay in treating congenital cataracts may lead to irreversible amblyopia.

5. A mydriatic agent (e.g., phenylephrine 2.5% tid or homatropine 2% tid) may be used as a temporizing measure, allowing peripheral light rays to pass around the lens opacity and reach the retina (rarely is this successful on a long-term basis).

Follow-up   Young infants not undergoing surgery are followed closely for cataract progression and amblyopia. Older children without amblyopia are less likely to develop it unless the cataract progresses, and they are followed on a 6-12 month basis.

NOTE   Children with rubella must be isolated from pregnant women.

9.7   Ophthalmia Neonatorum

(Newborn Conjunctivitis)

Critical Sign   Purulent, mucopurulent, or mucoid discharge from one or both eyes in the first month of life with diffuse conjunctival injection.

Other Signs   Eyelid edema, chemosis.

Etiology

- Chemical   (Seen within a few hours of instilling a prophylactic agent [e.g., silver nitrate], lasts no more than 24-36 hours.)
- Chlamydia trachomatis   (May see basophilic intracytoplasmic inclusion bodies in conjunctival epithelial cells, polymorphonuclear leukocytes [polys], or lymphocytes on Giemsa stain.)
- Neisseria gonorrhea   (May see gram-negative diplococci in polys on Gram's stain.)
- Bacteria (e.g., Staphylococci, streptococci, and gram-negative species— may be seen on Gram's stain)
- Herpes simplex virus   (May have typical herpetic vesicles on the eyelid margins, can see multinucleated giant cells on Giemsa stain.)

Differential Diagnosis

- Dacryocystitis   (Swelling and erythema of the inner canthus, purulent discharge may be expressed from the punctum by rolling a finger from the lacrimal sac to the punctum. Nasal conjunctival injection may be present, but diffuse injection is typically not present.)
- Nasolacrimal duct obstruction   (Tearing, may have a mild mucopurulent discharge from the punctum, minimal-to-no conjunctival injection or eyelid swelling.)

Work-up

1. History: Previous venereal disease in the mother? Were cervical cultures performed during pregnancy? If so, obtain the results.
2. Ocular examination with a penlight and then a blue light after fluorescein instillation, looking for corneal involvement.
3. Conjunctival scrapings for three slides: Gram's stain, Giemsa stain, and one slide to be held in reserve.
   Technique: Irrigate the discharge out of the fornices, place a drop of topical anesthetic (e.g., proparacaine) in the eye, and then scrape the palpebral conjunctiva of the lower eyelid with a flamed (sterilized) spatula after it cools off. Place the scrapings on the slides.
4. Conjunctival cultures for blood and chocolate agars (and Thayer-Martin cultures in cases highly suspicious for gonorrhea). Chocolate agar should be placed in an atmosphere of 2-10% carbon dioxide after being plated.
   Technique: Reanesthetize the eye if necessary, moisten a calcium alginate swab (a cotton-tipped applicator is a less desirable alternative) with liquid broth media and vigorously rub it along the inferior palpebral conjunctiva. Plate it directly on the culture dish. Repeat the procedure for additional cultures.
5. Viral culture: Moisten another cotton-tipped applicator and roll it along the palpebral conjunctiva. Break off the end of the applicator and place it into the viral transport medium.
6. Scrape the conjunctiva for the chlamydial immunofluorescent antibody test.

Treatment   Initial therapy is based on the results of the Gram's and Giemsa stains (if they can be examined immediately). Therapy is then modified according to the culture results and the clinical response.

A. No information from stains, no particular organism suspected: Erythromycin ointment qid plus erythromycin syrup 50 mg/kg/day[2] for 2-3 weeks.
B. Suspect chemical (e.g., silver nitrate) toxicity: No treatment—reevaluate in 24 hours.

---

[2]Erythromycin syrup is divided into 4 doses daily and placed into the baby's formula.

C. Suspect chlamydia: Erythromycin syrup 50 mg/kg/day[2] for 2-3 weeks plus erythromycin or sulfacetamide ointment qid.
    If confirmed by culture or immunofluorescent stain, treat the mother and her sexual partner(s) with:

    Tetracycline 250-500 mg po qid × 7 days (for men and mothers who are neither breast feeding nor pregnant)
    or
    Erythromycin 250-500 mg po qid × 7 days (for breast feeding or pregnant women)

    NOTE Inadequately treated chlamydial conjunctivitis in a neonate can lead to chlamydial pneumonia.

D. Suspect Neisseria gonorrhea: Treatment is not well established. We favor the following.
    1. Hospitalize.
    2. Ceftriaxone 50-100 mg/kg/day iv in 2 divided doses for 3-7 days. If the condition is improving, the IV antibiotic can be changed to an oral antibiotic (e.g., penicillin VK or cefaclor, depending on the sensitivities) to complete a 7-day course. In penicillin/cephalosporin allergic patients an infectious disease consult is obtained.
    3. Bacitracin ointment qid.
    4. Topical saline lavage to remove any discharge qid.
    5. Scopolamine ¼% tid if the cornea is involved.
    6. All neonates with gonorrhea should additionally be treated for chlamydia with erythromycin syrup 50 mg/kg/day[2] × 14 days.

    NOTE If confirmed by culture, the mother and her sexual partner(s) should be treated in accordance with the sensitivity results for 7 days. Additionally, chlamydia should be treated as outlined above.

E. Gram positive bacteria on Gram's stain, with no suspicion of gonorrhea and no corneal involvement: Erythromycin ointment qid × 2 weeks.
F. Gram negative bacteria on Gram's stain, but no suspicion of gonorrhea, and no corneal involvement: Gentamicin ointment qid × 2 weeks.
G. Bacteria on Gram's stain and corneal involvement: Hospitalize, work-up, and treat as per "Infectious Corneal Infiltrate/Ulcer," Section 4.12.
H. Suspect herpes simplex virus: Trifluorothymidine 1% drops (e.g., Viroptic) q 2 hours or vidarabine 3% ointment (e.g., Vira-A) 5×/day × 1 week then cut dosage in half × 1 week.

[2]Erythromycin syrup is divided into 4 doses daily and placed into the baby's formula.

Follow-up   Initially follow daily as an inpatient or outpatient. If the condition worsens (e.g., corneal involvement develops) reculture and hospitalize. As mentioned above, therapy is tailored according to the clinical response and the culture results. The frequency of follow-up visits may be reduced once improvement is clearly demonstrated.

REFERENCE

ULLMAN S, ROUSSEL TJ, FORSTER RK. Gonococcal keratoconjunctivitis. *Surv Ophthalmol* 32:199, 1987.

9.8   Congenital Nasolacrimal Duct Obstruction

Presentation   Persistent tearing, chronic low-grade discharge, matting of the eyelids.

Critical Signs   Wet-looking eye (tears flowing over the eyelid margin), may have crusting on the eyelashes (predominantly medially), and reflux of mucoid or mucopurulent material from the punctum when pressure is applied to the area over the lacrimal sac (where the lower eyelid abuts the nose).

Other Signs   Erythema (irritation) of the surrounding skin, redness and swelling of the medial canthus. Preseptal cellulitis can develop from dacryocystitis.

NOTE   Nasolacrimal duct obstruction may be associated with an otitis or pharyngitis.

Etiology   Usually due to an imperforate membrane at the distal end of the nasolacrimal duct.

Differential Diagnosis

• Conjunctivitis   (Red eye, discharge, usually acute, follicles or papillae may or may not be present on the inferior tarsal conjunctiva, tearing is usually not chronic.)
• Congenital anomalies of the upper lacrimal drainage system   (Atresia of the lacrimal puncta or canaliculus.)

- Other causes of tearing (e.g., entropion/trichiasis, corneal defects, foreign body under the upper eyelid, congenital glaucoma)

Work-up

1. Slit-lamp or penlight examination ruling out other causes of tearing: Make sure the corneal diameter is not large and ruptures in Descemet's membrane are not present (congenital glaucoma).
2. Palpation over the lacrimal sac observing for any mucoid or mucopurulent discharge from the punctum.
3. Intraocular pressure measurement if congenital glaucoma is suspected (Schiötz tonometry is often easiest in a child).

Treatment

1. Digital massage 2-4×/day (The mother is taught to place her index finger over the child's common canaliculus [inner corner of the eye] and to stroke downward slowly, several times in succession.)
2. Consider erythromycin ointment bid × 1 week if a significant mucopurulent discharge is present.
3. Warm compresses 2-4×/day are used to keep the eyelids clean when a discharge is present.
4. In the presence of acute dacryocystitis, a systemic antibiotic is needed, see "Dacryocystitis," Section 6.8.

The majority of cases will open spontaneously with this regimen by one year of age. If not:

5. Nasolacrimal duct probing is performed at 13 months of age (Some physicians will probe children between 6 and 12 months of age; we generally do not.) The majority will be corrected after the initial probing; others may require repeat probings. If patency is not established after three probings then consider placing sialastic tubing in the nasolacrimal duct, leaving it in place for weeks to months.

NOTE Children who develop recurrent or persistent infections of the lacrimal drainage apparatus despite antibiotics may need to be probed earlier than 13 months.

Follow-up Acute dacryocystitis should be treated as soon as possible and followed every day until significant improvement is noted; all other patients can be followed by monthly phone calls (the child returns if the situation is worse or if the parents are unsure).

REFERENCE

NELSON LB, CALHOUN JK, MENDUKE H. Medical management of congenital nasolacrimal duct obstruction. *Pediatrics* 76:172, 1985.

9.9 Congenital Glaucoma

Presentation   Photophobia, tearing, or eyelid squeezing (blepharospasm) most commonly in an infant. May have a red eye.

Critical Signs   Enlarged globe and corneal diameter (horizontal corneal diameter >12 mm before 1 year of age is suspicious), corneal edema, increased intraocular pressure (IOP), increased cup/disc ratio, commonly bilateral.

Other Signs   Linear tears in Descemet's membrane of the cornea (usually running horizontally or concentric to the limbus), corneal stromal scarring, conjunctival injection.

Etiology

- Primary congenital glaucoma   (Not associated with other ocular or systemic disorders.)
- Developmental anterior segment abnormality (Axenfeld's anomaly, Rieger's anomaly/syndrome, Peter's anomaly, others)   (Bilateral. Abnormalities of the cornea, iris, and anterior-chamber angle.)
- Lowe's syndrome (oculocerebrorenal syndrome)   (Cataract, glaucoma, and renal disease.)
- Rubella   (Glaucoma, cataracts, hearing and cardiac defects.)
- Phakomatoses   (Sturge-Weber, neurofibromatosis, others.)
- Others   (Aniridia, homocystinuria, persistent hyperplastic primary vitreous, etc.)

Differential Diagnosis

- Congenital megalocornea   (Large corneal diameter without corneal edema. IOP and cup/disc ratio are normal.)
- High myopia   (A large corneal diameter may be found along with a large eye; however, a highly myopic refractive error, tilted optic discs with adjacent myopic crescents, normal corneal thickness, and normal IOP are also found.)

- Birth trauma   (May produce tears in Descemet's membrane and corneal edema; however, the tears are typically vertical or oblique in orientation and the corneal diameter is normal. Birth trauma is generally unilateral and may often be obtained from the history.)
- Congenital hereditary endothelial dystrophy   (Bilateral corneal edema at birth with a normal corneal diameter and normal IOP.)
- Mucopolysaccharidoses and cystinosis   (Some inborn errors of metabolism produce cloudy corneas, but the corneal diameter and IOP are normal.)
- Nasolacrimal duct obstruction   (Tearing, sometimes with a mild mucopurulent discharge from the punctum. The cornea is clear and not enlarged. The IOP is normal.)

Work-up

1. History: Other systemic abnormalities? Infection during pregnancy? Birth trauma? Family history of congenital glaucoma?
2. Ocular examination, including a visual acuity assessment of each eye separately (can the child fixate and follow?), a penlight examination to detect corneal enlargement and haziness, and a refraction. An IOP measurement is attempted and a dilated fundus examination is performed to evaluate the optic disc and retina. (A hand-held portable slit lamp is sometimes used in uncertain cases to look for tears in Descemet's membrane and corneal edema.)
3. Gonioscopy may be attempted in cooperative children who are not expected to undergo examination under anesthesia.
4. Examination under anesthesia is performed in suspicious cases and in those in whom surgical treatment is planned. The horizontal corneal diameter and IOP are measured; retinoscopy, gonioscopy, and ophthalmoscopy are performed. Ultrasound is often employed to measure axial length.

NOTE   The IOP may be lowered substantially by general anesthesia (particularly halothane); an IOP of 20 mm Hg or greater under halothane anesthesia is suggestive of glaucoma. An exception is ketamine hydrochloride, which may increase the IOP. In general the IOP is measured as soon as possible after general anesthesia is induced to achieve as accurate a measurement as possible.

Treatment   Definitive treatment is usually surgical. Medical therapy is temporary and is started initially, pending surgery.

A. Medical (Any or all of the following may be used.)
  1. Topical beta-blocker (e.g., levobunolol ½% bid or timolol ¼-½% bid).
  2. Carbonic anhydrase inhibitor (e.g., acetazolamide 5 mg/kg po q 6 hours).

3. Epinephrine compound (e.g., dipivefrin 0.1% bid).

NOTE   Miotics are rarely effective in controlling (and may raise) the IOP, but sometimes are used to constrict the pupil in preparation for a surgical goniotomy.

B. Surgical
First choice   Goniotomy (incising the trabecular meshwork with a blade under gonioscopic visualization) or trabeculotomy (opening Schlemm's canal into the anterior chamber). These procedures are often repeated if they are unsuccessful at first.
Other   Trabeculectomy.

NOTE   Amblyopia may be superimposed upon glaucoma and should be treated by patching (see Section 9.5).

Follow-up   Repeat examinations, under anesthesia when needed, are necessary to follow corneal diameter, IOP, cup/disc ratio, and axial length. These patients need to be followed throughout life to monitor for progression.

9.10   Aniridia

Presentation   Decreased vision, photophobia, "jiggling" eyes.

Critical Signs   Bilateral near total absence of the iris from birth. The pupil appears to occupy the entire area of the cornea.

Other Signs   Childhood onset glaucoma, foveal hypoplasia, nystagmus, strabismus, cataract, progressive corneal opacification with pannus, and decreased vision. In sporadic cases, Wilms' tumor (tumor of the kidney in children <5 years old), genitourinary abnormalities (e.g., bilateral gonadoblastomas), and mental retardation may develop.

Inheritance   Autosomal dominant in ⅔. No inheritance (sporadic) in ⅓.

Differential Diagnosis

• Coloboma   (Absent segment of iris, typically inferiorly. Often associated with an absent retinal pigment epithelium and choroid inferiorly and an optic-nerve abnormality.)

Work-up

1. Family history: Examine other family members if possible.
2. Ophthalmic examination, including an intraocular pressure (IOP) check and gonioscopy of the anterior-chamber angle (if necessary, an examination under anesthesia should be performed).
3. Blood pressure measurement (may be elevated with a renal abnormality).
4. Referral to a pediatrician for frequent periodic physical examinations with special attention to the abdominal and genitourinary examination. Urinalysis may detect hematuria.
5. Chromosomal karyotype in sporadic cases. (There is an increased chance of Wilms' tumor with a deletion of the short arm of chromosome 11.)
6. Renal ultrasound in sporadic cases.
7. Consider intravenous pyelography if the renal ultrasound is suspicious for Wilms' tumor.

Treatment

1. Correct refractive errors and treat amblyopia; see Section 9.5. (NOTE A trial of patching is usually initiated if there is a difference in vision between the two eyes as superimposed amblyopia may be present in addition to the poor vision from aniridia.)
2. Glaucoma management if the IOP is elevated:
   a. Medical: Topical pilocarpine, epinephrine compounds, and beta-blockers are generally the first line drugs (see "Primary Open-Angle Glaucoma," Section 10.1). When topical medications fail, a carbonic anhydrase inhibitor may be used (e.g., acetazolamide 5 mg/kg po q 6 hours in children). NOTE If gonioscopy reveals trabecular meshwork obstruction, pilocarpine and epinephrine compounds will be ineffective.
   b. Surgery (often used initially in children): The surgery is difficult and the procedure of choice is controversial. We attempt trabeculectomy since goniotomy and trabeculotomy often fail.
   c. Cyclocryotherapy can be tried if surgery fails.
3. Cataract management: Must individualize cases by attempting to predict visual potential. Many patients will benefit from cataract extraction.
4. Corneal management: A corneal transplant should be considered in the presence of corneal scarring, but it often has poor results.
5. Consider contact lenses if better vision can be obtained.
6. Genetic counseling.
7. Systemic abnormalities, such as a Wilms' tumor, need to be managed by pediatric specialists.

Follow-up

1. Patients with aniridia need to have periodic ocular examinations (e.g., every 6-12 months) throughout life checking for increased IOP and glaucoma.
2. Renal ultrasound should be repeated every 3 months in sporadic cases until the age of 4-5 years if a deletion of the short arm of chromosome 11 is detected by the chromosome analysis, the patient is mentally retarded, or another genitourinary abnormality exists. The remainder of the sporadic cases undergo repeat renal ultrasound every 6 months until age 4-5 years.
3. Periodic physical examinations by a pediatrician, as mentioned above, including blood pressure checks, are also performed until age 4-5 years.

9.11 Developmental Anterior-Segment Abnormalities

Bilateral congenital abnormalities of the cornea, iris, and anterior-chamber angle which predispose to glaucoma. Specific disease entities include the following:

Axenfeld's anomaly Prominent, anteriorly displaced Schwalbe's line (posterior embryotoxon) with adherent iris processes. Autosomal dominant or sporadic.
Rieger's anomaly Above findings *plus* iris thinning with atrophic holes. The pupil may be displaced in the direction of a prominent peripheral tissue strand. Autosomal dominant or sporadic.
Rieger's syndrome Rieger's anomaly *plus* dental, craniofacial and skeletal abnormalities including short stature with growth hormone deficiency, umbilical hernia, cardiac defects, and mental retardation. Autosomal dominant or sporadic.
Peter's anomaly Central corneal opacity, usually with strands of iris stretching to the peripheral border of the opacity. Sometimes the anterior chamber is shallow and the lens adheres to the opacity. Autosomal recessive or sporadic.

Differential Diagnosis

- Iridocorneal endothelial (ICE) syndrome (Unilateral, onset in young adulthood, corneal endothelial abnormalities, no family history.)
- Posterior polymorphous dystrophy (Bilateral, corneal endothelial vesicles or bandlike changes, occasionally associated with iris-cornea adhesions.)

- Aniridia   (Bilateral, congenital, near total absence of the iris, often associated with glaucoma.)
- Ectopia lentis et pupillae   (Bilateral, lens displaced in one direction and the pupil displaced in the opposite direction, no anterior-chamber abnormalities.)

Work-up

1. History: Family history of ocular disease? Associated systemic abnormality?
2. Slit-lamp examination with intraocular pressure (IOP) measurement (may require an evaluation under anesthesia).
3. Gonioscopy of the anterior-chamber angle.
4. Optic-nerve examination, best with a slit lamp and a 60 diopter, Hruby, or fundus contact lens.
5. Stereo disc photographs.
6. Visual field test, preferably automated (e.g., Octopus or Humphrey)
7. A-scan ultrasound for axial length in infants if glaucoma is suspected.
8. Medical evaluation by an internist or pediatrician.

Treatment   No treatment is needed unless glaucoma is present or a corneal/lens opacity is significantly affecting the vision.

1. Treat glaucoma if present (Topical beta-blockers and systemic carbonic anhydrase inhibitors are often more effective than pilocarpine in this syndrome, see "Primary Open-Angle Glaucoma," Section 10.1.)
2. Goniotomy or trabeculotomy are used instead of medical management in congenital or infantile cases. See "Congenital Glaucoma," Section 9.9.
3. Consider trabeculectomy in adults in whom medical therapy has failed. Argon laser trabeculoplasty is ineffective and may lead to a marked rise in IOP.
4. Consider cataract extraction if a significant cataract is present, and a corneal transplant if a dense corneal opacity exists.
5. Treat amblyopia if present (see Section 9.5).

Follow-up   Every 3-6 months unless glaucoma develops (then every 1-3 months, depending on the clinical situation).

9.12   The Blind Infant

An infant whose visual skills are far below those expected (e.g., an inability to fix on and follow objects after several months of age) may have an obvious or inconspicuous ocular or neuro-ophthalmic disorder. Obvious causes include bilateral central corneal opacities, congenital cataracts, or infectious retinal problems with macular scarring. Below are listed conditions which may not be obvious on clinical examination.

I. Conditions which *usually* produce a searching nystagmus:
    A. Pupils react poorly to light:
        •   Leber's congenital amaurosis   (May have a normal-appearing fundus initially or pigmentary retinal changes which progress to a retinitis pigmentosa-like picture. Narrowing of the retinal vessels and optic disc pallor may be present early. The electroretinogram [ERG] is markedly abnormal or flat. Autosomal recessive.)
        •   Bilateral optic nerve hypoplasia   (Small optic discs often surrounded by a yellow-white ring, normal ERG. See "Optic Nerve Hypoplasia," Section 9.13.)
        •   Congenital optic atrophy   (Rare. Pale, normal sized optic disc often associated with mental retardation or cerebral palsy. Normal ERG. Autosomal recessive.)
    B. Pupils react briskly to light:
        •   Infantile nystagmus   (Some patients with this condition have a severe visual deficit. The iris is normal. It may be accompanied by a face turn and/or head nodding.)
        •   Albinism with delayed maturation   (Frequently have iris transillumination defects and foveal hypoplasia.)
II. No nystagmus present and pupils react normally to light:
    •   Diffuse cerebral dysfunction   (Infants do not respond to sound or touch and are neurologically abnormal. The vision may slowly improve with time.)
    •   Delayed maturation of the visual system   (Normal response to sound and touch and neurologically normal. The ERG is normal and vision usually develops between 4 and 12 months of age.)
    •   Extreme refractive error   (Diagnosed on cycloplegic refraction.)

Work-up

1. History: Premature? Normal development and growth? Maternal infection or drug use during pregnancy? Family history of eye disease?
2. Evaluate the infant's ability to fixate on an object and follow it with each eye individually (patch one eye and then the other).
3. Pupillary examination.
4. Look carefully for nystagmus.
5. Penlight examination of the anterior segment, checking especially for iris transillumination defects.
6. Dilated retinal evaluation.

7. Cycloplegic refraction.
8. ERG, especially if the cause of the poor vision is not known.
9. Consider a CT scan and/or MRI of the brain.
10. Consider a sweep visual evoked potential (VEP) for a vision measurement.
11. Consider eye movement recordings to evaluate the nystagmus wave form, if available.

Treatment

1. Parental counseling is necessary in all of the above conditions with respect to the infant's visual potential.
2. Information concerning educational services for the visually handicapped or blind may be helpful.
3. Genetic counseling.

9.13 Optic-Nerve Hypoplasia

Presentation Unilateral or bilateral poor vision since birth. When unilateral, the patient may be asymptomatic.

Critical Signs A small optic disc with peripapillary atrophy. When present, a "double ring sign" (a pigmented ring at the inner and outer edge of the peripapillary atrophy) is diagnostic.

Other Signs Severe cases may produce an afferent pupillary defect, strabismus, or nystagmus. Amblyopia may be superimposed upon the underlying optic-nerve abnormality, contributing to the poor vision.

Etiology Usually idiopathic. May be seen in infants of diabetic mothers or those who took certain drugs during pregnancy, including quinine, phenytoin, alcohol, and lysergic acid diethylamide (LSD).

Associated Abnormality

• Septo-optic dysplasia (de Morsier syndrome) (Midline abnormalities of the brain, sometimes leading to deficient secretion of growth hormone, thyroid hormone, or other tropic hormones. Growth retardation [which does not usually manifest itself until after age 3-4 years of life], seizures [often due to hypoglycemia], and diabetes insipidus may develop.)

Differential Diagnosis See "The Blind Infant," Section 9.12.

Work-up

1. History: Drugs during pregnancy? Normal growth and development?
2. Measure best corrected vision in each eye (in young children, determine whether each eye can fixate and follow well.)
3. Cycloplegic refraction.
4. Optic-nerve evaluation, best performed with a 60 diopter lens and a slit lamp if possible (a Hruby lens may be tried if the child is cooperative). A direct ophthalmoscope is next best.
5. Children of small stature or with a history of failure to thrive or developmental delay are referred for a pediatric endocrine evaluation. A CT scan (axial and coronal views) and/or MRI of the brain may be obtained, particularly in the presence of an associated neuro-ophthalmic abnormality.
6. The child's pediatrician should be informed of the condition and instructed to refer the patient for an endocrine evaluation if growth or development is or becomes delayed.

Treatment

1. Correct significant refractive errors.
2. A trial of patching over the better seeing eye is attempted to treat possible superimposed amblyopia (see Section 9.5).
3. Pituitary/hypothalamic disorders should be treated by an endocrinologist.

NOTE   Patients with very poor or no vision in one eye should be given polycarbonate protective lenses to wear at all times.

Follow-up   As described in "Amblyopia," Section 9.5, while patching; then every 6-12 months.

10

Glaucoma

10.1 Primary Open-Angle Glaucoma (POAG)

Symptoms Usually asymptomatic until the late stages, at which point decreased peripheral or central vision may be noted.

Critical Signs (four components)

1. A large or enlarging cup/disc ratio, often with asymmetry between the two eyes.
2. Visual field defects, commonly nasal, paracentral, or extending in an arcuate distribution from the blind spot to the horizontal raphé.
3. An elevated intraocular pressure (IOP), generally >22 mm Hg.
4. The anterior-chamber angle is open on gonioscopy and peripheral anterior synechiae are not present.

Other Signs The rim of the optic cup may be notched, the nerve may appear pale, the cup may be elongated vertically, and nerve fiber layer loss may be apparent. Large daily fluctuations in IOP (such that single IOP measurements may be misleading), absence of corneal edema, and a white uninflamed eye are characteristic.

Risk Factors Glaucoma in the fellow eye, family history of blindness or visual loss due to glaucoma, diabetes or hypertension (systemic vascular disease), black race, myopia.

Differential Diagnosis

- Low-tension glaucoma   (Findings of POAG, but IOP consistently not elevated.)
- Chronic angle-closure glaucoma   (Findings of POAG, but peripheral anterior synechiae are present on gonioscopy, closing part of the anterior-chamber angle. Patients with chronic angle-closure glaucoma do not typically develop the sudden painful acute rise in intraocular pressure seen with acute angle-closure glaucoma. It may be superimposed upon primary open-angle glaucoma).
- Secondary open-angle glaucoma   (Lens-induced, inflammatory, pseudoexfoliative, pigmentary, steroid-induced, developmental anterior-segment abnormalities, angle recession, iridocorneal endothelial (ICE) syndrome, glaucoma related to increased episcleral venous pressure [e.g., Sturge-Weber syndrome and carotid-cavernous fistula], glaucoma related to intraocular tumors or other ocular conditions). (See specific sections for more detailed information.)
- Optic atrophy   (Chiasmal tumors, syphilis, ischemic optic neuropathy, drugs, retinal vascular or degenerative disease, others. IOP is not elevated in these conditions, unless a secondary glaucoma is additionally present.)

Work-up

1. History: Known glaucoma or ocular disease? Family history of glaucoma? Medical problems, specifically diabetes, hypertension, asthma, congestive heart failure, heart block, renal stones, or allergies?
2. Ocular examination, with special attention to IOP, gonioscopic evaluation of the anterior-chamber angle, and optic-disc assessment (with a slit-lamp and a 60 diopter, Hruby, or fundus contact lens).
3. Stereo photographs of the optic discs are obtained in suspicious or definite cases to facilitate recognition of optic disc changes on future examinations.
4. Formal visual field examination, preferably automated—e.g., Humphrey or Octopus. (Goldmann visual fields are obtained in patients who lack the visual ability or intelligence required for automated visual fields.)
5. In atypical cases, a low-tension glaucoma work-up may be appropriate, see Section 10.2.

Treatment   The goal of therapy is to prevent further cupping and visual field loss by lowering IOP. There are no set rules as to when to institute therapy and what therapeutic modalities to use initially. The following guidelines may be used.

A. Patients with mildly elevated IOP (e.g., 22-27 mm Hg), normal optic discs, and normal visual fields: These patients may be followed as "glaucoma suspects," their IOP and optic nerve appearance monitored a few times per year, and a formal visual field rechecked yearly. Patients with risk factors for glaucoma (especially a positive family history) are sometimes given the option of treatment (particularly when the IOP is at the higher end of this range).

B. Patients with normal IOP, but suspicious optic nerves and questionable or unreliable visual fields: Followed as in (A).

C. Patients with optic nerves suggestive of glaucoma, mild-to-moderate visual field changes consistent with glaucoma and mild-to-moderately elevated IOP: These patients are generally started on one antiglaucoma medication in one eye on a 4-6 week trial basis. The IOP level of the two eyes is rechecked after the 4-6 week period (preferably at the same time of the day as the initial check), comparing the levels of the treated and untreated eyes to their levels prior to treatment. A decision of whether to maintain or discontinue the trial drug is based on whether the treated eye's IOP declined a significant amount compared to the untreated, fellow eye. If there is any hint of glaucoma in the fellow (untreated) eye, both eyes will be treated with a drug shown to be effective in that patient.

D. Patients with IOP >27 mm Hg (regardless of the disc and field changes): We generally treat these patients as in (C) to lower their risk of glaucomatous visual field loss.

E. Patients with marked optic-nerve cupping and a very high IOP upon presentation: These patients are treated aggressively with multiple antiglaucomatous medications initially, even prior to obtaining the visual field. A therapeutic trial is not performed if both eyes have advanced glaucoma and there is an impending risk of central visual loss. These patients are often followed sooner than the typical 4-6 week interval to evaluate the effect of treatment. If the IOP is well controlled with multiple medications, one drug at a time may be stopped to determine its antiglaucomatous efficacy.

Medications Drugs chosen for therapeutic trials must both lower the intraocular pressure and be tolerable. Patients who experience unpleasant side effects will not be compliant with their medication.

TYPICAL FIRST-LINE THERAPY

Topical medication

1. Beta-blockers (e.g., levobunolol ½% q day or bid or timolol ¼-½% bid): Often effectively lowers IOP, but cannot be given to patients with breathing problems (e.g., asthma), heart block, or congestive heart failure. The pulse is usually checked prior to and after initiating therapy with these drugs.

2. Miotics (e.g., pilocarpine qid): Generally used in low strengths initially (e.g., ½-1%) and then built up to higher strengths (e.g., 4-6%). Commonly

not tolerated in patients <40 years old due to accommodative spasm. Strong miotics are generally contraindicated in patients with retinal holes and should be used cautiously in patients at risk for retinal detachment (e.g., high myopes and aphakes). (NOTE Pilocarpine is also available in a 4% gel used nightly or as an ocular insert replaced once a week.)
3. Epinephrine compounds (e.g., dipivefrin 0.1% bid or epinephrine 0.5-2% bid): Rarely reduce IOP to the degree of the first two classes of drugs, but have very few side effects. May cause cystoid macular edema in aphakic patients.

SECOND-LINE THERAPY

(Generally reserved for patients who demonstrate progressive cupping or visual field loss on maximally tolerated topical medications. Topical medications are continued.)

1. Oral carbonic anhydrase inhibitors (e.g., methazolamide 25-50 mg po 2-3 × /day or acetazolamide 250 mg po qid or acetazolamide 500 mg sequel po bid): Cannot be given to patients with a sulfa allergy and probably should be avoided (or used cautiously) in patients with a history of renal stones. As these agents are also mild diuretics, potassium levels need to be monitored, especially if the patient is taking other diuretic agents or digitalis. Side effects are often intolerable. Rare, but severe, hematologic side effects have occurred.
2. Laser trabeculoplasty: Often effective, but sometimes not permanently. Side effects are few.

THIRD-LINE THERAPY

Glaucoma filtering surgery (e.g., trabeculectomy).

FOURTH-LINE THERAPY

(Any of the following) Repeat filtering surgery, shunt tube procedure (e.g., Shockett, Molteno), YAG laser cyclophotocoagulation, cyclodialysis, cyclo-cryotherapy.

Follow-up As mentioned above, patients are reseen 4-6 weeks after starting a new medication to evaluate its efficacy (in severe glaucoma the patient can be followed sooner). Once the IOP has been lowered substantially, patients are reevaluated in 3-6 month intervals for IOP and optic-nerve checks. Gonioscopy is performed yearly or after starting a new strength cholinergic agent (e.g., pilocarpine). Formal visual fields of the same type (e.g., Humphrey or Octopus) are rechecked every 6-12 months. Dilated retinal examinations should be performed yearly. If glaucomatous damage progresses despite compliance with medication, additional therapy is initiated. The goal of additional therapy is to lower the IOP beneath the range at which glaucomatous progression has occurred.

See the Drug Glossary for additional drug information.

10.2 Low-Tension Glaucoma

Description

1. A large or enlarging cup/disc ratio, often with asymmetry between the two eyes.
2. Visual field defects, usually paracentral, nasal, or extending in an arcuate fashion from the blind spot to the horizontal raphé.
3. Intraocular pressure (IOP) always ≤22 mm Hg.
4. Open angle on gonioscopy with no peripheral anterior synechiae.

Other Signs Splinter hemorrhages on or near the optic nerve, pallor of the optic nerve, nerve fiber layer loss.

Differential Diagnosis

- Primary open-angle glaucoma (POAG) (IOP >22 mm Hg in the past, or at other times of the day.)
- Angle-closure glaucoma (Narrow angles usually bilaterally, peripheral anterior synechiae. Often have a history of acute episodes of pain, photophobia, and red eye.)
- Previous glaucomatous damage (e.g., from steroids, uveitis, glaucomatocyclitic crisis)
- Previous ischemic damage to the optic nerve (e.g., a previous hypotensive event or ischemic optic neuropathy) (A history of acute visual loss can often be elicited. Visual field defects may be identical to glaucoma or may be altitudinal. Cupping and visual field abnormalities do not usually progress, but the other eye can become affected.)
- Hematologic disease (e.g., anemia or polycythemia vera)
- Syphilis (Positive FTA-ABS, may have a history or signs of prior iritis [e.g., synechiae], "ghost" vessels [blood vessels devoid of blood] in the cornea, or a "salt and pepper" appearance to the fundus.)
- Compressive optic neuropathy (Optic-nerve pallor greater than cupping, often from a tumor or aneurysm. Visual field defects are often atypical for glaucoma.)
- Congenital nerve defect (e.g., myopic discs, colobomas, optic nerve pits) (Cupping and visual field abnormalities do not usually progress.)

NOTE Low-tension glaucoma can develop as a consequence of any of the above. A compromised optic nerve may not tolerate an IOP in the teens.

Work-up

1. History: Acute episodes of eye pain? Steroid use? Acute visual loss? Surgery, trauma, heart attack, or other event which may have caused a hypotensive episode?
2. Slit-lamp examination with an IOP measurement.
3. Gonioscopy of the anterior-chamber angle.
4. Optic-nerve evaluation, preferably with a fundus contact, Hruby, or 60 diopter lens at the slit lamp.
5. Stereo optic disc photographs.
6. Visual field testing, preferably automated (e.g., Humphrey or Octopus).
7. Diurnal IOP curve (multiple IOP checks during the course of a day).
8. CBC, ESR, RPR, FTA-ABS, +/− ANA
9. CT scan (axial and coronal views) and/or MRI of the orbit and brain for atypical cases (e.g., unilateral cases, those in young patients, when visual field defects are uncharacteristic or are neurological [e.g., homonymous defects]) or when other neurological signs or symptoms are present.
10. Have the patient see their medical doctor for a complete cardiac evaluation.

Treatment/Follow-up In general, the goal of treatment is to lower the IOP beneath 10-12 mm Hg. See "Primary Open-Angle Glaucoma," Section 10.1 for a detailed treatment and follow-up regimen.

A. Treatment may be indicated for:
   1. Advanced optic-nerve cupping.
   2. A visual field defect threatening central vision (as determined by the visual field test).
   3. Glaucomatous cupping and field loss which cannot be accounted for by any disease other than low-tension glaucoma.
   4. Progression of cupping and/or field loss unexplained by progression of another disease process (e.g., cataract).
B. Observation (e.g., IOP and optic-nerve evaluation every 3-4 months; visual field examination every 6-12 months) may be indicated when:
   1. The diagnosis of glaucoma is in question (e.g., possible old nonarteritic ischemic optic neuropathy).
   2. An explanation for the glaucomatous changes is available (e.g., previous prolonged use of steroids or a previous episode of hypoperfusion).

10.3 Angle-Recession Glaucoma

Symptoms Usually asymptomatic until the late stages, at which point unilateral visual field or acuity loss may be noted. A history of trauma to the glaucomatous eye can usually be elicited (sometimes up to years prior).

Critical Signs Glaucoma (large or enlarging cup/disc ratio, characteristic visual field loss, and/or an elevated intraocular pressure [IOP]) in an eye with gonioscopic findings which include the following: A wide ciliary body band, torn iris processes, and a deep anterior-chamber angle (posterior iris insertion), all in the same quadrant(s) of the eye. In some cases, these findings and the angle recession extend 360 degrees. Comparison with corresponding angle structures of the normal fellow eye help in identification of recessed areas.

Other Signs The scleral spur may appear abnormally white on gonioscopy due to the recessed angle, other signs of previous trauma may be present (e.g., a cataract or iris sphincter tears).

Differential Diagnosis See ''Primary Open-Angle Glaucoma,'' Section 10.1.

Work-up
1. History: Trauma? Family history of glaucoma?
2. Slit-lamp examination, including an IOP measurement.
3. Gonioscopy of the anterior-chamber angle.
4. Optic-nerve evaluation with a slit lamp and 60 diopter, Hruby, or fundus contact lens.
5. Stereo photographs of the optic discs for a baseline.
6. Formal visual field examination, preferably automated (e.g., Humphrey or Octopus) in cases suspicious for, or with definite, glaucoma.

Treatment Similar to primary open angle glaucoma (see Section 10.1) with the exception that miotics (e.g., pilocarpine) may be ineffective (or even cause an elevation of IOP due to a reduction of uveoscleral outflow). Argon laser trabeculoplasty is effective less often in this condition than in other forms of glaucoma.

Follow-up Patients with angle recession without glaucoma are followed yearly. Those with glaucoma are followed according to the guidelines of ''Primary Open-Angle Glaucoma,'' Section 10.1. Follow-up should carefully monitor both eyes, as there is a high incidence of open-angle glaucoma in the uninvolved eye as well as the traumatized eye.

10.4 Inflammatory Open-Angle Glaucoma

Symptoms   Pain, photophobia, decreased vision; symptoms may be minimal.

Critical Signs   Increased intraocular pressure (IOP), significant amount of aqueous white blood cells and flare, open angle on gonioscopy.

Other Signs   Miotic pupil, peripheral anterior synechiae, keratic precipitates on the posterior corneal surface or trabecular meshwork, conjunctival injection, ciliary flush.

NOTE   An acute IOP elevation is distinguished from a chronic IOP elevation by the presence of corneal edema, pain, and the symptoms of halos around light.

Etiology

- Anterior uveitis
- Intermediate and posterior uveitis
- Panuveitis
- Kerato-uveitis   (Corneal pathology present in addition to uveitis.)
- Following trauma or intraocular surgery.

Differential Diagnosis

- Glaucomatocyclitic crisis (Posner-Schlossman syndrome)   (Markedly elevated IOP (usually 40-60 mm Hg), open angle and absence of synechiae on gonioscopy, *mild* anterior-chamber reaction with few fine keratic precipitates, and minimal-to-no conjunctival injection. Unilateral with recurrent attacks.)
- Acute angle-closure glaucoma   (Angle closed in the involved eye and usually narrow in the fellow eye, mid-dilated pupil which reacts poorly to light, corneal edema, mild anterior-chamber reaction without keratic precipitates.)
- Pigmentary glaucoma   (Acute rise in IOP often after exercise or pupillary dilatation; *pigment* cells in the anterior chamber, on the trabecular meshwork, and along the posterior corneal surface. The angle is open and radial iris transillumination defects are often present.)
- Neovascular glaucoma   (Iris and anterior chamber-angle neovascularization are present.)
- Fuchs' heterochromic iridocyclitis   (Asymmetry of the iris color, *mild* iritis in the eye with the lighter-colored iris, usually unilateral, often associated

with a cataract and/or glaucoma. Conjunctival injection and ciliary flush are minimal. See "Anterior Uveitis," Section 13.1.)

Work-up

1. History: Recent dilating drops or a systemic anticholinergic agent (suggests angle-closure glaucoma)? Previous attacks? Systemic disease (e.g., juvenile rheumatoid arthritis, ankylosing spondylitis, sarcoidosis, AIDS)? Previous corneal disease?
2. Slit-lamp examination: Assess the degree of conjunctival injection and aqueous cell and flare.
3. IOP measurement.
4. Gonioscopy of the anterior-chamber angle (Is the angle open? Synechiae present? Neovascular membrane present?)
5. Evaluation of the optic nerve.

Treatment

1. Topical steroid (e.g., prednisolone acetate 1%) q 1-6 hours, depending on the severity of the anterior-chamber cellular reaction.

   NOTE Topical steroids are not used, or are used with extreme caution, in patients with an infectious process, particularly a fungal or herpes simplex infection.

2. Mydriatic/cycloplegic (e.g., scopolamine ¼% tid or atropine 1% tid).
3. Topical beta-blocker (e.g., timolol ½% bid or levobunolol ½% bid).

One or more of the following pressure-lowering agents can be used in addition, depending on the IOP and the status of the optic nerve:

4. Carbonic anhydrase inhibitor (e.g., methazolamide 25-50 mg po 2-3 ×/day or acetazolamide 250 mg po qid or 500 mg sequel po bid).
5. Topical epinephrine compound (e.g., epinephrine 0.5-2% bid or dipivefrin 0.1% bid).
6. Hyperosmotic agent when the IOP is acutely elevated (e.g., mannitol 20% 1-2 g/kg iv over 45 minutes. NOTE A 500 cc bag of 20% mannitol contains 100 grams of mannitol).
7. Manage the underlying problem.
8. When the IOP remains dangerously elevated despite maximum medical therapy (a rare event), glaucoma filtering surgery may be indicated.

NOTE Miotics (e.g., pilocarpine) are contraindicated in inflammatory glaucoma.

Follow-up Patients are seen every 1-7 days at first. The higher the IOP and the greater the amount of glaucomatous damage already present (e.g., the larger the optic nerve cup and the paler the nerve) the more frequent the follow-up. Steroids are tapered as the inflammation subsides. Antiglaucoma medications are discontinued as the IOP returns to normal. Steroid-induced glaucoma should always be considered in unresponsive cases, see Section 10.5.

10.5 Steroid-Response Glaucoma

Critical Signs Increased intraocular pressure (IOP) with steroid use, usually within a few weeks of starting topical (eye drops or skin cream), repository, or systemic steroids (although the IOP rise may develop from a few days to a few months after initiating therapy). The IOP usually returns to normal within days to weeks of stopping the steroid.

Other Signs Signs of primary open-angle glaucoma may develop, including optic-nerve cupping and field loss in an eye with an open anterior-chamber angle.

NOTE Patients with primary open-angle glaucoma or a predisposition to develop glaucoma (i.e., positive family history, diabetes, and high myopia) are more likely to develop a steroid response and subsequent glaucoma.

Differential Diagnosis

- Inflammatory open-angle glaucoma (Increased IOP due to anterior-chamber inflammation. As steroids are used to treat ocular inflammation, it may be difficult to determine the cause of the increased IOP.)
- Neovascular glaucoma (Abnormal iris and/or anterior-chamber angle vessels may develop in the presence of ocular inflammation, producing open- and, later closed-angle glaucoma.)

Work-up

1. History: Duration of steroid use? Previous steroid use or an eye problem from steroid use? Glaucoma or family history of glaucoma? Diabetes?
2. Complete ocular examination, evaluating the degree of ocular inflammation and determining whether iris and/or angle neovascularization (by gonioscopy) is present. Measure the IOP and inspect the optic nerve.

3. Optic disc photographs and formal visual fields (e.g., Humphrey or Octopus) are obtained when the optic nerve appears damaged or when the duration of IOP elevation is prolonged or unknown.

Treatment   Any or all of the following may be necessary to reduce the IOP.

1. Discontinue the steroid or reduce the frequency of its administration (steroids should not be stopped abruptly, but rather tapered).
2. Reduce the concentration or dosage of the steroid (e.g., topical prednisolone acetate 1% can be changed to topical prednisolone acetate 0.12%).
3. Switch from a potent steroid with a greater propensity to produce a steroid response (e.g., prednisolone acetate) to one with a lesser propensity (e.g., fluorometholone).
4. Start antiglaucoma therapy: See "Inflammatory Open-Angle Glaucoma," Section 10.4, for options of medical therapy.

NOTE

1. When a high IOP is found in a patient on topical steroids for inflammatory glaucoma, it may be difficult to determine the cause of the increased IOP (i.e., whether it is due to the inflammatory reaction or the steroids). If the inflammation is moderate to severe, we usually will increase the steroids initially to reduce the inflammation while initiating antiglaucoma (e.g., topical beta-blocker) therapy. If the inflammation subsides, but the IOP remains elevated, the glaucoma is assumed to be steroid-induced and the treatment regimen above is followed.
2. When a dangerously high IOP, uncontrollable with medication, develops after a depot steroid injection, the steroid may need to be excised.

10.6   Pigmentary Glaucoma

Symptoms   May be asymptomatic or experience episodes of blurred vision, eye pain, and colored halos around lights after exercise or pupillary dilatation. Typically occurs in young adult men.

Critical Signs   Mid-peripheral spokelike iris transillumination defects, a dense homogeneous pigment band on the trabecular meshwork for 360 degrees (seen on gonioscopy), and glaucoma (optic-nerve cupping, glaucomatous visual field loss, and/or increased intraocular pressure [IOP]). The anterior-chamber angle is open.

Other Signs A vertical pigment band on the corneal endothelium (Krukenberg's spindle), pigment deposition on Schwalbe's line and sometimes along the iris (which can produce iris heterochromia), myopia, and typically large fluctuations in IOP. During IOP spikes, pigment cells may be seen to be floating within the anterior chamber, corneal edema may be present, and patients may be symptomatic as described above.

Differential Diagnosis

- Pseudoexfoliative glaucoma   (Trabecular meshwork pigmentation, but no mid-peripheral iris transillumination defects. White flaky material may be seen on the pupillary border and anterior lens capsule.)
- Inflammatory open angle glaucoma   (White blood cells and flare in the anterior chamber, typically no iris transillumination defects. Central corneal endothelial pigment deposits sometimes appear.)
- Iris melanoma   (Pigmentation of the angular structures accompanied by either a raised pigmented lesion on the iris or a diffusely darkened iris. No iris transillumination defects.)

Work-up

1. History: Previous episodes of decreased vision or halos?
2. Slit-lamp examination, particularly checking for iris transillumination: Shine a small slit beam directly into the pupil to obtain a red reflex. Look at the iris, searching for an iris defect.
3. Check the IOP.
4. Gonioscopy of the anterior-chamber angle.
5. Optic-nerve evaluation.
6. Dilated retinal examination.
7. Stereo disc photographs.
8. Visual field examination, preferably automated (e.g., Humphrey or Octopus).

Treatment Depends on the IOP, status of the optic nerve, visual field changes, and the extent of the symptoms. A stepwise approach to control IOP is usually taken when mild-to-moderate glaucomatous changes are present. When advanced glaucoma is discovered on initial examination, maximal medical therapy may be instituted initially. (See "Primary Open-Angle Glaucoma," Section 10.1.)

1. Miotic drops (the first line of therapy because they eliminate irido-zonular contact that produces pigmentary release into the anterior chamber). Any one of the following may be used:

- Pilocarpine 1-4% qid (start with weaker preparations and slowly increase as needed.)
- Pilocarpine 4% gel qhs (sometimes tolerated better than drops, but patients need to be started on low-strength drops initially before they will tolerate a 4% gel.)
- Pilocarpine inserts (e.g., Ocusert) inserted every week (may produce less fluctuation in myopia.)

(Less commonly used miotics: Echothiophate iodide 0.03% or carbachol ¾-3.0% tid.)

NOTE These drops may need to be used cautiously because of the risk of retinal detachment in myopic patients.

2. Other antiglaucoma medications (e.g., beta-blockers, epinephrine compounds, carbonic anhydrase inhibitors) may be required in addition. (See "Primary Open-Angle Glaucoma," Section 10.1.)
3. Consider argon laser trabeculoplasty (these patients usually respond well).
4. Consider trabeculectomy, when medical and laser therapy fail.

Follow-up Every 1-6 months with a formal visual field test every 6-12 months, depending on the severity of the symptoms and the glaucoma.

NOTE Some patients have the "pigment dispersion syndrome" without glaucoma. These patients are at risk to develop glaucoma and are examined every 6-12 months.

10.7 Pseudoexfoliative Glaucoma

Symptoms Usually asymptomatic.

Critical Signs White flaky material on the pupillary margin, anterior lens capsular changes (central zone of exfoliation material, often with rolled-up edges, middle clear zone, and a peripheral cloudy zone), and glaucoma (optic-nerve cupping, glaucomatous visual field loss, and/or increased intraocular pressure [IOP]).

Other Signs Irregular pigment deposition on the trabecular meshwork and along Schwalbe's line (Sampaolesi's line) seen on gonioscopy. Unilateral or bilateral.

Differential Diagnosis

- Pigmentary glaucoma   (Pigmented trabecular meshwork accompanied by mid-peripheral iris transillumination defects. May have a vertical pigment band on the corneal endothelium.)
- True exfoliation syndrome   (No glaucomatous changes. Trauma, exposure to intense heat [e.g., glass blower], or severe uveitis can cause a thin membrane to peel off of the anterior lens capsule.)
- Primary amyloidosis   (Amyloid material can deposit along the pupillary margin or anterior lens capsule. Gonioscopic findings are similar and glaucomatous changes can occur.)

Work-up

1. History: Occupational exposure to heat?
2. Slit-lamp examination with an IOP measurement (often need to dilate the pupil to see the anterior lens capsular changes).
3. Gonioscopy of the anterior-chamber angle (best before dilatation).
4. Optic-nerve evaluation.
5. Stereo disc photographs.
6. Visual field test, preferably automated (e.g., Humphrey or Octopus).

Treatment

1. Medical therapy, see "Primary Open-Angle Glaucoma," Section 10.1.
2. Consider argon laser trabeculoplasty (higher success rate than in primary open-angle glaucoma) when medical therapy fails.
3. Consider trabeculectomy, when medical/laser therapy fails.

NOTE   Cataract extraction does not eradicate the glaucoma. Cataract extraction may be complicated by weakened zonular fibers and synechiae between the iris and peripheral anterior lens capsule.

Follow-up   Every 1-3 months, depending on the severity of the glaucoma.

NOTE   Some patients have pseudoexfoliation without glaucoma. These patients are reexamined every 6-12 months as they are at risk for glaucoma, but are not treated unless glaucoma develops.

10.8   Phacolytic Glaucoma

Definition   Leakage of lens material from a cataract through an intact lens capsule leads to trabecular meshwork outflow obstruction.

Symptoms   Unilateral pain, decreased vision, red eye, tearing, photophobia.

Critical Signs   Markedly increased intraocular pressure (IOP) accompanied by iridescent particles and white material within the anterior chamber or on the anterior surface of the lens capsule. A hypermature (liquefied) or mature cataract is typical (although an immature cataract may be present).

Other Signs   Corneal edema, anterior-chamber cells and significant flare, pseudohypopyon, and conjunctival injection. Gonioscopy reveals an open anterior-chamber angle.

Differential Diagnosis   All of the following can produce an acute rise in IOP to high levels, but none display iridescent particles and white material in the anterior chamber.

- Inflammatory glaucoma   (Acute increased IOP due to a severe anterior uveitis.)
- Pigmentary glaucoma   (Acute IOP spike due to dispersion of pigment cells into the anterior chamber.)
- Glaucomatocyclitic crisis   (Recurrent idiopathic attacks of increased IOP with an open anterior-chamber angle and mild iritis.)
- Acute angle-closure glaucoma   (Increased IOP due to sudden closure of the anterior-chamber angle, confirmed by gonioscopy.)
- Lens-particle glaucoma   (''Fluffed-up'' lens material is seen in the anterior chamber, but a history of traumatic lens damage or cataract extraction in the involved eye is characteristic.)

Work-up

1. History: Recent trauma or ocular surgery? Recurrent episodes? Uveitis in the past?
2. Slit-lamp examination, looking for iridescent or white particles as well as cells and flare within the anterior chamber. Evaluate for a cataract and an elevated IOP producing corneal edema.
3. Gonioscopy of the anterior chamber angles of *both* eyes (topical glycerin may be placed on the cornea to clear it temporarily if it is edematous).
4. Retinal and optic-disc examination if possible (the degree of optic-nerve cupping helps determine how long the elevated IOP may be tolerated).
5. If the diagnosis is in doubt, a paracentesis can be performed to detect macrophages bloated with lens material on microscopic examination.
6. B-scan ultrasound prior to cataract extraction when there is no fundus view (to rule out an intraocular tumor or retinal detachment).

Treatment The goal of therapy is to lower the IOP immediately and to reduce the inflammation. The cataract is removed as soon as possible.

1. Topical beta-blocker (e.g., levobunolol ½% or timolol ¼-½% × 1 initially and then bid).
2. Carbonic anhydrase inhibitor (e.g., acetazolamide 250 mg tab po × 2 [taken at the same time] and then 250 mg po qid).
3. Hyperosmotic agent (e.g., mannitol 1-2 g/kg iv over 45 minutes. Note that a 500 cc bag of mannitol 20% contains 100 grams of mannitol).
4. Topical steroid (e.g., prednisolone acetate 1% q 15 minutes × 4 then q 1 hour).
5. Topical cycloplegic (e.g., scopolamine ¼% tid).
6. Cataract extraction is performed after the IOP is under control and the inflammation has been reduced. It is generally performed within 24-36 hours. If the IOP cannot be controlled medically, the patient may need hospitalization and urgent cataract extraction.

Follow-up If patients are not hospitalized they should be seen the following day. Patients are usually hospitalized after their cataract surgery to monitor their IOP over the ensuing 24 hours. If the IOP returns to normal after the procedure, the patient should be rechecked within one week.

10.9 Lens-Particle Glaucoma

Definition Lens material liberated by trauma or surgery which obstructs aqueous outflow channels.

Symptoms Pain, blurred vision, red eye, tearing, photophobia. A history of recent ocular trauma or cataract surgery can be obtained.

Critical Signs White, fluffy pieces of lens cortical material in the anterior chamber combined with increased intraocular pressure (IOP). A break in the lens capsule may be observed in post-traumatic cases.

Other Signs Anterior chamber cells and flare, conjunctival injection, or corneal edema. The anterior-chamber angle is open on gonioscopy.

Differential Diagnosis (See also the differential diagnosis of "Phacolytic Glaucoma," Section 10.8.) (In phacolytic glaucoma the cataractous lens has not been extracted nor traumatized.)

- Infectious endophthalmitis (Unless lens cortical material can be unequivocally identified in the anterior chamber and there is nothing atypical about the presentation, endophthalmitis must be ruled out.)
- Phacoanaphylactic endophthalmitis (Follows trauma or intraocular surgery, producing anterior-chamber inflammation and sometimes a high IOP. The inflammation is often granulomatous, and fluffy lens material is not present in the anterior chamber.)

Work-up

1. History: Recent trauma or ocular surgery?
2. Slit-lamp examination: Search the anterior chamber for lens cortical material and measure the IOP.
3. Gonioscopy of the anterior-chamber angle.
4. Optic-nerve evaluation (the degree of optic-nerve cupping helps determine how long the elevated IOP can be tolerated.)

Treatment

1. Topical beta-blocker (e.g., levobunolol ½% bid or timolol ¼-½% bid).
2. Carbonic anhydrase inhibitor (e.g., methazolamide 25-50 mg po 2-3 ×/day or acetazolamide 250 mg po qid or 500 mg sequel po bid).
3. Topical cycloplegic (e.g., scopolamine ¼% tid).
4. Topical steroid (e.g., prednisolone acetate 1% qid).

- If the IOP is markedly elevated (e.g., >45 mm Hg in a previously healthy eye or less in a patient with previous optic nerve damage), a hyperosmotic agent is added to acutely lower the pressure (e.g., mannitol 1-2 g/kg iv over 45 minutes. Note that a 500 cc bag of mannitol 20% contains 100 grams of mannitol).
- If medical therapy fails to control the IOP, the residual lens material needs to be removed surgically.

Follow-up Depending on the IOP and the health of the optic nerve, patients are reexamined within 1-7 days.

10.10 Acute Angle-Closure Glaucoma

Symptoms Pain, blurred vision, colored halos around lights, decreased visual acuity, frontal headache, nausea and vomiting.

Critical Signs Closed angle in the involved eye, acutely elevated intraocular pressure (IOP), and corneal microcystic edema.

Other Signs Conjunctival injection, a fixed mid-dilated pupil, and a shallow anterior chamber.

Etiology

- Pupillary block (More common in hyperopic eyes. May be precipitated by topical mydriatics, systemic anticholinergics [e.g., antihistamines or anti-psychotics], or dim illumination [e.g., movie theater]. Posterior synechiae from previous ocular inflammation also predisposes to pupillary block. The angle is usually narrow or occludable in the fellow eye.)
- Angle crowding due to an abnormal iris configuration (e.g., plateau iris syndrome—angle closure occurs despite a patent peripheral iridectomy.)
- Neovascular or inflammatory membrane pulling the angle closed (Abnormal misdirected blood vessels along the pupillary margin and/or the trabecular meshwork are seen.)
- Mechanical closure of the angle secondary to anterior displacement of the lens-iris diaphragm:
  a. Lens-induced (Pupillary occlusion due to a large lens [phacomorphic].)
  b. Choroidal detachment (serous or hemorrhagic) (Generally follows surgery; diagnose by indirect ophthalmoscopy and/or B-scan ultrasonography.)
  c. Choroidal swelling following extensive retinal laser surgery or after placement of a tight encircling band in retinal detachment surgery
  d. Posterior segment tumor (e.g., choroidal/ciliary body melanoma)
  e. Malignant glaucoma (Aqueous misdirection.)

NOTE A secondary mechanical cause of angle-closure glaucoma should be suspected when the fellow eye's angle is wide open.

Differential Diagnosis (Other causes of an acute IOP rise, but with an open angle.)

- Glaucomatocyclitic crisis (Posner-Schlossman syndrome) (Recurrent IOP spikes in one eye, *mild* cell and flare $+/-$ fine keratic precipitates; the eye is generally not inflamed and not painful.)
- Inflammatory open-angle glaucoma (Moderate-to-severe anterior-chamber reaction.)
- Retrobulbar hemorrhage or inflammation (Proptosis and restriction of ocular motility.)
- Traumatic (hemolytic) glaucoma (History of trauma, red blood cells in the anterior chamber.)

- Pigmentary glaucoma   (Pigment cells floating in the anterior chamber, often after exercise or pupillary dilatation, radial iris transillumination defects.)
- Phacolytic glaucoma   (A cataract and anterior-chamber iridescent particles or white material are present.)

Work-up

1. History: Retinal problem? Recent laser treatment or surgery? Medications?
2. Slit-lamp examination, looking for keratic precipitates, posterior synechiae, iris neovascularization, a swollen lens, anterior-chamber cells and flare or iridescent particles, and a shallow anterior chamber.
3. Measure the IOP.
4. Gonioscopy of both anterior-chamber angles (You may want to initially avoid gonioscopy of the involved eye when there is a significant amount of corneal edema and the diagnosis is fairly well established; gonioscopy of an edematous cornea predisposes to a corneal abrasion. Gonioscopy of the involved eye after the IOP is lowered is essential in determining whether the angle has opened up.)
5. Evaluate the optic nerve (without dilating).

Treatment   (See "Malignant Glaucoma," Section 10.16, "Neovascular Glaucoma," Section 10.13, and "Postoperative Glaucoma," Section 10.15 for specific treatment of these conditions.)

1. Attempt corneal compression with a gonioprism if the attack is of recent onset and no corneal edema is present (this may be of help in opening the angle and reducing the IOP).
2. Topical beta-blocker (e.g., levobunolol ½% or timolol ½%) × 1.
3. Carbonic anhydrase inhibitor (e.g., acetazolamide 250-500 mg iv or 250 mg tab × 2 po at once)
4. Osmotic agent (e.g., isosorbide 50-100 grams po or mannitol 1-2 g/kg iv over 45 minutes. NOTE   500 cc of mannitol 20% contains 100 grams of mannitol).
5. Topical steroid (e.g., prednisolone acetate 1%) q 15-30 minutes × 4 and then hourly.
6. When due to:
   a. Phakic pupillary block or angle crowding: Pilocarpine 1-2% q 15 minutes × 2 and pilocarpine ½% to the fellow eye × 1.
   b. Aphakic or pseudophakic pupillary block or mechanical closure of the angle: Do *not* use pilocarpine. A mydriatic/cycloplegic agent (e.g., cyclopentolate 2% and phenylephrine 2.5% q 15 minutes × 4) is used when laser or surgery is not being initially employed due to corneal edema and/or inflammation.

7. In cases of phacomorphic glaucoma, the lens needs to be removed urgently.

Recheck the IOP in 1 hour.

- If the IOP drops significantly *and* the angle is determined to be open by gonioscopy, definitive treatment is performed once the cornea is clear and the anterior chamber is quiet (see below). In most cases, this requires waiting 1-3 days for the inflammation to resolve. Patients are discharged on the following medications and followed daily.

  Prednisolone acetate 1% qid
  Acetazolamide 500 mg sequel po bid
  Topical beta-blocker (e.g., levobunolol ½% bid or timolol ½% bid)
  Pilocarpine 1-2% qid (in cases of phakic pupillary block or angle crowding)
  Pilocarpine ½% qid to the fellow eye if the angle is narrow or occludable.

- If the IOP is still elevated or the angle is still closed, medical treatment is continued or definitive treatment is implemented (despite ocular inflammation).

Definitive Treatment

A. *Pupillary block (all forms) or angle crowding*
   1. Laser peripheral iridectomy (PI) (argon or YAG) to the involved eye.
   2. Laser PI to the fellow eye if it is occludable. (Only one eye is lasered in one sitting. If corneal edema prohibits laser in the involved eye at the time of initial treatment, the fellow eye can be lasered first.)
   3. Surgical iridectomy if a laser PI is not possible.
   4. Consider a trabeculectomy when the IOP remains high despite an iridectomy and maximal medical treatment, especially in presence of significant optic-nerve cupping.
B. *Mechanical angle closure*
   1. Consider argon laser gonioplasty to open the angle, particularly in cases due to extensive retinal laser surgery, a tight encircling band from retinal detachment surgery, or nanophthalmos.
   2. Treat the underlying problem.

Follow-up   After definitive treatment to one or both eyes, patients are reevaluated in weeks to months initially and then less frequently. Visual fields (e.g., Humphrey or Octopus) and stereo disc photographs are obtained for baseline purposes.

NOTES

1. The patient's cardiovascular status and electrolyte balance must be considered when contemplating osmotic agents, carbonic anhydrase inhibitors, and beta-blockers.
2. When mechanical angle-closure glaucoma is suspected, a B-scan ultrasound may be helpful in diagnosis.
3. If a repeat attack of angle closure occurs despite a patent iridectomy, a plateau iris syndrome may be present (see Section 10.11).

10.11   Plateau Iris

Symptoms   Usually asymptomatic unless acute angle-closure glaucoma develops (decreased vision, throbbing pain, nausea, and vomiting, see Section 10.10).

Critical Signs   Flat iris plane and normal anterior-chamber depth centrally, convex peripheral iris with an anterior iris insertion seen on gonioscopy.

Other Signs   With acute angle-closure associated with a plateau iris, the axial anterior-chamber depth remains normal, but the peripheral iris bunches up to occlude the angle. (See Section 10.10 for other associated signs.)

Types

Plateau iris configuration   Due to the anatomic configuration of the angle, these patients may develop acute angle-closure glaucoma from only a mild degree of pupillary block. These angle-closure attacks are cured by peripheral iridectomy (PI), as it relieves the pupillary block.
Plateau iris syndrome   The peripheral iris can bunch up in the anterior-chamber angle and obstruct aqueous outflow without any element of pupillary block. The diagnosis is made when angle-closure glaucoma occurs despite a patent PI.

Differential Diagnosis

- Acute angle-closure glaucoma associated with pupillary block   (The central anterior-chamber depth is decreased and the entire iris has a convex appearance.)
- Malignant glaucoma   (Marked flattening of the anterior chamber, often following cataract extraction or glaucoma surgery.)

• For other disorders see "Acute Angle-Closure Glaucoma," Section 10.10.

Work-up

1. Slit-lamp examination (specifically checking for the presence of a patent PI and the critical signs above).
2. Measure the intraocular pressure (IOP).
3. Gonioscopy of both anterior-chamber angles. In cases of angle-closure glaucoma and significant corneal edema, gonioscopy may be deferred in the involved eye until the IOP is lowered.
4. Undilated optic-nerve evaluation.

NOTE If dilatation needs to be performed in a patient suspected of having a plateau iris, then warn the patient that this may provoke an acute angle-closure attack. Dilate with tropicamide ½% only. Recheck the IOP every few hours until the pupil returns to normal size. Have the patient notify you immediately if symptoms of acute angle-closure develop.

Treatment

1. Treat acute angle-closure glaucoma medically if present (see Section 10.10).
2. A laser PI is performed within 1-2 days if the angle-closure attack can be controlled medically. If the attack cannot be controlled, a laser or surgical PI may need to be done emergently.
3. A week after the laser PI, the eye should be dilated with a weak mydriatic (e.g., tropicamide ½%). If the IOP rises, plateau iris syndrome is diagnosed and should be treated with a weak miotic (e.g., pilocarpine ½-1% 3-4 ×/day chronically).
4. If angle-closure glaucoma develops despite a patent PI, then the plateau iris syndrome exists and should be treated with a weak miotic chronically as above.
5. Consider a laser gonioplasty (iridoplasty) in refractile cases, or to break an acute attack not responsive to medical treatment and a PI.
6. As in many forms of acute angle-closure glaucoma, a prophylactic laser PI is often indicated in the fellow eye (usually within 1-2 weeks of the first attack). The development of a plateau iris syndrome in one eye suggests the need for chronic pilocarpine therapy in addition to a laser PI in the fellow eye.

Follow-up

1. Following a laser PI for an attack of acute angle-closure glaucoma, patients are reevaluated in 1 week, 1 month, and 3 months and then every 3-6 months. IOP and gonioscopy should be checked at each visit and signs of

increasing angle closure looked for. The PI should be examined for patency. In patients *not* receiving pilocarpine, periodic tests for the plateau iris syndrome should be performed with topical tropicamide ½%.

2. Patients suspected of having a plateau iris configuration who have never had an acute angle-closure attack are followed every 6 months. At each visit the IOP is measured and gonioscopy is performed, looking for peripheral anterior synechiae formation and further narrowing of the anterior-chamber angle.

10.12   Glaucomatocyclitic Crisis

(Posner-Schlossman Syndrome)

Symptoms   Mild pain, decreased vision, and the observation of colored rainbows around lights. Often a history of similar episodes is obtained. Usually unilateral.

Critical Signs   Markedly elevated intraocular pressure (IOP) (usually 40-60 mm Hg), open angle without synechiae on gonioscopy, minimal conjunctival injection (white eye), and a very mild anterior-chamber reaction (few aqueous cells and little flare).

Other Signs   Corneal epithelial edema, ciliary flush, pupillary constriction, iris hypochromia, few fine keratic precipitates on the corneal endothelium or trabecular meshwork.

Differential Diagnosis

- Inflammatory open-angle glaucoma   (Significant amount of aqueous cells and flare, conjunctival injection, and pain. Synechiae may be present. May be bilateral.)
- Acute angle-closure glaucoma   (Closed angle in the involved eye and usually a narrow angle in the fellow eye, painful, conjunctival injection, corneal edema; may have history of recent dilatation with drops or use of systemic anticholinergic medication.)
- Pigmentary glaucoma   (Acute rise in IOP often after exercise or pupillary dilatation, *pigment* cells in the anterior chamber, open-angle, radial iris transillumination defects, vertically oriented pigmented cells on the posterior

corneal surface [Krukenberg's spindle], and pigment in the trabecular meshwork seen on gonioscopy.)

- Neovascular glaucoma (Iris and/or angle neovascularization is present.)
- Fuchs' heterochromic iridocyclitis (Asymmetry of iris color, mild iritis in the eye with the lighter-colored iris, usually unilateral, often associated with a cataract and/or glaucoma. The IOP rise is rarely as acute. See "Anterior Uveitis," Section 13.1.)

Work-up

1. History: Recent dilating drops, systemic anticholinergic agents, or exercise? Previous attacks? Corneal or systemic disease?
2. Slit-lamp examination: Assess the degree of conjunctival injection and aqueous cell and flare. Measure the IOP.
3. Gonioscopy of the anterior-chamber angle: Angle open? Synechiae, neovascular membrane, or keratic precipitates present?
4. Optic-nerve evaluation.

Treatment

1. Topical beta-blocker (e.g., timolol ½% bid or levobunolol ½% bid).
2. Topical steroid (e.g., prednisolone acetate 1% qid).
3. Add a carbonic anhydrase inhibitor (e.g., methazolamide 25-50 mg po 2-3 ×/day or acetazolamide 250 mg po qid or 500 mg sequel po bid) if the IOP is significantly elevated.
4. Hyperosmotic agents (e.g., mannitol 20% 1-2 g/kg iv over 45 minutes) are used acutely when the IOP is determined to be dangerously high for the involved optic nerve. NOTE 500 cc of mannitol 20% contains 100 grams of mannitol.
5. Consider a cycloplegic agent (e.g., cyclopentolate 2% tid) if the patient is symptomatic.

Follow-up Patients are seen every few days at first, then weekly until the episode resolves. Attacks usually subside within a few hours to a few weeks. No medical (or surgical) therapy is required between attacks. Steroids are tapered rapidly if they are used for one week or less, and slowly if they are used for longer. Note that both eyes are at risk of developing chronic open-angle glaucoma.

10.13 Neovascular Glaucoma

Symptoms May be asymptomatic or may complain of pain, red eye, photophobia, and decreased vision.

Critical Signs

Stage 1 Abnormal misdirected blood vessels along the pupillary margin and/or the trabecular meshwork. No signs of glaucoma.

Stage 2 Stage 1 plus increased intraocular pressure (IOP) (open-angle neovascular glaucoma).

Stage 3 Angle-closure glaucoma either partial or complete, due to a fibrovascular membrane covering the trabecular meshwork. Peripheral anterior synechiae and florid iris neovascularization are common.

Other Signs Mild anterior-chamber cells and flare, conjunctival injection, corneal edema (when an acute rise in IOP occurs), hyphema, eversion of the pupillary margin allowing visualization of the iris pigment epithelium (ectropion uvea), optic-nerve cupping, and visual field loss.

Etiology

- Diabetic retinopathy.
- Central retinal vein occlusion, particularly the ischemic type.
- Central retinal artery occlusion.
- Ocular ischemic syndrome (carotid occlusive disease).
- Others (Branch retinal vein occlusion, chronic uveitis, chronic retinal detachment, intraocular tumors, trauma, and other ocular vascular disorders.)

Differential Diagnosis

- Inflammatory glaucoma (Increased IOP, abundant anterior-chamber cells and marked flare, and dilated normal iris blood vessels may be seen. No neovascular vessels. Normal iris blood vessels run radially, have a sense of direction, and are usually symmetrical 360 degrees around the pupillary margin. The angle is open.)
- Primary acute-angle closure glaucoma (No signs of new iris blood vessels. Usually a narrow angle in the fellow eye.)

Work-up

1. History: Determine the underlying etiology.
2. Complete ocular examination, including an IOP measurement and gonioscopic evaluation of the anterior-chamber angle (to determine what degree

of the angle is closed, if any). A dilated retinal evaluation is essential in determining the cause of the iris neovascularization.

3. Fluorescein angiogram as needed to identify an underlying retinal abnormality or in preparation for retinal laser treatment (panretinal photocoagulation).
4. Carotid noninvasive studies to rule out carotid disease when no retinal pathology can be found accountable for the neovascularization.
5. B-scan ultrasound is indicated when the retina cannot be visualized (to rule out an intraocular tumor or retinal detachment).

Treatment

1. Control the IOP if it is elevated (any or all of the following medications are used):
   a. Topical beta-blocker (e.g., levobunolol ½% bid or timolol ½% bid).
   b. Systemic carbonic anhydrase inhibitor (e.g., methazolamide 25-50 mg po 2-3 × /day or acetazolamide 500 mg po bid).
   c. Hyperosmotic agent (e.g., mannitol 20% 1-2 g/kg iv over 45 minutes. Note that a 500 cc bag of mannitol 20% contains 100 grams of mannitol.)

NOTE   Miotics (e.g., pilocarpine) and epinephrine compounds are generally ineffective and not often used.

2. Reduce inflammation and pain: Topical steroid (e.g., prednisolone acetate 1% q 1-6 hours) and a cycloplegic (e.g., atropine 1% tid). (Atropine may lower IOP when the angle is closed by increasing uveoscleral outflow.)
3. If retinal ischemia is thought to be responsible for the iris neovascularization, then treat with panretinal photocoagulation (PRP) (if the retina can be visualized) or panretinal cryoablation (if it cannot be well seen). These procedures are used if the angle is open or if the patient is going to have filtration surgery (whether the angle is open or closed).
4. Goniophotocoagulation (laser photocoagulation of new vessels in the angle) may be used in addition to the above treatment in patients with significant angle neovascularization, but minimal to no angle closure. This procedure reduces the risk of angle closure during the time interval required for the PRP to take effect (often several weeks).
5. Glaucoma filtration surgery (e.g., trabeculectomy) is often performed when the neovascularization is inactive and the IOP cannot be controlled with medical therapy. Shunt tube procedures or YAG laser cyclophotocoagulation are helpful to control IOP in selective cases.

In eyes without useful vision, topical steroids and cycloplegics, beta-blockers, YAG laser cyclophotocoagulation, cyclocryotherapy, or a retrobulbar alcohol injection may be required to reduce pain (see "The Blind, Painful Eye," Section 15.9).

6. Treat the underlying disorder (see the appropriate section).

Follow-up The presence of iris neovascularization, especially when accompanied by a high IOP, requires urgent therapeutic intervention, usually within 1-2 days. Angle closure can proceed relatively rapidly (within days to weeks).

NOTE   Iris neovascularization without glaucoma is managed in a similar manner as to that described above; however, there is no need for antiglaucomatous therapy unless the IOP rises.

10.14   Iridocorneal Endothelial (ICE) Syndrome

Symptoms Usually asymptomatic, but may note an irregular iris appearance, blurred vision, or pain in one eye. Patients are typically young to middle-aged adults.

Critical Signs Corneal endothelial changes ("fine, hammered-metal" appearance), peripheral anterior synechiae which often extend beyond Schwalbe's line, and iris alterations as follows:

Essential iris atrophy Marked iris thinning often leading to iris holes and displacement and distortion of the pupil.

Chandler's syndrome Mild iris thinning and pupil distortion. (The corneal changes are most marked in this variant.)

Iris nevus (Cogan-Reese) syndrome Pigmented nodules on the iris surface, variable iris atrophy.

Other Signs Corneal edema, increased intraocular pressure (IOP), optic-nerve cupping, or visual field loss. Typically unilateral, although mild changes consistent with this syndrome are sometimes found in the fellow eye.

Differential Diagnosis

- Axenfeld-Rieger syndrome   (Prominent, anteriorly displaced Schwalbe's line [posterior embryotoxon], peripheral iris strands extending to Schwalbe's line, iris thinning with atrophic holes, may have dental, craniofacial and skeletal abnormalities. Bilateral and congenital.)
- Posterior polymorphous dystrophy   (Bilateral, corneal endothelial vesicles or bandlike lesions, occasionally associated with iridocorneal adhesions.)

- Fuchs' endothelial dystrophy   (Bilateral corneal edema and endothelial guttata, the iris and anterior-chamber angle are normal.)
- Iris melanoma   (Pigmented iris lesion[s] noted to enlarge over time.)

Work-up

1. Family history: ICE syndrome is not inherited; Axenfeld-Rieger syndrome and posterior polymorphous dystrophy are often autosomal dominant.
2. Slit-lamp examination: Assess the cornea and iris and measure the IOP.
3. Gonioscopy of the anterior-chamber angle.
4. Optic-nerve examination, best with a Hruby, fundus contact, or 60 diopter lens.
5. Stereo disc photographs.
6. Visual field test, preferably automated (e.g., Humphrey or Octopus).

Treatment   No treatment is needed unless glaucoma or corneal edema is present, at which point one or more of the following treatments is used:

1. Antiglaucomatous medications for corneal edema or glaucoma (see "Primary Open-Angle Glaucoma," Section 10.1). The IOP may need to be lowered beneath a critical level to rid the cornea of edema. This critical level may become lower as the patient ages.
2. Hypertonic saline solutions (e.g., sodium chloride 5% drops qid and ointment qhs) to reduce corneal edema.
3. Consider trabeculectomy when medical therapy fails to maintain the IOP low enough to prevent corneal edema or progression of optic-nerve damage. (Argon laser trabeculoplasty is usually ineffective.)
4. Consider a corneal transplant in cases of advanced chronic corneal edema in the presence of good IOP control.

Follow-up   Every 3-12 months, unless glaucoma is present, then every 1-3 months depending on the severity of the glaucoma.

10.15   Postoperative Glaucoma

Early Postoperative Glaucoma

Intraocular pressure (IOP) tends to rise 6-7 hours postoperatively and generally returns to normal within one week. Most normal eyes can tolerate an IOP less than 30 mm Hg for this short a duration. However, eyes with preexisting optic-nerve damage require antiglaucoma medications (e.g., levobunolol ½% bid, timolol ½% bid, or methazolamide 25-50 mg po 2-3 × /day) for any significant pressure rise. Any eye with an IOP greater than 30 mm Hg should likewise be treated. If inflammation is excessive, increase the topical steroid dose (see "Inflammatory Open-Angle Glaucoma," Section 10.4).

Aphakic/Pseudophakic Pupillary Block

Signs Increased IOP, a flat anterior chamber, and the absence of a patent peripheral iridectomy (PI).

Treatment

A. If the cornea is clear and the eye is not significantly inflamed, then a PI (usually by laser), is performed.
B. If the cornea is hazy, the eye is inflamed, or a PI cannot be performed immediately, then:
   1. Mydriatic agent (e.g., cyclopentolate 2% and phenylephrine 2.5% q 15 minutes × 4).
   2. Carbonic anhydrase inhibitor (e.g., acetazolamide 250 mg po × 2 or 500 mg iv).
   3. Topical beta-blocker (e.g., timolol ½%) × 1.
   4. Consider a hyperosmotic agent (e.g., mannitol 1-2 g/kg iv over 45 minutes. NOTE   500 cc of mannitol 20% contains 100 grams of mannitol.)
   5. Topical steroid (e.g., prednisolone acetate 1% q 15-30 minutes × 4).
   6. PI (preferably laser) as soon as available and the eye is less inflamed. If the cornea is edematous and cloudy, topical glycerin may be used to clear it temporarily.

Uveitis, Glaucoma, Hyphema (UGH) Syndrome

Signs Anterior chamber cells and flare, increased IOP, often with a hyphema. Usually secondary to irritation from an intraocular lens.

Treatment

1. Atropine 1% tid.
2. Topical steroid (e.g., prednisolone acetate 1% qid—more often if the uveitis is severe).
3. Carbonic anhydrase inhibitor (e.g., acetazolamide 250 mg po qid, or 500 mg sequel po bid, or methazolamide 25-50 mg po 2-3 × /day).
4. Topical beta-blocker (e.g., timolol ½% bid or levobunolol ½% bid).

5. Consider argon laser treatment to control the hemorrhage if a bleeding site can be identified.
6. Consider surgical removal of the intraocular lens (especially if peripheral anterior synechiae are forming).

Malignant Glaucoma   (See Section 10.16.)

Steroid-Induced Glaucoma   (See Section 10.5.)

Follow-up   Patients should generally not be sent out of the office/emergency room with an IOP greater than 35-40 mm Hg. If the patient is monocular or has significant optic-nerve damage, then the IOP should be even lower. For aphakic/pseudophakic pupillary block, be certain that the angle is open and the block is relieved (use gonioscopy). If the above criteria are met, the patient needs to be reevaluated in 1-7 days, depending on the particular situation.

10.16   Malignant Glaucoma

Symptoms   Pain, red eye, photophobia, often after surgical treatment of angle-closure glaucoma or cataract extraction.

Critical Signs   Shallow or flat anterior chamber plus elevated intraocular pressure (IOP) in the presence of a patent iridectomy and in the absence of a choroidal detachment.

Etiology   It is believed that aqueous is "misdirected" and accumulates within or posterior to the vitreous, displaces the vitreous forward, and causes a collapse of the anterior chamber.

Differential Diagnosis

• Acute angle-closure glaucoma   (The anterior chamber is shallow and the angle is closed, the IOP is elevated, but a patent iridectomy is not present.)
• Choroidal detachment   (Shallow or flat anterior chamber, but the IOP is typically low. A choroidal detachment is seen on funduscopic examination or by B-scan ultrasound in most cases.)
• Suprachoroidal hemorrhage   (Shallow or flat anterior chamber, often elevated IOP, but a choroidal detachment may be seen on funduscopic examination or B-scan ultrasound.)

Work-up

1. History: Previous eye surgery?
2. Slit-lamp examination: Determine if a patent iridectomy is present. Pupillary block is unlikely in the presence of a patent iridectomy (unless it is plugged with vitreous or totally bound down or unless plateau iris syndrome is present).
3. Gonioscopy of the anterior-chamber angle.
4. Dilated retinal examination if a patent iridectomy is present (and phakic angle closure is ruled out).
5. Consider a B-scan ultrasound to rule out a choroidal detachment and suprachoroidal hemorrhage if they cannot be ruled out by ophthalmoscopy.

Treatment

1. If an iridectomy is not present or you cannot be sure whether an existing one is patent, pupillary block cannot be ruled out and a peripheral iridectomy (PI) should be performed (see "Acute Angle-Closure Glaucoma," Section 10.10).

If signs of malignant glaucoma are still present with a patent iridectomy:
2. Atropine 1% + phenylephrine 2.5% qid topically.
3. Carbonic anhydrase inhibitor (e.g., acetazolamide 500 mg iv or 250 mg × 2 po, then 250 mg po qid).
4. Hyperosmotic agent (e.g., mannitol 20% 1-2 g/kg iv over 45 minutes. NOTE 500 cc of mannitol 20% contains 100 grams of mannitol).
5. Topical beta-blocker (e.g., timolol ½% bid or levobunolol ½% bid).

If the block is broken (the anterior chamber deepens and the IOP returns to normal), maintain atropine 1% q day indefinitely.

If steps 1-5 are unsuccessful consider one or more of the following:
6. YAG laser disruption of the anterior hyaloid face/posterior capsule if the patient is aphakic or pseudophakic.
7. Argon laser treatment of the ciliary processes.
8. Surgery (core vitrectomy and reformation of the anterior chamber).

NOTE A choroidal detachment may be present yet undetectable. Therefore, a sclerotomy to drain a choroidal detachment may be advisable prior to vitrectomy.

9. PI to the fellow eye if the angle appears occludable (generally performed at a later date).

Follow-up Variable, depending upon the therapeutic modality employed. A PI is generally performed in an occludable fellow eye one week after treatment of the involved eye.

11

Neuro-
ophthalmology

11.1 Anisocoria

Definition   The two pupils are unequal in size.

Etiology

A. The abnormal pupil is constricted.
- Unilateral use of miotic drops (green-top eye drops) (e.g., pilocarpine)
- Iritis   (Eye pain, redness, and anterior-chamber cells and flare.)
- Horner's syndrome   (Mild ptosis is usually present on the side of the small pupil, [+] cocaine test.)
- Argyll Robertson (syphilitic) pupil   (The pupil is irregular in shape, reacts poorly [or not at all] to light, but constricts normally during convergence. Although the disease is typically bilateral, a mild degree of anisocoria is often present [+] FTA-ABS).
- Longstanding Adie's pupil   (The pupil is initially dilated, but over time may constrict. At the slit lamp, it can be seen to react slowly and irregularly to a bright light. It is supersensitive to pilocarpine 1/8% or methacholine 2.5%, constricting even further.)
B. The abnormal pupil is dilated.
- Iris sphincter muscle damage from trauma   (Torn pupillary margin or iris transillumination defects seen on slit-lamp examination.)

- Adie's tonic pupil (The pupil is irregular, reacts minimally to light and slowly to convergence, but is supersensitive to weak cholinergic agents such as pilocarpine 1/8% or methacholine 2.5%.)
- Third-nerve palsy (Associated ptosis plus extraocular muscle palsies. The pupil will not react to weak cholinergic agents, but will constrict to regular strength miotic drops [e.g., pilocarpine 1%].)
- Unilateral use of a dilating drop (red-top eye drop) (e.g., atropine) (If the drop has been instilled recently, the pupil will not react to pilocarpine 1% drops. If the effect of the drop is wearing off [e.g., the atropine was used 1-2 weeks previously], the eye may be dilated and partly reactive to the pilocarpine.)

C. Physiologic anisocoria (Pupil size disparity is the same in light as in dark and the pupils react normally to light. The size difference is usually ≤1 mm in diameter, but not always.)

Work-up

1. History: When was the anisocoria first noted? Any associated symptoms or signs? History of ocular trauma? Use of any eye drops or ointments? History of syphilis?
2. Ocular examination: Try to determine which is the abnormal pupil by observing the pupillary size. Younger patients tend to have pupillary diameters of 4-5 mm on average, whereas elderly patients often have slightly smaller pupils. If it is uncertain which is the abnormal pupil compare pupil sizes in light and in dark. Anisocoria greater in light suggests the abnormal pupil is the larger pupil; anisocoria greater in dark suggests the abnormal pupil is the smaller pupil. Test the pupillary reaction to light (and that to convergence if the light reaction is abnormal). Look for ptosis, evaluate ocular motility, and examine the pupillary margin with a slit lamp.

- If the abnormal pupil is small and anisocoria is thought to be worse in darkness, a diagnosis of Horner's syndrome may be confirmed by a cocaine test (see Section 11.2). In the presence of ptosis and unequivocal worsening of anisocoria in dim illumination, a cocaine test may be unnecessary as the diagnosis is made clinically.
- If the abnormal pupil is large and there is no sphincter muscle damage nor extraocular motility restriction or ptosis consistent with a third-nerve palsy, the pupils may be tested with one drop of pilocarpine ⅛% or methacholine 2.5%. Within 10-15 minutes, an Adie's pupil will usually have constricted significantly more than the fellow pupil (see Section 11.4).

NOTE Soon after the development of an Adie's pupil, the pupil may be *unreactive* to a weak cholinergic agent.

- If the pupil does not constrict with pilocarpine 1/8% or methacholine 2.5% and/or pharmacologic dilatation is suspected, pilocarpine 1% is instilled in both eyes. A normal pupil constricts sooner and to a greater extent than the pharmacologically dilated pupil. An eye which recently received a strong mydriatic agent such as atropine will usually not constrict at all.

See "Horner's Syndrome" (Section 11.2), "Argyll Robertson Pupil" (Section 11.3), "Adie's Tonic Pupil" (Section 11.4), and "Isolated Third-Nerve Palsy" (Section 11.5) for more information regarding diagnosis and treatment.

11.2 Horner's Syndrome

Symptoms Droopy eyelid, pupil size disparity, often asymptomatic.

Critical Signs Anisocoria which is greater in dim illumination (especially during the first few seconds the room light is dimmed) because of a small pupil which does not dilate as well as the normal, larger pupil; usually mild ptosis and lower eyelid elevation on the same side as the small pupil.

Other Signs All of the following may occur on the side of the Horner's syndrome: Lower intraocular pressure, lighter iris color in congenital cases (iris heterochromia), loss of sweating ability (anhidrosis), increase in accommodation (older patients can be noted to hold their reading card closer in the Horner's eye). Light and near reactions are intact.

Differential Diagnosis See "Anisocoria," Section 11.1.

Etiology

First-order neuron disorder Stroke (e.g., vertebrobasilar artery insufficiency or infarct), tumor, rarely severe osteoarthritis of the neck with bony spurs.
Second-order neuron disorder Tumor (e.g., lung carcinoma, metastasis, thyroid adenoma, and neurofibroma). Patients with arm pain should be suspected of having a Pancoast tumor.
Third-order neuron disorder Headache syndrome (e.g., cluster, migraine, or Raeder's paratrigeminal syndrome), herpes zoster virus, otitis media, or Tolosa Hunt syndrome.
Congenital Horner's syndrome Trauma (e.g., during delivery.)

Work-up

1. If the diagnosis is uncertain, it may be confirmed with a cocaine test: Cocaine 10% one drop is placed into both eyes and then repeated 1 minute later. Check the pupils in 15 minutes. If no change in pupillary size is noted, repeat one set of drops and recheck the pupils in another 15 minutes. A Horner's pupil dilates less well than the normal pupil.
2. Hydroxyamphetamine 1% (e.g., Paredrine) is used to distinguish a third-order neuron disorder from a first- and second-order neuron disorder: Place one drop of hydroxyamphetamine 1% into each eye, repeating the drop one minute later. Check the pupils in 30 minutes. Failure of the Horner's pupil to dilate to an equivalent degree as the fellow eye indicates a third-order neuron lesion.

NOTES

1. Hydroxyamphetamine should not be administered within 24 hours of cocaine or they will interfere with each other's action.
2. Both tests require an intact corneal epithelium and no prior eye drop administration for accurate results.

3. Determine the duration of the Horner's syndrome from the patient's history and an examination of old photographs. A new-onset Horner's syndrome requires a more extensive diagnostic work-up. An old Horner's syndrome is more likely to be benign.
4. History: Headaches? Arm pain? Previous stroke? Previous surgery that may have damaged the sympathetic chain, including cardiac, thoracic, thyroid or neck surgery?
5. Physical examination (especially check for supraclavicular nodes, thyroid enlargement, or a neck mass).

Depending on the duration of the Horner's syndrome and the results of the hydroxyamphetamine test, none or all of the following tests may be ordered (a more aggressive work-up is performed for new-onset Horner's syndromes, first- or second-order neuron disorders, and those with a history or physical examination that might indicate a tumor):

6. Chest x-ray with special views of the apex of the lung.
7. CT scan (axial and coronal views) or MRI of the brain.
8. X-rays of the cervical spine.
9. CBC with differential.
10. Lymph node biopsy when lymphadenopathy is present.

Treatment

1. Treat the underlying disorder if possible.
2. Ptosis surgery may be performed as needed.

Follow-up Acute Horner's syndromes should be worked up as soon as possible to rule out life-threatening causes. Chronic Horner's syndromes can be evaluated with less urgency. With the exception of possible amblyopia in children (which only occurs when the eyelid covers the visual axis), there are no ocular complications that necessitate close follow-up.

11.3 Argyll Robertson Pupil

Symptoms Usually asymptomatic.

Critical Signs Small, irregular pupil which reacts poorly (or not at all) to light but constricts normally during convergence. By definition, vision is normal.

Other Signs The pupil does not dilate well. Initially it may be unilateral, but it becomes bilateral (although it may be asymmetric).

Etiology Tertiary syphilis (positive FTA-ABS).

Differential Diagnosis See "Anisocoria," Section 11.1.

Work-up

1. Test the pupillary reaction to light and convergence, and test for an afferent pupillary defect. (To test the reaction of the pupil to convergence, patients are asked to look first at a distant target and then at their own finger, which the examiner holds in front of them and slowly brings in toward their face).
2. Slit-lamp examination, looking for interstitial keratitis.
3. Dilated fundus examination, searching for chorioretinitis, papillitis, and uveitis.
4. FTA-ABS or MHA-TP, RPR or VDRL.
5. Consider a lumbar puncture if the diagnosis of syphilis is established (see Section 14.2).

Treatment The decision to treat is based on whether active disease is present and whether the patient has been treated appropriately in the past. See "Acquired Syphilis,'' Section 14.2 for treatment indications and specific antibiotic therapy.

Follow-up This is not an emergency, but a diagnostic work-up and determination of syphilitic activity should be undertaken within a few days of detecting an Argyll Robertson pupil.

11.4 Adie's Tonic Pupil

Symptoms Difference in the size of the pupils, blurred vision, or asymptomatic.

Critical Signs An irregularly dilated pupil exhibiting minimal or no reaction to light, slow constriction to convergence, and slow redilatation. It is typically unilateral and found most often in young women. The pupil demonstrates supersensitivity to weak cholinergic agents (e.g., pilocarpine 1/8% or methacholine 2.5%).

Other Signs It may develop acutely and may be bilateral. The pupil dilates normally to mydriatic agents. Deep tendon reflexes (knees and ankles) are often absent. The involved pupil may become smaller than the normal pupil over time.

NOTE Supersensitivity may not be present soon after the development of an Adie's pupil and may need to be tested a few weeks later.

Etiology Idiopathic, orbital trauma or infection, herpes zoster infection, diabetes, autonomic neuropathies, Guillian-Barré syndrome, and others.

Differential Diagnosis See "Anisocoria," Section 11.1.

NOTE Parinaud's syndrome may produce bilateral mid-dilated pupils which react poorly to light, but constrict normally during convergence. Eyelid retraction and paralysis of up-gaze with retraction nystagmus may additionally be present. A pinealoma or other midbrain abnormality needs to be ruled out by CT scan or MRI.

Work-up See "Anisocoria," Section 11.1, for a general work-up when the diagnosis is uncertain.

1. Observe the suspect pupil with the slit lamp, shining a bright light on it. The pupil will be seen to contract slowly and irregularly in Adie's condition.

2. Test for a supersensitive pupil: Have the patient fixate at distance and measure the pupil size of each eye. Instill one drop of methacholine 2.5% or pilocarpine 1/8% in each eye and recheck the pupil size in 10-15 minutes. Do not allow the patient to do near work during this interval. The tonic pupil constricts significantly more than the fellow pupil in Adie's condition.

NOTE   The methacholine/pilocarpine test may occasionally be positive in an Argyll Robertson pupil and in familial dysautonomia.

3. If Adie's pupil and/or supersensitivity is present and the patient is less than one year old, refer him to a pediatric neurologist to rule out familial dysautonomia (Riley-Day syndrome).

Treatment   None indicated.

Follow-up   If the diagnosis is established with certainty, follow-up is routine.

11.5   Isolated Third-Nerve Palsy

Symptoms   Double vision which disappears when one eye is closed, droopy eyelid, $+/-$ pain.

Critical Signs

A. *Complete palsy:* Limitation of ocular movement in all fields of gaze except temporally, ptosis, may have a dilated unreactive pupil (pupil-involved).
B. *Superior-division palsy:* Ptosis plus an inability to look up.
C. *Inferior-division palsy:* Inability to look nasally or inferiorly, pupil-involved.

Other Signs   Aberrant regeneration   (Elevation of the upper eyelid with gaze down or nasally; sometimes pupil constriction [usually segmental] when looking up, down, or nasally), exotropia, hypotropia.

NOTE   Aberrant regeneration may occur spontaneously (primary regeneration), without a preceding third-nerve palsy. This is usually caused by a cavernous sinus tumor or aneurysm.

Etiology

A. *Pupil-involved*

More common   Aneurysm (particularly a posterior communicating artery aneurysm).

Less common   Microvascular disease (typically due to diabetes or hypertension), tumor, trauma, congenital.

Rare   Uncal herniation, cavernous sinus mass lesion, orbital disease, herpes zoster, leukemia.

B. *Pupil-sparing*

More common   Microvascular disease.

Less common   Cavernous sinus syndrome.

C. *Aberrant regeneration present:* Trauma, aneurysm, tumor, congenital. *Not* microvascular.

Differential Diagnosis

- Myasthenia gravis   (Diurnal variation of symptoms and signs, pupil not involved, increased eyelid droop after sustained up-gaze, weak orbicularis oculi muscle, positive edrophonium chloride [e.g., Tensilon] test.)
- Thyroid eye disease   (Eyelid lag, stare, injection over the rectus muscles, proptosis, resistance on forced duction testing, abnormal CT scan of the orbits, no ptosis.)
- Chronic progressive external ophthalmoplegia   (Bilateral, slowly progressive ptosis and limitation of ocular motility, pupil spared, often no double vision.)
- Orbital inflammatory pseudotumor   (Pain and proptosis are usually present.)
- Midbrain lesion   (Inability to look up and/or down, pupils react slowly to light and briskly to convergence, no ptosis, $+/-$ eyelid retraction, $+/-$ retraction nystagmus. Bilateral.)

Work-up

1. Complete ocular examination, checking for pupillary involvement, the directions of motility restriction (in both eyes), ptosis, a visual field defect (visual fields by confrontation), proptosis, resistance to retropulsion, and eyelid fatigue with sustained up-gaze. Look carefully for signs of aberrant regeneration (discussed above).
2. Full neurological examination, carefully assessing the other cranial nerves on both sides. (The ipsilateral fourth nerve can be assessed by focusing with the slit lamp on a superior conjunctival blood vessel and asking the patient to look down and nasally. The eye should intort and the blood vessel turn down and toward the nose.)

3. Edrophonium chloride (e.g., Tensilon) test when the pupil is not involved (rule out myasthenia, see Section 11.9).
4. *Immediate* CT scan of the brain (axial and coronal views) and/or MRI is indicated for:
   a. Pupil-involved (relatively or completely involved) third-nerve palsies.
   b. Pupil-spared third-nerve palsies in . . .

      • Patients <50 years old (unless there is known long-standing diabetes or hypertension.)
      • Patients with incomplete third-nerve palsies (e.g., sparing of some muscle function.)
      • Patients whose third-nerve palsy is >2-3 months old, but has not improved.
      • Patients with an additional cranial nerve or neurologic abnormality.

   c. All patients who develop aberrant regeneration with the exception of regeneration following traumatic third-nerve palsies.
   (A CT scan is generally not required in pupil-spared third-nerve palsies which do not fit the above criteria, especially when patients have known vasculopathic risk factors such as diabetes or hypertension.)
5. CBC with a differential in children.
6. Cerebral angiography is indicated for all patients >20 years old who fit one of the criteria mentioned in (4) above *and* whose CT scan and/or MRI is normal. This should be obtained as soon as possible.

Treatment

1. Treat the underlying abnormality or vasculopathic risk factors if present.
2. If the third-nerve palsy is causing double vision, a patch may be placed over the involved eye. Patching is generally not performed in children less than 9-11 years of age due to the risk of amblyopia.

Follow-up

A. Patients classified in groups 4a, 4b, or 4c: Immediate hospitalization and work-up as described above.
B. Pupil-spared third-nerve palsies not classified in groups 4a, 4b, or 4c: Recheck every 6 weeks. Patients should regain the function lost from their third-nerve palsy within three months. If the palsy does not reverse by this time or if an additional neurologic abnormality develops, an MRI is obtained.

NOTE Some physicians recommend reexamining the patient with a pupil-spared third-nerve palsy within 5 days of onset, checking for delayed pupillary involvement. If the pupil becomes affected, the patient is worked-up as described above for pupil involvement.

REFERENCE

TROBE JD. Third-nerve palsy and the pupil (Editorial). *Arch Ophthalmol* 106: 602, 1988.

11.6   Isolated Fourth-Nerve Palsy

Symptoms   Binocular vertical diplopia (double vision which disappears when one eye is occluded; one image appears on top of or up and to the side of the second image with both eyes open), difficulty reading, or a sensation that objects appear tilted. Some patients are asymptomatic.

Critical Signs   Deficient movement of an eye when attempting to look down and in. The "three-step test" isolates a palsy of the superior oblique muscle (see below).

Other Signs   The involved eye is higher (hypertropic) when looking straight. The hypertropia increases when looking in the direction of the uninvolved eye or tilting the head toward the ipsilateral shoulder. The patient often maintains a head tilt toward the contralateral shoulder to eliminate double vision.

Etiology

  More common   Trauma, vascular infarct (often due to underlying diabetes or hypertension), congenital, idiopathic, and demyelinating disease.
  Rare   Tumor, hydrocephalus, aneurysm.

Differential Diagnosis   All of the following may produce binocular vertical diplopia and/or hypertropia.

  • Myasthenia gravis   (Double vision worse toward the end of the day when fatigued, usually accompanied by ptosis, positive edrophonium chloride [e.g., Tensilon] test.)
  • Thyroid eye disease   (May have proptosis, eyelid lag, stare, or injection over the involved rectus muscles. Positive forced duction test.)
  • Orbital inflammatory pseudotumor   (Pain and proptosis are common.)

- Skew deviation (The three-step test does not isolate a particular muscle. Need to rule out a posterior fossa lesion by CT scan or MRI of the brain if the above conditions are ruled out.)
- Vertical hypertropia (One eye is higher than the other in all fields of gaze by a constant amount, no torsional component.)

Work-up

1. History: Onset and duration of the diplopia? Misaligned eyes or a head tilt since early childhood? Trauma? Stroke?
2. Examine old photographs to determine whether the head tilt is old (indicating an old or congenital fourth-nerve palsy).

   NOTE   A congenital fourth-nerve palsy can often be distinguished from an acquired fourth-nerve palsy by measuring the vertical fusional amplitudes. A patient with an acquired fourth-nerve palsy will have a normal vertical fusional amplitude of 1-3 prism diopters. On the other hand, a patient with a congenital fourth-nerve palsy has greater than 1-3 prism diopters (often up to 10-15 prism diopters) of fusional amplitude. This is detected using vertical prism bars. If a patient can fuse greater than 1-3 prism diopters, then the fourth-nerve palsy is probably congenital.

3. Three-step test:

   STEP 1   Determine which eye is deviated upward in primary gaze (looking straight). This is best seen with the cover-uncover test (see Appendix 2). The higher eye comes down after being uncovered.

   STEP 2   Determine whether the upward deviation is greater when the patient looks to the left or to the right.

   STEP 3   Determine whether the upward deviation is greater when tilting the head to the left shoulder or right shoulder.

   (As mentioned above, patients with a superior oblique paresis have a hyperdeviation which is worse when turning their elevated eye nasally and when tilting their head toward the shoulder ipsilateral to the elevated eye.)

   (Patients with a bilateral fourth-nerve palsy demonstrate a hypertropia of the right eye when looking left, a hypertropia of the left eye when looking right, and a "V"-pattern esotropia. That is, the eyes cross more when looking down.)

4. Perform a double Maddox rod test[1] if a bilateral fourth-nerve palsy is suspected.
5. Edrophonium chloride (e.g., Tensilon) test if myasthenia gravis is suspected, see "Myasthenia Gravis," Section 11.9.
6. Fasting blood sugar and/or glucose tolerance test.
7. CT scan (axial and coronal views) or MRI of the brain for:
   a. A fourth-nerve palsy accompanied by other cranial nerve or neurological abnormalities (i.e., not an isolated palsy).
   b. Children with a symptomatic fourth-nerve palsy.

Treatment

1. Treat the underlying disorder.
2. A patch may be placed over one eye or tape can be applied to one lens if the patient has symptomatic double vision. Patching is generally not performed in children less than 9-11 years old due to the risk of amblyopia.
3. Surgery may be indicated for bothersome double vision in primary or reading position or for cosmetic purposes. We generally wait at least 6 months after the onset of the palsy since many palsies resolve spontaneously.

Follow-up

Acquired fourth-nerve palsy If the work-up is negative and no previous head tilt is observed in old photographs, reexamine the patient in three months, checking for the development of any new neurologic abnormality (CT scan or MRI of the brain would be indicated for any new development). Patients are instructed to return immediately if they notice a new deficit.
Congenital fourth-nerve palsy As needed.

11.7   Isolated Sixth-Nerve Palsy

Symptoms Binocular horizontal diplopia (double vision producing side-by-side images; single vision is restored when one eye is closed or covered), worse

---

[1] A white Maddox rod is placed before one eye and a red one before the other eye in a trial frame, aligning the axes of each rod along the 90-degree (vertical) mark. While looking at a white light at distance, the patient is asked if both the white and red lines seen through the Maddox rods are horizontal and parallel to each other (sometimes placing a six-prism diopter base-down in front of one eye helps the patient determine if the lines are parallel, but this should not be performed in the presence of a hypertropia). When the lines are not horizontal and parallel, the patient is asked to rotate the Maddox rod(s) until they are parallel. If he rotates the vertical axis outward (away from the nose) for more than 10 degrees (total for the two eyes), then a bilateral superior oblique paresis exists.

for distance than near, most pronounced in the direction of the paretic lateral rectus muscle.

Critical Sign One eye does not turn outwardly (temporally).

Other Signs No restriction on forced duction testing. No significant proptosis.

Differential Diagnosis All of the following may produce limitation of abduction.

- Thyroid eye disease (Proptosis, injection of blood vessels over the restricted muscle, restriction on forced duction testing.)
- Myasthenia gravis (Symptoms worse towards the end of day when fatigued, orbicularis oculi weakness, $+/-$ ptosis, positive edrophonium chloride [e.g., Tensilon] test.)
- Orbital inflammatory pseudotumor (Proptosis, pain, restriction on forced duction testing.)
- Orbital trauma causing entrapment of the ipsilateral medial rectus (Restriction on forced duction testing.)
- Duane's syndrome (Congenital, narrowing of the palpebral fissure and retraction of the globe on adduction.)
- Convergence spasm (The pupils constrict on attempted abduction.)
- Möbius' syndrome (Congenital, bilateral facial paralysis present.)

Etiology

ADULTS

More common	*Less common*
Trauma	Increased intracranial pressure
Diabetes	Giant-cell arteritis
Hypertension	Cavernous sinus mass (e.g., meningioma, aneurysm, metastasis)
	Multiple sclerosis
	Sarcoidosis/Vasculitis
	Postmyelography or lumbar puncture
	Stroke (usually not isolated)

CHILDREN

Benign post-viral condition
Gradenigo's syndrome (Petrositis causing 6th and often seventh- $+/-$ eighth- $+/-$ fifth-cranial-nerve involvement on the same side.)

Pontine glioma
Trauma

Work-up

ADULTS

1. History: Do the symptoms fluctuate during the day? Past history of cancer, diabetes, or thyroid disease?
2. Complete neurologic and ophthalmic examinations, paying careful attention to the function of the other cranial nerves and the appearance of the optic disc. (It is especially important to evaluate the fifth cranial nerve; corneal sensation [supplied by the first division] can be tested by touching a wisp of cotton or a tissue to the unanesthetized corneas.) Measure ocular motility in each field of gaze by the alternate cover test using prisms (see Appendix 2). Consider a forced duction test when the diagnosis is uncertain. (See Appendix 6.)
3. Check blood pressure.
4. Fasting blood sugar and ESR (an ESR is obtained only if the patient is greater than 50-55 years old).
5. CT scan (axial and coronal views) or MRI of the brain is indicated if the sixth-nerve palsy is accompanied by any other neurologic or neuro-ophthalmic sign or by severe pain. Additionally, it should be obtained in any patient with a history of cancer.

CHILDREN

1. Complete ocular examination as above.
2. Neurologic (and otoscopic by a pediatrician) examination.
3. CT scan (axial and coronal views) or MRI of the brain in all children.

Treatment   Any underlying problem revealed by the work-up is treated; otherwise, patients are managed by observation.

- In patients greater than 9-11 years of age with bothersome diplopia, the paretic eye can be occluded with a patch or opaque glasses until the condition resolves. The nonparetic eye can be patched instead if its visual acuity is much worse.
- In patients less than 9-11 years of age, patching is avoided. These patients are monitored closely for the development of amblyopia (see Section 9.5).

Follow-up   Reexamine every 6 weeks following the onset of the palsy until it resolves. A CT scan or MRI of the head is indicated if:

- Any neurologic or neuro-ophthalmic signs or symptoms develop during the follow-up period.

- The ocular movement becomes more restricted.
- The isolated sixth-nerve palsy does not resolve in 3-6 months.

11.8   Cavernous Sinus / Superior Orbital Fissure Syndrome

(Multiple Ocular Motor Nerve Palsies)

Symptoms   Double vision, eyelid droop, facial pain or numbness.

Critical Signs   Limitation of eye movement corresponding to any combination of a third-, fourth-, or sixth-cranial-nerve palsy on one side; facial pain or numbness corresponding to one or more branches of the fifth cranial nerve; a droopy eyelid and a small pupil (Horner's syndrome). All signs involve the same side of the face when one cavernous sinus/superior orbital fissure is involved.

NOTE   The pupil is often not involved when the third nerve is damaged in the cavernous sinus (and a Horner's syndrome is not present).

Other Signs   There may be a partial third-nerve palsy (e.g., superior division—eyelid droop and limitation of up-gaze; inferior division—limitation of down-gaze and adduction, and a dilated, nonreactive pupil); proptosis may be present when the superior orbital fissure is involved.

Etiology

- Arteriovenous fistula (carotid-cavernous or dural-cavernous)   (Prominent exophthalmos and chemosis, dilated episcleral and conjunctival blood vessels, often a bruit which may be heard by the patient and sometimes by the physician during ocular auscultation. Abnormal pulsations of the globe are often present, but difficult to observe. CT scan or MRI shows an enlarged superior ophthalmic vein.)
- Cavernous sinus thrombosis   (Proptosis, chemosis, and eyelid edema. Usually bilateral. Fever, nausea, vomiting, and an altered level of consciousness often develop. Commonly due to spread of infection from the face, mouth, throat, sinus, or orbit. Less commonly noninfectious resulting from trauma or surgery.)
- Metastatic tumors to the cavernous sinus (e.g., leukemia, lymphoma)

- Perineural spread of a periocular skin malignancy (e.g., squamous cell carcinoma) (Resected tumors may invade the cavernous sinus years after resection.)
- Pituitary apoplexy (Acute onset of the critical signs listed above; often bilateral with severe headache, decreased vision, and possibly bilateral blindness. An enlarged sella turcica is seen on CT scan or MRI of the brain.)
- Intracavernous aneurysm (Usually unruptured. If one does rupture, the signs of a carotid-cavernous fistula develop.)
- Mucormycosis (Must be suspected in all diabetics, particularly those in ketoacidosis, and any debilitated or immunocompromised individual with multiple cranial-nerve palsies, $+/-$ proptosis. Onset is acute. Nasal discharge of blood may be present and nasal examination may reveal a black crusty material. This condition is life-threatening.)
- Herpes zoster (Patients with the typical zoster rash may develop ocular motor nerve palsies as well as a mid-dilated pupil which reacts better to convergence than light.)
- Tolosa-Hunt syndrome (Acute inflammation of the superior orbital fissure or anterior cavernous sinus. Orbital pain often precedes restriction of eye movements. Recurrent episodes are common. This is a diagnosis of exclusion.)
- Others (Meningioma, sphenoid sinus carcinoma, mucocele, or other infections.)

Differential Diagnosis

- Myasthenia gravis (Eyelid droop and limitation of eye movements [especially when fatigued], weakness of the orbicularis oculi muscle, positive edrophonium chloride [e.g., Tensilon] test. No pupillary abnormality, no pain, no proptosis.)
- Chronic progressive external ophthalmoplegia (Slowly progressive, painless, bilateral limitation of eye movements with ptosis. The pupils are normal and the orbicularis oculi muscles are usually weak.)
- Orbital lesions (e.g., tumor, thyroid disease, pseudotumor) (Proptosis and resistance to retropulsion are usually present in addition to motility restriction. Forced duction tests are abnormal [see Appendix 6]. May have an afferent pupillary defect if the optic nerve is involved.)
- Brain stem disease (Tumors and vascular lesions of the brainstem can produce multiple ocular motor nerve palsies. MRI of the brain is best for making this diagnosis.)
- Carcinomatous meningitis (Diffuse seeding of the leptomeninges by metastatic tumor cells can produce a rapidly sequential bilateral cranial-nerve disorder. Diagnosis is made by lumbar puncture $\times$ 3.)

- Nasopharyngeal carcinoma   (Most commonly affects the sixth cranial nerve, but the third, fourth, and fifth cranial nerves may be involved as well. Typically, one cranial nerve after another is affected. The patient may have cervical lymphadenopathy, nasal obstruction, ear pain or ear popping due to serous otitis media or blockage of the eustachian tube, weight loss, or exophthalmos.)
- Parinaud's syndrome (dorsal midbrain syndrome)   (Deficient upward gaze, retraction-convergence nystagmus on attempted upward gaze, can have mid-dilated pupils which react better to convergence than to light; some patients have accompanying deficient downgaze.)
- Progressive supranuclear palsy   (Vertical limitation of eye movements, initially downward gaze restriction, with dementia and rigidity of the neck and trunks. All eye movements are eventually lost.)
- Rare   (Myotonic dystrophy, ophthalmoplegic migraine, the bulbar variant of the Guillian-Barré syndrome [Miller-Fisher variant], intracranial sarcoidosis, others.)

Work-up

1. History: Diabetes? Prior cancer (including skin cancer)? Weight loss? Ocular bruit? Recent infection? Severe headache? Diurnal variation of symptoms?
2. Ophthalmic examination, with special attention to pupils, extraocular motility, Hertel exophthalmometry, and resistance to retropulsion.
3. Examine the periocular skin for malignant lesions.
4. CT scan (axial and coronal views) and/or MRI of the sinuses, orbit, and brain.

If the CT scan and MRI are normal, consider any or all of the following:
5. Repeat the CT scan or MRI if the cavernous sinus area is not well visualized.
6. Lumbar puncture × 3 to rule out carcinomatous meningitis.
7. Nasopharyngeal examination +/− a blind nasopharyngeal biopsy to rule out nasopharyngeal carcinoma.
8. Lymph node biopsy when lymphadenopathy is present.
9. CBC with differential, ESR, ANA, rheumatoid factor (rule out infection, malignancy, or systemic vasculitis).
10. Chest x-ray.
11. Cerebral arteriogram (rarely required to rule out an aneurysm or arteriovenous fistula since most of these are seen by CT scan or MRI).

If cavernous sinus thrombosis is being considered, obtain blood cultures × 2-3 and culture the presumed primary source of the infection.

Treatment/Follow-up

ARTERIOVENOUS FISTULA

1. Many fistulas will close spontaneously or after arteriography. Others may require neurosurgical or invasive neuroradiologic techniques.
2. Treat secondary glaucoma with a topical beta-blocker (e.g., timolol ¼-½% bid or levobunolol ½% bid) +/− a carbonic anhydrase inhibitor (e.g., methazolamide 50 mg po bid). Drugs which increase outflow facility (e.g., epinephrine and pilocarpine) are generally not as effective due to increased episcleral venous pressure.

CAVERNOUS SINUS THROMBOSIS

1. For possible infectious cases (usually due to Staph. aureus) hospitalize and treat with intravenous antibiotics for several weeks:
   Nafcillin 1-2 g iv q 4 hours or cefazolin 1 g iv q 8 hours
   (alternatively can use vancomycin 1 g iv q 12 hours if penicillin allergic)
   + Ceftazidime 1-2 g iv q 8 hours
   Blood culture results usually dictate later therapy.
2. Intravenous fluid replacement is usually required.
3. For aseptic cavernous sinus thrombosis, consider systemic anticoagulation (heparin followed by warfarin) or aspirin 600 mg po q day. Systemic anticoagulation therapy may require collaboration with a medical internist.
4. Exposure keratopathy needs to be treated with lubricating ointment tid and qhs (e.g., Refresh PM) (See Section 4.4.)
5. Treat glaucoma as described above for arteriovenous fistulas.

METASTATIC DISEASE TO THE CAVERNOUS SINUS

Often requires systemic chemotherapy (if a primary is found) +/− radiation therapy to the metastasis.

PITUITARY APOPLEXY

Refer to a neuro-specialist for surgical consideration.

INTRACAVERNOUS ANEURYSM

Hospitalize and refer to a neuro-specialist.

MUCORMYCOSIS

1. Hospitalize and treat the underlying disorder.
2. Consultation with a medical, infectious disease and/or an ear, nose, and throat specialist may be helpful.
3. Surgical debridement of all necrotic tissue with irrigation of the involved sinuses with amphotericin B is usually necessary.
4. Amphotericin B 0.25-0.30 mg/kg iv in D5W slowly over 3-6 hours on the first day, 0.5 mg/kg iv on the second day, and then 45-50 mg iv daily. The duration of treatment is determined by the clinical condition.

5. BUN and creatinine levels are obtained every other day, watching for renal compromise.

TOLOSA-HUNT SYNDROME

Prednisone 100 mg po q day, tapering rapidly as the pain subsides. If pain persists despite steroid therapy, reinvestigation may be necessary to rule out other disorders.

REFERENCES

KOHN R, HEPLER R. Management of Limited Rhino-orbital Mucormycosis without Ex-enteration. *Ophthalmology* 92: 1440, 1985.
LEVINE SR, TWYMAN RE, GILMAN S. The Role of Anticoagulation in Cavernous Sinus Thrombosis. *Neurology* 38: 517, 1988.

11.9 Myasthenia Gravis

Symptoms   Droopy eyelid and/or double vision worse toward the end of the day or when the individual is fatigued, may have weakness of facial muscles, limb muscles, or difficulty swallowing or breathing.

Critical Signs   Worsening of the eyelid droop with sustained up-gaze or double vision on continued eye movements, weakness of the orbicularis muscle on the affected side (cannot close the eyelid as forcefully as the unaffected side), no pupillary abnormalities.

Other Signs   Can have complete limitation of ocular movements.

Etiology   Autoimmune disease sometimes triggered by an underlying thymoma, thyroid disease, or infection.

Differential Diagnosis

- Eaton-Lambert syndrome   (A myasthenialike condition which is due to a carcinoma located elsewhere in the body. Isolated eye signs do *not* occur in this condition, although eye signs may accompany systemic signs of weakness. Unlike myasthenia, muscle strength increases after exercise. Electromyography distinguishes the two. Specifically look for lung cancer.)
- Myasthenialike syndrome due to medication (e.g., penicillamine and aminoglycosides)

- Chronic progressive external ophthalmoplegia (CPEO) (No diurnal variation of symptoms or relation to fatigue, usually a negative edrophonium chloride [e.g., Tensilon] test, but not always.)
- Kearns-Sayre syndrome (CPEO + retinal pigmentary degeneration in a young person; heart block develops a few years later. See Section 11.10.)
- Third-nerve palsy (Pupil may be involved, no orbicularis weakness, no fatigability, no diurnal variation.)
- Horner's syndrome (Miosis accompanies the ptosis. Pupil does not dilate well in darkness.)
- Levator muscle dehiscence/disinsertion (High eyelid crease on the side of the droopy eyelid, no variability of eyelid droop, no orbicularis weakness.)
- Thyroid eye disease (No ptosis. May have eyelid retraction or eyelid lag, $+/-$ exophthalmos, no diurnal variation of double vision.)
- Orbital inflammatory pseudotumor (Proptosis, pain with ocular movements, inflammation.)
- Myotonic dystrophy (May have ptosis and rarely gaze restriction. After a handshake, these patients are often unable to release their grip.)

Work-up

1. History: Do the signs fluctuate with the time of the day and fatigue? Any systemic weakness? Difficulty swallowing, chewing, or breathing? Medications?
2. Have the patient focus on your finger in up-gaze for one minute. Observe whether the eyelid droops more than expected.
3. Test for double vision in up-gaze (hold the eyelid back so each eye can see your finger).
4. Assess orbicularis function by asking the patient to squeeze the eyelids shut while you attempt to force them open.
5. Test pupillary function.
6. Edrophonium chloride (e.g., Tensilon) test to confirm the diagnosis:
   a. Inject Tensilon 0.2 ml iv. Observe one minute. If an improvement in eyelid droop or double vision (whichever was present initially) is noted, the test is positive and may be stopped at this point. If no improvement nor untoward reaction to the medication develops, continue.
   b. Tensilon 0.4 ml iv. Observe for 30 seconds for a response or side effect. If neither develops, proceed.
   c. Tensilon 0.4 ml iv. If no improvement is noted within two additional minutes, the test is negative.

Improvement within the stated time period is diagnostic of myasthenia gravis (rarely a patient with CPEO, an intracavernous tumor, or some other rare disorder will give a false positive result). A negative test does *not* exclude myasthenia.

NOTE   Cholinergic crisis, syncopal episode and respiratory arrest, although rare, may be precipitated by a Tensilon test. Treatment includes atropine 0.4 mg iv while monitoring vital signs.

7. Check swallowing function.
8. Thyroid function tests (T3, T4, TSH).
9. CT scan of the chest (rule out thymoma).
10. Consider a blood test for acetylcholine receptor antibodies.
11. Consider ANA, rheumatoid factor, other tests to rule out other autoimmune disease.

Treatment   Consider collaborating with a neurologist or medical physician familiar with this disease.

1. If the patient is having difficulty swallowing or breathing, hospitalization with a consideration for plasmapheresis and/or ventilatory support may be indicated.
2. If the condition is mild and not disturbing to the patient, therapy need not be instituted (the patient may patch one eye as needed).
3. If the condition is disturbing or more than mild, an oral anticholinesterase agent (e.g., pyridostigmine 60 mg po qid) should be given. The dosage must be adjusted according to the response. (Patients rarely benefit from greater than 120 mg po q 3 hours of pyridostigmine.) Overdosage may produce cholinergic crisis.
4. If symptoms persist consider systemic steroids. (There is no uniform agreement concerning the dosage. One way is to start with prednisone 20 mg po q day, increasing the dose slowly until the patient is receiving 100 mg/day. These patients are monitored in the hospital for several days when the steroids are started.) See Appendix 5 for a systemic steroid work-up.
5. Rarely, immunosuppressive therapy may be helpful.
6. Treat any underlying thyroid disease or infection.
7. Surgical removal of a thymoma is usually performed. Thymectomy on people without a thymoma occasionally helps.

Follow-up   If systemic symptoms are present or the ocular involvement is acute, patients need to be followed closely at first (every 1-4 days) until improvement is demonstrated. Patients who have had their isolated ocular abnormality for an extended time period (e.g., months) need not be seen again for weeks (assuming no worsening of the condition develops). Patients should always be warned to return immediately if swallowing or breathing difficulties arise.

NOTE   Myasthenia should be looked for in newborns of myasthenic mothers. Poor sucking reflex, ptosis, or an ocular motility disturbance may be seen.

11.10 Chronic Progressive External Ophthalmoplegia (CPEO)

Symptoms Gradual onset of a droopy eyelid +/− double vision +/− other muscle weakness; ocular involvement is usually bilateral, there is no diurnal variation, and there may be a positive family history.

Critical Signs Ptosis, limitation of ocular motility (sometimes complete limitation), normal pupils.

Other Signs Weak orbicularis oculi muscles, weakness of limb and facial muscles, exposure keratopathy.

Differential Diagnosis See "Myasthenia Gravis," Section 11.9, for a complete list. Below are four syndromes which need to be ruled out when CPEO is diagnosed. All of them may have CPEO as part of their clinical picture:

- Kearns-Sayre syndrome (Onset before age 20 years, ptosis, retinal pigmentary degeneration with a "salt and pepper" appearance, heart block that generally occurs years after the ocular signs and may cause sudden death. There is usually no double vision. Other signs may include hearing loss, mental retardation, cerebellar signs, short stature, delayed puberty, vestibular abnormalities, elevated cerebrospinal fluid protein, and characteristic findings on muscle biopsy.)
- Abetalipoproteinemia (Bassen-Kornzweig syndrome) (Retinal pigmentary degeneration similar to retinitis pigmentosa, diarrhea, ataxia and other neurologic signs, acanthocytosis of red blood cells seen on peripheral blood smear, increased cerebrospinal fluid protein. See "Retinitis Pigmentosa," Section 12.24, for treatment.)
- Refsum's disease (Retinitis pigmentosa + increased blood phytanic acid level. May have polyneuropathy, ataxia, hearing loss, anosmia, others. See Section 12.24 for treatment.)
- Ocular pharyngeal dystrophy (Difficulty swallowing sometimes leading to aspiration of food; may have autosomal dominant inheritance.)

Work-up

1. Careful history, determining the rate of onset (gradual versus sudden as in cranial-nerve disease).
2. Family history.
3. Examine the pupils and ocular motility carefully.
4. Test orbicularis oculi strength.

5. Fundus examination, looking for diffuse pigmentary changes.
6. Check swallowing function.
7. Edrophonium chloride (e.g., Tensilon) test to rule-out myasthenia gravis, see Section 11.9.

NOTE   Sometimes patients with CPEO are supersensitive to Tensilon.

8. Consider electromyography for a more definitive diagnosis.
9. Consider a lumbar puncture (if Kearns-Sayre syndrome is a possibility).
10. Yearly electrocardiograms by a cardiologist if Kearns-Sayre syndrome is possible.
11. Lipoprotein electrophoresis and peripheral blood smear to check for acanthocytes if abetalipoproteinemia is suspected.
12. Serum phytanic acid level if Refsum's disease is suspected.

Treatment   There is no proven cure as of yet for CPEO. The following will help:

1. Treat exposure keratopathy with lubricants at night (e.g., Refresh PM ointment) and artificial tears during the day (e.g., Refresh 4-8 × /day) (See "Exposure Keratopathy," Section 4.4, for additional treatments.)
2. Base-down prisms within reading glasses may help reading when downward gaze is restricted.
3. In Kearns-Sayre syndrome, a pacemaker may be required.
4. In ocular pharyngeal dystrophy, dysphagia and aspirations may require cricopharyngeal surgery.
5. In severe ptosis, consider surgical repair (but watch for worsening exposure keratopathy).
6. Genetic counseling.

Follow-up   Depends on ocular and systemic findings.

11.11   Internuclear Ophthalmoplegia (INO)

Symptoms   Double vision which disappears when one eye is occluded.

Critical Signs   Weakness or paralysis of inward (medial) eye movement with nystagmus of the opposite eye when it attempts to look outward (temporally).

Other Signs A skew deviation (either eye is turned upward, but the three-step test cannot isolate a specific muscle, see "Isolated Fourth-Nerve Palsy," Section 11.6), and upbeat nystagmus in upgaze. The involved eye can sometimes turn in when attempting to read (intact convergence). Unilateral or bilateral. Bilateral disease can give an exotropia.

Etiology

- Multiple sclerosis (more common in young patients)
- Ischemic vascular disease of the brainstem (more common in elderly patients)
- Brainstem mass lesion (e.g., tumor, aneurysm)

Differential Diagnosis (Weakness of inward eye movement.)

- Myasthenia gravis (May closely mimic an INO, however, ptosis and orbicularis oculi weakness are common. Symptoms worsen toward the end of the day when the patient is fatigued. An edrophonium chloride [e.g., Tensilon] test is usually positive.)
- Orbital disease (e.g., tumor, thyroid disease, inflammatory pseudotumor) (Proptosis, globe displacement, or pain may be present additionally. Nystagmus is usually not present. Orbital CT scan is abnormal.)

Work-up

1. History: Age? Are symptoms always present or only towards the end of the day when fatigued? Previous episode of optic neuritis, urinary incontinence, numbness or paralysis of an extremity, or another unexplained neurologic event (multiple sclerosis)?
2. Complete ocular examination, including a careful evaluation of eye movement.

   NOTE Ocular motility can appear full, but a muscle weakness can be detected by observing slower eye movement in the involved eye compared with the fellow eye. The ability of the right eye to look medially is assessed by holding one of the fingers of your left hand lateral to the patient's right eye. The patient is asked to first look at your finger being held up and then at your nose. If a right INO is present, the right eye will show slower eye movement from the finger to the nose than the left eye. The left eye may be tested in a similar fashion, by holding a finger from your right hand lateral to the patient's left eye.

3. Edrophonium chloride (e.g., Tensilon) test when the diagnosis of myasthenia gravis cannot be ruled out, see Section 11.9.
4. MRI of the brainstem and midbrain.

Treatment/Follow-up

- Patients with the diagnosis of a stroke within 72 hours of the acute onset of symptoms are admitted to the hospital for neurological evaluation and observation.
- Otherwise patients are managed by physicians familiar with the underlying disease.

11.12 Papilledema

Definition   Optic disc swelling produced by increased intracranial pressure.

Symptoms   Episodes of transient, often bilateral, visual loss (lasting seconds), headache, double vision, nausea, vomiting, and rarely a decrease in visual acuity (a mild decrease in visual acuity can occur in the acute setting if associated with a macular disturbance). Visual field defects and severe loss of central visual acuity can occur with chronic papilledema.

Critical Signs   Bilaterally swollen, hyperemic discs (in early papilledema, disc swelling may be asymmetric) with blurring of the disc margin often obscuring the blood vessels. The nerve-fiber layer is also usually involved.

Other Signs   Papillary or peripapillary retinal hemorrhages (often flame-shaped), loss of venous pulsations (NOTE   20% of the normal population do not have venous pulsations), dilated, tortuous retinal veins, cotton wool spots, normal pupillary response, normal color vision, and an enlarged physiologic blind spot by formal visual field testing.

As chronic papilledema progresses to optic atrophy the hemorrhages and cotton wool spots resolve, peripapillary gliosis and sheathing and narrowing of the peripapillary retinal vessels occur, and optociliary shunt vessels may develop around the disc. Loss of color vision, central visual acuity, and peripheral field, especially inferonasally, also occur.

NOTE   A unilateral or bilateral sixth-cranial-nerve palsy may also result from increased intracranial pressure.

Etiology

- Primary and metastatic intracranial tumors.
- Aqueductal stenosis.

- Pseudotumor cerebri   (Often young, overweight females.)
- Subdural and epidural hematomas   (From trauma.)
- Subarachnoid hemorrhage   (Severe headache, may have preretinal hemorrhages.)
- Arteriovenous malformation.
- Brain abscess   (Often high fever.)
- Meningitis   (Fever, stiff neck, headache, etc.—e.g., syphilis, TB, Lyme disease, bacterial.)
- Encephalitis   (Often mental status abnormalities.)
- Sagittal sinus thrombosis.

Differential Diagnosis   (Other causes of disc swelling.)

- Pseudopapilledema (e.g., optic disc drusen)   (Not true disc swelling. Vessels overlying the disc are not obscured, the disc is not hyperemic, and the surrounding nerve-fiber layer is normal. Spontaneous venous pulsations are often present.)
- Papillitis   (An afferent pupillary defect and decreased color vision are often present, white blood cells are seen in the posterior vitreous, pain with eye movement, decreased visual acuity in most cases, usually unilateral. See "Optic Neuritis," Section 11.14.)
- Malignant hypertensive retinopathy   (Blood pressure extremely high, narrowed arterioles, hemorrhages +/− cotton wool spots extend to the peripheral retina.)
- Central retinal vein occlusion   (Hemorrhages extend far beyond the peripapillary area, generally unilateral, acute loss of vision in most cases.)
- Ischemic optic neuropathy   (Disc swelling is pale, not hyperemic; initially unilateral with sudden, sometimes severe, visual loss.)
- Optic-disc vasculitis   (Unilateral disc swelling in a young patient. There may be flame-shaped hemorrhages in the periphery.)
- Infiltration of the optic disc (e.g., sarcoid or tuberculous granuloma, leukemia, metastasis, or other inflammatory disease or tumor)   (Other ocular or systemic abnormalities may be present, the disc may have an irregular outline, usually unilateral.)
- Leber's optic neuropathy   (Usually males in the second to third decade, initially unilateral, rapid, progressive visual loss, disc swelling associated with peripapillary telangiectasias. Optic atrophy later develops.)
- Orbital optic-nerve tumors   (Unilateral disc swelling, +/− proptosis.)
- Diabetic papillitis   (Benign disc edema in a diabetic, usually bilateral.)

NOTE   Optic-disc swelling in a patient with a history of leukemia is usually a visually threatening sign of leukemic infiltration of the optic nerve. Immediate radiation therapy is usually required to preserve vision.

Work-up

1. History and physical examination (including a blood pressure measurement).
2. Ocular examination, including a pupillary and color vision (using color plates) assessment, posterior vitreous evaluation to check for white blood cells, and a dilated fundus examination using indirect ophthalmoscopy. The optic disc is best examined with a slit lamp and Hruby, fundus contact, or 60 diopter lens.
3. Emergent CT scan (axial and coronal views) and/or MRI of the head and orbit.
4. Lumbar puncture if the CT and/or MRI do not reveal the cause of the papilledema.

Treatment   Treatment should be directed at the underlying cause of the elevated intracranial pressure.

11.13   Pseudotumor Cerebri

Symptoms   Headache (usually worse in the morning), transient episodes of visual loss (typically lasting seconds), double vision (objects appear side by side; the double vision resolves when one eye is covered), tinnitus, dizziness, nausea, or vomiting. Occurs predominantly in females.

Critical Signs   By definition a patient with pseudotumor cerebri will display:

1. Increased intracranial pressure with papilledema.
2. Normal head CT scan (or MRI).
3. Normal cerebral spinal fluid composition.

Other Signs   See "Papilledema," Section 11.12.

Etiology   Associated factors include obesity, pregnancy, and various medications including oral contraceptives, tetracycline, nalidixic acid, and vitamin A. Systemic steroid withdrawal may also be causative.

Differential Diagnosis   See "Papilledema," Section 11.12.

Work-up

1. History: Inquire specifically about medications.
2. Ocular examination, including a pupillary assessment, color vision test (color plates), and optic-nerve evaluation.
3. Systemic examination, including blood pressure and temperature.
4. CT scan (axial and coronal views) or MRI of the orbit and brain. Any patient who presents with papilledema needs to be imaged as soon as possible. If normal, the patient should have a thorough neuro-ophthalmologic evaluation including a lumbar puncture to rule out treatable causes of papilledema (see Section 11.12).
5. Visual field test (e.g., Octopus, Humphrey, Goldmann, or other).

Treatment Pseudotumor cerebri may be a self-limited process. Treatment is indicated for:

1. Severe intractable headache or
2. Evidence of progressive visual acuity or visual field loss.

Methods of treatment include:

1. Weight loss if overweight.
2. Diuretics (e.g., acetazolamide 250 mg po qid initially, building up to 500 mg qid if tolerated).
3. Discontinuation of any causative medication.

If unsuccessful, one of the following may be tried:

4. Systemic steroids (controversial).
5. Optic-nerve decompression surgery (our choice).
6. Lumbo-peritoneal shunt.

Follow-up Every 1-2 weeks initially, monitoring for visual loss, especially visual field loss. Then every 2-6 weeks depending on the response to treatment.

11.14 Optic Neuritis

Symptoms Loss of vision, deteriorating over hours (rarely) to days (most commonly), with the nadir about one week after onset. Visual loss may be subtle or profound.

- Usually unilateral, but may be bilateral.
- Age typically 18-45 years.
- Orbital pain, especially with eye movement.
- Acquired loss of color vision.
- Reduced perception of light intensity.
- Occasionally Uhtoff's sign (visual deficit with exercise or increase in body temperature).
- May have neurologic symptoms or an antecedent viral syndrome (upper respiratory, gastrointestinal, etc.).

Critical Signs   Relative afferent pupillary defect (RAPD) (in unilateral or asymmetric cases), decreased color vision, central, cecocentral, or arcuate visual field defects.

Other Signs   Swollen disc with or without peripapillary flame hemorrhages (papillitis—most commonly seen in children and young adults) or a normal disc (retrobulbar optic neuritis—more common in adults). Posterior vitreous cells are often observed. Can rarely be associated with nervous obstructive disease.

Etiology

- Idiopathic.
- Multiple sclerosis.
- Childhood infections (e.g., measles, mumps, chicken pox).
- Other viral infections (e.g., mononucleosis, herpes zoster, encephalitis).
- Contiguous inflammation of the meninges, orbit or sinuses.
- Granulomatous inflammations (e.g., tuberculosis, syphilis, sarcoidosis, cryptococcus).
- Intraocular inflammations.

Differential Diagnosis

- Ischemic optic neuropathy (ION)   (Visual loss is sudden, no pain with ocular motility, optic nerve swelling tends to be pale. Visual field defects are most commonly inferior altitudinal. In ION due to giant-cell arteritis, the age is >55 years. In nonarteritic ION, the age is typically 40-60 years.)
- Acute papilledema   (No RAPD, no decreased color vision, no decreased visual acuity, no pain with ocular motility, no vitreous cells. Spontaneous venous pulsations are almost always absent. An enlarged blind spot is often noted on visual field testing.)
- Severe systemic hypertension   (Bilateral disc edema, elevated blood pressure, flame-shaped retinal hemorrhages, and cotton wool spots.)

- Orbital tumor compressing the optic nerve (Unilateral, often proptosis or restriction of extraocular motility is evident; there are no vitreous cells even when disc swelling is present.)
- Intracranial tumor compressing the afferent visual pathway (Normal disc, positive afferent pupillary defect, decreased color vision, mass evident on CT scan or MRI of the brain.)
- Leber's optic neuropathy (Usually males in the second or third decade, positive family history, rapid visual loss of one eye then the other eye within days to months, may have peripapillary telangiectasias. Disc swelling is followed by optic atrophy.)
- Toxic/metabolic optic neuropathy (Progressive painless bilateral visual loss, may be secondary to alcohol, malnutrition, various toxins [e.g., ethambutol, chloroquine, isoniazid, chlorpropamide, heavy metals], anemia, and others.)

Work-up

1. History: Determine the patient's age and the rapidity of onset of the visual loss. Associated symptoms? Previous episode?
2. Complete ophthalmic and neurologic examinations, including a pupillary assessment, a color vision evaluation with color plates, an evaluation of the vitreous for cells, and a dilated retinal examination with an optic nerve assessment.
3. Check blood pressure.
4. Visual field test (preferably automated, e.g., Octopus or Humphrey).
5. Blood tests: CBC, RPR, FTA-ABS, $+/-$ ANA, $+/-$ ESR.
6. Chest x-ray.
7. CT scan and/or MRI of the orbits and brain in atypical cases (e.g., out of the typical age range, no vitreous cells in the presence of disc swelling, etc.) or if above tests are negative or the condition is not improving after 3 months.

Treatment Controversial and unknown at the present time. Any one of the following is appropriate treatment:

1. Observation.
2. Prednisone 1 mg/kg/day po $\times$ 2 weeks. Then taper over 1-2 weeks.
3. Pulse steroids: Methylprednisolone 250 mg iv q 6 hours $\times$ 12 doses in the hospital, followed by prednisone 1 mg/kg/day po $\times$ 11 days. Then taper over 1-2 weeks.

NOTES

1. See Appendix 5 for a systemic steroid work-up.
2. An anti-ulcer medication (e.g., ranitidine 150 mg po bid) is given along with steroids.

Follow-up In general, follow every 1-3 months. Patients being treated with steroids need to be followed more closely due to the risk of intraocular pressure rise.

11.15 Arteritic Ischemic Optic Neuropathy

(Giant-Cell Arteritis) (GCA)

Symptoms Sudden, painless, nonprogressive visual loss, initially unilateral, but rapidly may become bilateral; age >50 years (usually ≥55 years); antecedent or simultaneous headache, jaw claudication (pain with chewing), scalp tenderness (tenderness with hair combing), proximal muscle and joint aches (polymyalgia rheumatica), anorexia, weight loss, or fever may occur.

Critical Signs Afferent pupillary defect, devastating visual loss (counting fingers or worse), pale, swollen disc, often with flame hemorrhages. Later optic atrophy occurs as the edema resolves. The ESR may be markedly elevated.

Other Signs Visual field defect (commonly altitudinal or involving the central field); a palpable, tender, and nonpulsatile temporal artery; a central retinal artery occlusion or a cranial-nerve palsy (especially a sixth-nerve palsy) may occur.

Differential Diagnosis

- Nonarteritic ischemic optic neuropathy (Patients may be younger, usually have less severe visual loss, do not have the accompanying symptoms listed above, and usually have normal ESRs.)
- Inflammatory optic neuritis (papillitis) (Younger age group, typically less severe and sudden onset of visual loss, pain with eye movements, optic-disc swelling is more hemorrhagic, posterior vitreous cells are often present, no symptoms of GCA.)
- Compressive optic nerve tumor (Slowly progressive visual loss, few-to-no symptoms in common with GCA.)
- Central retinal vein occlusion (Severe visual loss may be accompanied by an afferent pupillary defect and disc swelling, but the retina shows diffuse retinal hemorrhages extending out to the periphery.)
- Central retinal artery occlusion (Sudden, painless, severe visual loss with an afferent pupillary defect, but the disc is not swollen and retinal edema with a cherry red spot is frequently observed.)

Work-up

1. History: Attempt to elicit the symptoms above. Age is critical.
2. Complete ocular examination, particularly a pupillary assessment, a dilated retinal examination (ruling out retinal causes of severe visual loss), and an optic-nerve evaluation.
3. Stat ESR (Westergren is the most reliable method). A guideline for top normal ESRs: men = ½ × age, women = ½ × (age + 10).
4. Perform a temporal artery biopsy if GCA is suspected from the symptoms, signs, or ESR. The ESR does not have to be elevated.

   NOTE The biopsy should be performed within one week after starting systemic steroids, but a positive result may be seen up to one month later. A biopsy is especially important in patients in whom steroids are relatively contraindicated (e.g., diabetics).

5. Consider ocular pneumoplethysmography (OPG) if available, as an aid in diagnosis.

Treatment Systemic steroids should be given immediately once GCA is the suspected diagnosis. We give methylprednisolone 250 mg iv q 6 hours for 12 doses in the hospital and then switch to prednisone 80-100 mg po q day. A temporal artery biopsy is obtained while in the hospital.

- If the temporal artery biopsy is positive for GCA, then the patient needs to be maintained on prednisone 80-100 mg po q day.
- If the biopsy is negative on an adequate (2-cm) section, then the likelihood of GCA is small. However, in highly suspicious cases a biopsy of the contralateral artery is performed. Steroids are usually discontinued when the disease is not found on adequate biopsies.

NOTES

1. Without steroids (and occasionally on adequate steroids), the fellow eye can become involved within 24 hours.
2. An H2 blocker (e.g., ranitidine 150 mg po bid) or another anti-ulcer medication is given along with the steroids.

Follow-up Patients suspected of having GCA need to be evaluated and treated emergently. After the diagnosis is confirmed by biopsy, the initial steroid dosage is maintained for 2-4 weeks until the symptoms reverse and ESRs normalize. The dosage is then tapered slowly, repeating the ESRs with each dosage change or monthly to ensure that the new steroid dosage is enough to suppress the disease. If the ESR increases or symptoms return, the dosage must be increased. Treatment should last at least 3-6 months and sometimes for a year or more. The smallest dose that suppresses the disease is used.

11.16 Nonarteritic Ischemic Optic Neuropathy

Symptoms Sudden, painless, nonprogressive visual loss of moderate degree, initially unilateral, but may become bilateral. Age typically 40-60 years.

Critical Signs Afferent pupillary defect, pale disc swelling, often involving only a segment of the disc, flame hemorrhages. Normal ESR.

Other Signs Reduced color vision, altitudinal or central visual field defect, optic atrophy (after the edema resolves).

Etiology Idiopathic (Arteriosclerosis, diabetes, and hypertension are thought to be causative, but have never been proven to be.)

Differential Diagnosis See "Arteritic Ischemic Optic Neuropathy," Section 11.15.

Work-up Same as "Arteritic Ischemic Optic Neuropathy," Section 11.15. A medical evaluation by an internist is also obtained to rule out cardiovascular disease, diabetes, and hypertension.

Treatment None indicated.

Follow-up One month.

11.17 Miscellaneous Optic Neuropathies

Toxic/Metabolic Optic Neuropathy

Symptoms Painless, progressive, bilateral loss of vision.

Critical Signs Bilateral cecocentral or central visual field defects, signs of alcoholism or poor nutrition.

Other Signs   Visual acuity 20/50-20/200, reduced color vision testing, temporal disc pallor, optic atrophy or normal-appearing disc.

Etiology

- Tobacco/alcohol abuse.
- Severe malnutrition with thiamine (vitamin B-1) deficiency.
- Pernicious anemia   (Usually due to a problem with vitamin B-12 absorption.)
- Toxic   (Often from chloramphenicol, ethambutol, isoniazid, digitalis, chloroquine, streptomycin, chlorpropamide, ethchlorvynol [e.g., Placidyl], disulfiram [e.g., Antabuse], and lead.)

Work-up

1. History: Drug or substance abuse? Medications?
2. Complete ocular examination, including pupillary evaluation, color testing with color plates, and an optic-nerve examination.
3. Formal visual field test (e.g., Goldmann).
4. CBC.
5. Serum vitamin B-12 level (consider a GI consult for a possible Schilling test if the vitamin B-12 level is low).
6. Consider a heavy-metal (i.e., lead, thallium) screen.

Treatment

1. Thiamine 100 mg po bid.
2. Folate 0.1 mg po q day.
3. Multivitamin tablet q day.
4. Eliminate any causative agent (e.g., alcohol, medication, etc.).
5. Vitamin B-12 1000 ug im every month for pernicious anemia (usually coordinated by the patient's internist).

Follow-up   Every month at first, then every 6-12 months.

Compressive Optic Neuropathy

Symptoms   Slowly progressive visual loss, although occasionally acute or noticed acutely.

Critical Signs   Central visual field defect, relative afferent pupillary defect.

Other Signs   The optic nerve can be normal, pale, or, occasionally, swollen; proptosis; optociliary shunt vessels (small vessels around the disc which shunt blood from the retinal to the choroidal venous circulation).

Etiology

- Optic-nerve glioma   (Age usually less than 20 years, often associated with neurofibromatosis.)
- Optic-nerve meningioma   (Usually adult women. Orbital CT scan may show an optic-nerve mass, diffuse optic-nerve thickening, or a "railroad track" sign [increased contrast of the periphery of the nerve].)
- Malignant optic glioma   (Rare, usually adults, painful, involvement of the other eye may soon follow, poor prognosis.)

Work-up   All patients with progressive visual loss and optic-nerve dysfunction should have a CT scan (coronal and axial views) or an MRI of the orbit and brain.

Treatment/Follow-up   Depends on the etiology. Treatments of optic-nerve glioma and meningioma are controversial. These lesions are often followed unless there is evidence of intracranial involvement, at which point surgical excision may be indicated. There is no satisfactory treatment of malignant optic glioma.

Leber's Optic Neuropathy

Symptoms   Rapidly progressive visual loss of one eye, then the other eye within days to months of each other, painless.

Critical Signs   Mildly swollen optic disc progessing over weeks to optic atrophy; small telangiectatic blood vessels near the disc, usually in young males (age 15-30 years) (less commonly females in their twenties to thirties).

NOTE   The telangiectatic blood vessels near the disc do not leak fluorescein on intravenous fluorescein angiography.

Other Signs   Visual acuity 20/200 to counting fingers, cecocentral visual field defect.

Transmission   By mitochondrial DNA, so it is transmitted by females to give 50% of their sons the disease and all of their daughters the carrier state (10% of daughters will get the disease). Males do not transmit the disease.

Treatment   No effective treatment is available. Genetic counseling should be offered. A cardiology consult may be indicated as patients have a higher incidence of cardiac conduction defects.

Dominant Optic Neuropathy

Mild-to-moderate bilateral visual loss (20/40-20/200) usually presenting about age 4-8 years, slow progression, temporal disc pallor, cecocentral visual field defect, tritanopic color defect on Farnsworth-Munsell 100 hue test, strong family history, no nystagmus.

Complicated Hereditary Optic Atrophy

Bilateral optic atrophy with spinocerebellar degenerations (e.g., Friedreich's, Marie's, Behr's), polyneuropathy (e.g., Charcot-Marie-Tooth), or inborn errors of metabolism.

Radiation Optic Neuropathy

Delayed effect (usually 1-5 years) after radiation therapy to the eye, orbit, sinus, nasopharynx, and occasionally brain with acute or gradual stepwise visual loss. Disc swelling and/or retinopathy may or may not be present.

11.18   Nystagmus

Nystagmus may be congenital or acquired.

Symptoms   Asymptomatic unless acquired after age eight, at which point the environment may be noted to oscillate horizontally, vertically, or torsionally or vision may seem blurred or unstable.

Critical Sign   Repetitive oscillations of the eye horizontally, vertically, or torsionally.

Jerk nystagmus = The eye slowly drifts in one direction (slow phase) and then abruptly returns to its original position (fast phase), only to drift off again and repeat the cycle.
Pendular nystagmus = A smooth back-and-forth movement of the eye.

A. Congenital

Onset at age 2-3 months with wide, swinging eye movements. At age 4-6 months small amplitude pendular eye movements are added, and at 6-12 months of age jerk nystagmus with a null point (a position of gaze where the nystagmus is minimized) develops. Compensatory head nodding develops at any point up to age 20 years. Congenital nystagmus is usually horizontal and typically dampens with convergence.

Etiology

- Idiopathic.
- Albinism   (Iris transillumination defects and foveal hypoplasia are common.)
- Aniridia   (Bilateral near total absence of the iris from birth.)
- Leber's congenital amaurosis   (Markedly abnormal or flat electroretinogram.)
- Others   (Bilateral optic-nerve hypoplasia, rod monochromatism [achromatopsia], bilateral congenital cataracts, optic-nerve or macular disease.)

Differential Diagnosis

- Opsoclonus   (Repetitive, irregular, multidirectional eye movements associated with cerebellar or brainstem disease, postviral encephalitis, or neuroblastoma.)
- Spasmus nutans   (Head nodding and head turn with vertical, horizontal, or torsional nystagmus appearing between age 6 months and 3 years and resolving between age 2 and 8 years. It may be unilateral or bilateral. A glioma of the optic chiasm may produce an identical clinical picture and needs to be ruled out by CT scan or MRI.)

Work-up

1. History: Age of onset? Head nodding? Known ocular or systemic abnormality? Medications? Family history?
2. Complete ocular examination, carefully observing the eye movements, checking for iris transillumination, and inspecting the optic disc and macula for disease. Slit-lamp or optic-disc observation may help detect subtle cases of nystagmus.
3. Consider obtaining an eye-movement recording if the diagnosis of congenital nystagmus is uncertain.
4. When opsoclonus cannot be ruled out, obtain a urinary vanillylmandelic acid and consider an abdominal CT scan.
5. In select cases, a CT scan (axial and coronal views) or MRI of the brain may be obtained to rule out organic pathology.

Treatment   Patients with congenital nystagmus seldom benefit from base out prism glasses, but do benefit from maximally pushing plus lens in their refraction and carefully correcting all of their astigmatism.

B. Acquired

Etiology

- Toxic/metabolic (e.g., alcohol intoxication, lithium, barbiturates, phenytoin, salicylates, benzodiazepines, phencyclidine, other anticonvulsants or sedatives, Wernicke's encephalopathy, and thiamine deficiency.)
- Central nervous systemic disorders (e.g., thalamic hemorrhage, tumor, stroke, multiple sclerosis, trauma.)
- Cone dystrophy
- Nonphysiologic (Voluntary, rapid, horizontal, small oscillatory movements of the eyes which usually cannot be sustained more than 30 seconds without fatigue.)
- Others (e.g., blind eye, myasthenia gravis)

Below are listed types of acquired nystagmus with localizing neuroanatomic significance:

- See-saw (One eye rises and intorts while the other descends and extorts. Most commonly the lesion involves the chiasm and/or third ventricle. Rarely it may be congenital.)
- Convergence retraction (Convergencelike eye movements are accompanied by retraction of the globe into the orbit when the patient attempts to look up. There is limitation of upward gaze, eyelid retraction, and large, unreactive pupils. Papilledema may be present. Usually a pineal gland tumor or other midbrain abnormality is responsible.)
- Upbeat (The fast phase of nystagmus is up. Most commonly the lesion involves the brainstem or vermis of the cerebellum.)
- Rebound (Triggered by changing directions of gaze. The fast phase is in the direction of gaze, but fatigues with sustained gaze, and then changes direction. When gaze is returned to primary position, the fast phase increases in the direction the eye takes in returning to the primary position. Most commonly the lesion involves the cerebellum.)
- Gaze-evoked (Not present when the individual looks straight, but appears as the eyes look to the side. Slow frequency. Most commonly due to alcohol intoxication or cerebellar disease, less commonly brainstem disease.)
- Downbeat (The fast phase of nystagmus is down. Most commonly the lesion is at the cervicomedullary junction [e.g., Arnold-Chiari malformation].)

- Periodic alternating (Fast eye movements are in one direction [with head turn] for 60-90 seconds, and then reverses direction for 60-90 seconds. The cycle repeats continuously. May be congenital or rarely due to blindness. Acquired forms not due to blindness are most commonly due to lesions of the cervicomedullary junction.)
- Vestibular (May have a rotatory component. Vertigo, tinnitus, or deafness may accompany it. Commonly it is due to inner ear disease [e.g., labyrinthitis]. Unless the cerebellum is impaired, it clears within two weeks. If associated with interstitial keratitis it is called Cogan's syndrome.)

Differential Diagnosis

- Superior oblique myokymia (Small unilateral vertical and torsional movements of one eye can be seen with a slit lamp or ophthalmoscope. Symptoms and signs are more pronounced when the involved eye looks inferonasally. It is usually benign, resolving spontaneously. It can be treated with carbamazepine [e.g., Tegretol] 200 mg po tid. A medical consult for hematologic evaluation is obtained prior to carbamazepine use, and periodic evaluation during therapy is recommended.)

Work-up

1. History: Nystagmus, strabismus, or amblyopia in infancy? Oscillopsia? Drug or alcohol use or abuse? Episodes of weakness/numbness/loss of vision in the past (multiple sclerosis)? Vertigo?
2. Family history: Nystagmus? Albinism? Eye disorder?
3. Complete ocular examination, paying close attention to the eye movements. Slit-lamp or optic-disc observation may be helpful in subtle cases. Iris transillumination should be performed (rule out albinism).
4. Obtain an eye movement recording when congenital nystagmus is being considered, if available.
5. Visual field examination, particularly with see-saw nystagmus.
6. Consider a drug/toxin/dietary screen of the urine and/or serum.
7. CT scan (axial and coronal views) or MRI as needed (Make sure the scan carefully evaluates the area which most commonly causes the particular nystagmus.)

NOTE The cervicomedullary junction and cerebellum are usually best evaluated with MRI.

Treatment The underlying etiology must be treated. The nystagmus of periodic alternating nystagmus may respond to baclofen. Baclofen is given in three divided doses, starting with a total daily dose of 15 mg po and increasing by 15 mg every 3 days until a desired therapeutic effect is obtained. Do not exceed 80 mg/day. If there is no improvement on the maximum tolerated dose, the dosage should be tapered slowly. Baclofen is not recommended for use in children.

Follow-up   A work-up should be instituted as soon as available to rule out a central nervous system abnormality.

11.19   Vertebrobasilar Artery Insufficiency

Symptoms   Transient bilateral blurred vision lasting from a few seconds to a few minutes, sometimes accompanied by flashing lights. Ataxia, vertigo, dysarthria or dysphasia, hemiparesis or hemisensory loss may accompany the visual symptoms. History of "drop attacks"—the patient suddenly falls to the ground without warning or loss of consciousness. Recurrent attacks are common.

Signs   Normal ocular examination.

Differential Diagnosis   Causes of transient visual loss.

- Papilledema   (Bilateral visual loss lasts 5-15 seconds.)
- Migraine   (Visual loss from 10-45 minutes, often with history of migraine or car sickness, or a family history of migraine. May or may not be followed by a headache.)
- Amaurosis fugax   (Monocular, usually lasts minutes, appears as if a curtain drops down in front of the eye.)
- Giant-cell arteritis (GCA)   (Can cause transient visual loss in patients >50-55 years old. Usually associated with a temporal headache, scalp tenderness, pain with chewing, weight loss, fever, and anorexia.)

Work-up

1. History: Associated symptoms of vertebrobasilar insufficiency? History of car sickness or migraine? Symptoms of GCA?
2. Dilated fundus examination, looking for retinal emboli or papilledema.
3. Blood pressure (in each arm looking for the subclavian steal syndrome).
4. Cardiac auscultation (rule out arrhythmia).
5. EKG and Holter monitor × 24 hours (looking for sick sinus syndrome, ventricular ectopy).

6. Consider carotid noninvasive flow studies.
7. CBC (rule out anemia and polycythemia) +/− ESR (if suspect giant-cell arteritis).
8. Consider cervical spine x-rays (rule out compressive cervical spine disease) if arthritis of the neck is present.

Treatment

1. Aspirin 80 mg po q day.
2. Control hypertension, diabetes, and hyperlipidemia if present (as per medical internist).
3. Reduce fat and cholesterol intake; stop smoking.
4. Correct any underlying problem revealed by the work-up.

Follow-up   One week to check test results.

11.20 Cortical Blindness

Symptoms   Bilateral complete or severe loss of vision. Patients may deny they are blind (Anton's syndrome).

Critical Signs   Markedly decreased vision and visual field in both eyes (sometimes no light perception) with normal pupillary responses.

Etiology

Most common   Bilateral occipital lobe infarctions.
Less common   Neoplasms (e.g., metastases and meningiomas)

Work-up

1. Test the vision with a near card (sometimes patients with bilateral occipital lobe infarcts appear completely blind, but actually have a very small residual visual field and are unable to locate a distant eye chart.)
2. Complete ocular and neurological examinations.
3. Rule out functional visual loss by appropriate testing (see "Nonphysiologic Visual Loss," Section 11.21).
4. Cardiac auscultation (rule out arrhythmia).
5. Check blood pressure.
6. CT scan and/or MRI of the brain.
7. CBC (to rule out polycythemia in cases of stroke).

8. Referral to a neurologist or internist for evaluation of stroke risk factors.

Treatment

1. Patients diagnosed with a stroke within 72 hours of the onset of symptoms are admitted to the hospital for neurological evaluation and observation.
2. If possible, treat the underlying condition.
3. Arrange for services to help the patient function at home and in the environment.

Follow-up As per the internist or neurologist.

11.21 Nonphysiologic Visual Loss

Symptoms Loss of vision. Malingerers frequently are involved with an insurance claim or are looking for some other form of financial gain. Hysterics truly believe they have lost vision.

Critical Signs No ocular or neuro-ophthalmic findings which would account for the decreased vision. Normal pupillary light reaction.

Differential Diagnosis The following must be considered in anyone with a normal neuro-ophthalmic examination:

• Amblyopia (Poor vision in one eye since childhood, rarely both eyes. Patient often has strabismus [eye misalignment best seen with a cover test] or anisometropia [one eye is usually more far-sighted or astigmatic or very near-sighted]. May have a history of eye patching as a child. Vision is no worse than counting fingers, especially in the temporal periphery of an amblyopic eye.)
• Cortical blindness (Bilateral complete or severe visual loss with normal pupils. CT scan or MRI of the brain shows bilateral occipital lobe infarcts in most cases.)
• Retrobulbar optic neuritis (Afferent pupillary defect present.)
• Cone-rod dystrophy (Positive family history, decreased color vision, abnormal dark adaptation studies and electroretinogram [ERG].)
• Chiasmal tumor (Visual loss may precede optic atrophy. Pupils usually react sluggishly to light and an afferent pupillary defect is usually present. Visual fields are abnormal.)

Work-up (Fooling the malingerer or hysteric into seeing better than he admits to seeing). The following tests may be used to deceive a patient with non-physiologic visual loss. U = may be used to test patients feigning unilateral decreased vision. B = may be used to test patients feigning bilateral visual loss.

PATIENTS CLAIMING NO LIGHT PERCEPTION

Determine whether each pupil reacts to light (U): When one eye has no light perception, its pupil will not react to light. The pupil should *not* appear dilated unless the patient has bilateral no light perception or third-nerve involvement.

PATIENTS CLAIMING HAND-MOTION TO NO LIGHT PERCEPTION

1. Test for an afferent pupillary defect (U): A defect should be present in unilateral visual loss to this degree. If not, the diagnosis of nonphysiologic visual loss is clinched.
2. Mirror test (U or B): If the patient claims unilateral visual loss, cover the better seeing eye with a patch; otherwise leave both uncovered. Ask the patient to hold eyes still and slowly move a large mirror from side to side in front of the eyes, holding it beyond the patient's range of hand-motion vision). If the eyes move, the patient can see better than hand motion.
3. Optokinetic test (U or B): Patch the uninvolved eye when unilateral visual loss is claimed. Ask the patient to look straight ahead, and slowly move an optokinetic tape in front of the eyes (or rotate an optokinetic drum). If nystagmus can be elicited, vision is better than hand motion.

PATIENTS CLAIMING 20/40-20/400

1. Visual acuity testing (U or B): Start with the 20/10 line and ask the patient to read it. When the patient claims incompetence, look amazed and then offer reassurance. Inform the patient you will go to an easier line and show the 20/15 line. Again, force the patient to work to see this line. Slowly proceed up the chart, asking the patient to read each line as you pass it (including the three or four 20/20 lines). Make the patient feel incompetent. By the time the 20/30 or 20/40 lines are reached, the patient may in fact read one or two letters correctly. You may stop now and record the visual acuity.
2. Retest visual acuity in the "poorly seeing eye" at 10 feet from the chart (U or B). Vision should be twice as good (e.g., a patient with 20/100 vision at 20 feet should read 20/50 at 10 feet). If it is better than expected, record the better vision. If it is worse, be assured the patient has nonphysiologic visual loss.
3. Test near vision. If normal vision can be documented at near, nonphysiologic visual loss (or myopia) has been documented.
4. Visual field testing (U or B): Goldmann visual field tests often reveal inconsistent responses and nonphysiologic field losses.

CHILDREN

1. Tell the child that there is an eye abnormality, but the strong drops about to be administered will cure it. Dilate the child's eyes (e.g., tropicamide 1%), and retest the visual acuity in 40 minutes. Children, as adults, sometimes need a "way out."
2. Test as above.

Treatment Patients are usually told that no ocular abnormality can be found that accounts for their decreased vision. Hysterical patients often benefit from being told that everything is going to be all right and that their vision can be expected to return to normal by their next visit. Psychiatric referral is sometimes indicated.

Follow-up If nonphysiologic visual loss is highly suspected but cannot be proven, reexamine in 1-2 weeks. Consider obtaining an ERG, a fluorescein angiogram, and/or a CT scan or MRI of the brain. If functional visual loss can be documented, have the patient return as needed.

NOTE Always try to determine the patient's vision and document your findings.

12
Retina

12.1 Central Retinal Artery Occlusion (CRAO)

Symptoms Unilateral painless acute loss of vision (counting fingers to light perception in 90% of eyes) occurring over seconds; may have a history of amaurosis fugax.

Critical Signs Superficial opacification or whitening of the retina in the posterior pole and a "cherry red spot" in the center of the macula.

Other Signs A marked afferent pupillary defect; narrowed retinal arterioles; and boxcarring, or segmentation of the blood column, in the arterioles. Occasionally retinal arteriolar emboli or cilioretinal artery sparing of the foveola is evident.

Differential Diagnosis

- Acute ophthalmic artery occlusion (Usually no cherry red spot in the foveola; the entire retina appears whitened. The treatment is the same as for a CRAO.)
- Inadvertent intraocular injection of gentamicin (Recent injection.)
- Arteritic ischemic optic neuropathy (Age ≥55 years, acute severe visual loss, a history of temporal headache with scalp tenderness, jaw claudication,

muscle pains, weakness, and weight loss, a significant afferent pupillary defect, pale optic disc swelling, and a markedly elevated ESR are typical.)
- Other causes of a "cherry red spot" (e.g., Tay-Sachs or other storage diseases) (Present in early life, other systemic manifestations, usually bilateral.)

Etiology

- Embolus (especially carotid or cardiac).
- Thrombosis.
- Giant-cell arteritis (GCA) (May produce a CRAO or an ischemic optic neuropathy. See above for concomitant symptoms.)
- Collagen vascular disease other than giant-cell arteritis (e.g., systemic lupus erythematosus and polyarteritis nodosa).
- Hypercoagulation disorders (e.g., oral contraceptives, polycythemia).
- Rare causes (e.g., migraine, Behçet's disease, syphilis, sickle-cell disease).
- Trauma.

Treatment To be instituted immediately after the diagnosis is made, before the work-up, *if* the CRAO is <24 hours old.

1. Immediate ocular massage (fundus contact lens or digital massage).
2. Anterior-chamber paracentesis (Fig. 12.1): Place a drop of topical anesthetic (e.g., cocaine 2-4%) in the eye and anesthetize the base of the medial rectus muscle by holding a cotton-tipped applicator dipped in the topical anesthetic against the muscle for 1 minute. Next, retract the eyelid with an eyelid speculum and, using an operating microscope or slit-lamp (a microscope is easier), grasp the base of the medial rectus muscle with fixation forceps (where you just anesthetized). With a 30-gauge short needle on a TB syringe, enter the eye temporally at the limbus with the bevel of the needle pointing up, away from the eye. Make sure you keep the tip of the needle over the iris (not the lens) when entering the anterior chamber. Withdraw fluid until the chamber shallows slightly (usually 0.1-0.2 cc). Withdraw the needle and place a drop of antibiotic on the eye (e.g., gentamicin).
3. Acetazolamide 500 mg iv or 250 mg × 2 po and/or a topical beta-blocker (e.g., timolol ½% bid or levobunolol ½% bid) is used to lower the intraocular pressure.
4. Consider admission to the hospital for Carbogen (95% oxygen, 5% carbon dioxide) therapy, 10 minutes every 2 hours around the clock for 48 hours. The patient's blood pressure, pulse, and mental status need to be monitored.

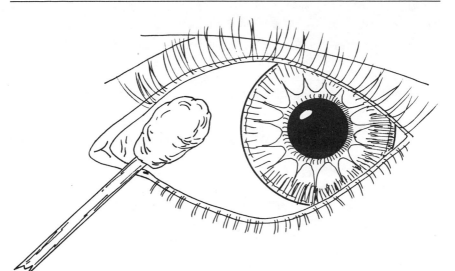

(a)

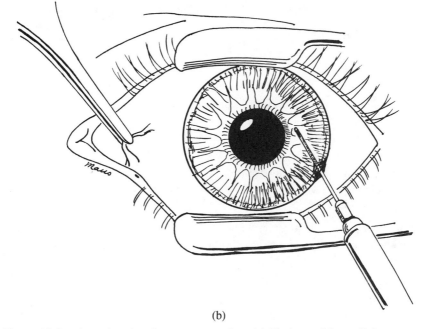

(b)

Figure 12.1. Anterior-chamber paracentesis. (a) The base of the medial rectus muscle is anesthetized with a cotton-tipped applicator dipped in cocaine 2-4%. (b) While fixating the globe with forceps, a 30-gauge needle is passed through the cornea into the anterior chamber. The needle should stay over the iris.

Work-up

1. Immediate ESR to rule out giant-cell arteritis if the patient is ≥55 years old. (This is obtained immediately after the paracentesis. If the patient's history and/or ESR are consistent with GCA, high-dose systemic steroids are started. See "Arteritic Ischemic Optic Neuropathy," Section 11.15, for further details.)
2. Check the blood pressure.
3. Other blood tests: Fasting blood sugar (FBS) (3-hour glucose tolerance test if the FBS is negative), CBC with differential and platelets, lipid profile, PT/PTT, ANA, rheumatoid factor, and FTA-ABS. Consider a serum protein electrophoresis and hemoglobin electrophoresis.
4. Carotid artery evaluation (Doppler and ultrasound of the carotid arteries).
5. Cardiac evaluation (echocardiogram and Holter monitor).
6. Fluorescein angiogram and/or electroretinogram to confirm the diagnosis.

Follow up   The patient is discharged from the hospital after 2-3 days and is seen by an internist to complete the medical work-up above. A repeat eye examination is performed in 3-6 weeks, checking for neovascularization of the iris.

12.2   Branch Retinal Artery Occlusion (BRAO)

Symptoms   Unilateral painless abrupt loss of partial visual field, a history of transient visual loss (amaurosis fugax) may be elicited.

Critical Sign   Superficial opacification or whitening along the distribution of a branch retinal artery. The affected retina becomes edematous.

Other Signs   Narrowed branch retinal artery; boxcarring, or segmentation of the blood column, or emboli are sometimes seen in the branch retinal artery. Cotton wool spots may appear in the involved area.

Etiology   See "Central Retinal Artery Occlusion," Section 12.1.

Work-up   See "Central Retinal Artery Occlusion," Section 12.1. An electroretinogram, however, is not obtained.

Treatment

1. No ocular therapy of proven value is available. Ocular massage (and rarely anterior-chamber paracentesis) may dislodge a cholesterol embolus (cholesterol emboli appear as bright reflective crystals, generally at a vessel bifurcation).
2. Treat any underlying medical problem.

Follow-up   Patients need to be evaluated urgently to treat any underlying disorders (especially giant-cell arteritis). Reevaluate every 3-6 months after concluding the work-up.

12.3   Central Retinal Vein Occlusion (CRVO)

Symptoms   Painless loss of vision, usually unilateral.

Critical Signs   Diffuse retinal hemorrhages in all quadrants of the retina and dilated tortuous retinal veins.

Other Signs   Cotton wool spots, disc edema and hemorrhages, retinal edema, optociliary shunt vessels on the disc, or neovascularization of the optic disc, retina, or iris.

Types

Ischemic   Multiple cotton wool spots (usually > 10), extensive retinal hemorrhage, and widespread capillary nonperfusion on fluorescein angiogram.
Non-ischemic   Mild fundus changes.

Etiology

• Atherosclerosis of the adjacent central retinal artery   (The artery compresses the central retinal vein in the region of the lamina cribrosa.)
• Hypertension.
• Optic-disc edema.
• Glaucoma (open- or narrow-angle).
• Optic-disc drusen.

- Hypercoagulable state (e.g., polycythemia, lymphoma, leukemia, sickle-cell disease, multiple myeloma, cryoglobulinemia, Waldenström's macro-globulinemia, etc.)
- Vasculitis (e.g., sarcoid, syphilis, systemic lupus erythematosus).
- Drugs (e.g., oral contraceptives, diuretics).
- Abnormal platelet function (e.g., mitral valve prolapse).
- Retrobulbar external compression (e.g., thyroid disease, orbital tumor, etc.)
- Migraine   (Rare.)

Differential Diagnosis

- Ocular ischemic syndrome (carotid occlusive disease)   (Veins are usually dilated and irregular in caliber, but are not usually tortuous; disc edema does not usually occur; hemorrhages are not usually present on the disc, although neovascularization of the disc is present in one-third of cases; hemorrhages tend to be in the mid-periphery; patients may have a history of amaurosis fugax, transient ischemic attacks, or orbital pain. Intraocular pressure [IOP] is often low.)
- Diabetic retinopathy   (Hemorrhages and microaneurysms are usually concentrated in the posterior pole, exudate is more prominent, and the condition is typically bilateral. Fluorescein angiography may be required to distinguish.)
- Papilledema   (Bilateral disc swelling with flame hemorrhages surrounding the disc, but not extending out to the peripheral retina; secondary to increased intracranial pressure.)

Work-up

1. History: Medical problems, medications, eye diseases?
2. Complete ocular examination, including an IOP measurement, slit-lamp and gonioscopic examinations to rule out iris and angle neovascularization or the presence of a narrow angle, and a dilated fundus examination.
3. Fluorescein angiogram.
4. Check the blood pressure.
5. Blood tests: Fasting blood sugar, CBC with differential, platelets, serum protein electrophoresis, lipid profile, FTA-ABS, and ANA. (Other tests which may be considered include hemoglobin electrophoresis, PTT, PT, ESR, VDRL, and cryoglobulins.)
6. Chest x-ray (when an underlying medical problem is to be ruled out).
7. Complete medical evaluation (especially to rule out cardiovascular disease).
8. If the diagnosis is uncertain, oculopneumoplethysmography (OPG) or ophthalmodynamometry may help to distinguish a CRVO from carotid disease (ophthalmic artery pressure is low in carotid disease, but normal to elevated in a CRVO).

Treatment

1. Discontinue oral contraceptives; change diuretics to other antihypertensive medications if possible.
2. Lower IOP if elevated (e.g., >20 mm Hg) in either eye (see "Primary Open-Angle Glaucoma," Section 10.1).
3. Treat underlying medical disorders.
4. If neovascularization of the iris, retina, or optic nerve is present or if the CRVO is ischemic, laser therapy (panretinal photocoagulation [PRP]) is performed.
5. Aspirin 60-360 mg po q day.

Follow-up

Nonischemic   Every 4 weeks for the first 6 months; if the fundus picture worsens and can be categorized as ischemic, treat as ischemic.

Ischemic   Every 2-3 weeks after treatment for the first 6 months; watch for neovascularization of the iris.

12.4   Branch Retinal Vein Occlusion (BRVO)

Symptoms   Blind spot in the visual field or loss of vision, generally unilateral.

Critical Signs   Superficial hemorrhages in a sector of the retina along a retinal vein. The hemorrhages almost never cross the horizontal raphé (midline).

Other Signs   Cotton wool spots, retinal edema, a dilated and tortuous retinal vein, narrowing and sheathing of the adjacent artery, retinal neovascularization, or a vitreous hemorrhage.

Etiology   Disease of the adjacent arterial wall (usually due to hypertension, arteriosclerosis, or diabetes) compresses the venous wall at a crossing point.

Differential Diagnosis

• Diabetic retinopathy   (Dot and blot hemorrhages and microaneurysms extend across the horizontal raphé. Nearly always bilateral.)

- Hypertensive retinopathy (Narrowed retinal arterioles. Hemorrhages are not confined to a sector of the retina and usually cross the horizontal raphé. Bilateral in most.)

Work-up

1. History: Systemic disease, particularly hypertension or diabetes?
2. Complete ocular examination, including a dilated retinal examination with indirect ophthalmoscopy looking for retinal neovascularization and a macular examination using a slit-lamp and a Hruby, 60 or 90 diopter, or a fundus contact lens to detect macular edema.
3. Check the blood pressure.
4. Consider obtaining a fasting blood sugar, CBC with differential and platelets, PT/PTT, ESR, ANA, rheumatoid factor, and chest x-ray.
5. Medical examination (usually performed by an internist to check for cardiovascular disease).
6. A fluorescein angiogram is obtained after the hemorrhages have cleared or sooner if neovascularization is suspected.

Treatment

1. Retinal laser photocoagulation is indicated for:
   a. Chronic macular edema (3-6 months duration) reducing vision below 20/40.
   b. Retinal neovascularization.
2. Underlying medical problems are treated.

Follow-up Every 1-2 months at first then every 3-12 months, checking for neovascularization and/or macular edema.

12.5 Hypertensive Retinopathy

Symptoms Usually asymptomatic, although may have decreased vision.

Critical Sign Generalized or localized retinal arteriolar narrowing, almost always bilateral.

Other Signs Arteriovenous crossing changes, retinal arteriolar sclerosis ("copper" or "silver" wiring), cotton wool spots, hard exudates often in a "macular star" configuration, flame hemorrhages, retinal edema, arterial macroaneurysms, chorioretinal atrophy ("Elschnig spots" of choroidal nonperfusion).

Rarely, retinal detachment, vitreous hemorrhage, central or branch occlusion of an artery or vein, or neovascular complications can develop.

Signs of "malignant hypertension": Swelling of the optic-nerve head (disc edema) plus other signs listed above.

NOTE When hypertensive changes are only found in one eye, suspect carotid artery obstruction on the side of the normal appearing eye (sparing the retina from the effects of the hypertension).

Etiology

- Essential hypertension   (No known underlying cause.)
- Secondary hypertension   (Typically due to preeclampsia/eclampsia, pheochromocytoma, kidney disease, adrenal disease, or coarctation of the aorta.)

Differential Diagnosis

- Diabetic retinopathy   (Hemorrhages are generally dot and blot, microaneurysms are common, vessel attenuation is less common.)
- Collagen vascular disease   (May show multiple cotton wool spots, but few-to-no other fundus findings characteristic of hypertension.)
- Anemia   (Hemorrhage predominates without marked arterial changes.)
- Radiation retinopathy   (Can appear similar to hypertension. A history of irradiation to the eye or an adnexal structure such as the brain, sinus, or nasopharynx can usually be elicited. It may develop anytime after the radiation therapy, but most commonly within a few years.)
- Central or branch retinal vein occlusion   (Unilateral, multiple hemorrhages, venous dilatation and tortuosity, no arteriolar narrowing. May be secondary to hypertension.)

Work-up

1. History: Known hypertension, diabetes, or adnexal radiation?
2. Complete ocular examination, particularly a dilated retinal examination.
3. Check blood pressure.
4. Refer to a medical internist or the emergency room of a hospital. (The urgency generally depends on the blood pressure reading and whether the patient is symptomatic. As a general rule, a diastolic blood pressure >110-120 mm Hg or the presence of chest pain, difficulty breathing, headache, or blurred vision with optic disc swelling require immediate medical attention.)

Treatment Control the hypertension (as per the internist).

Follow-up   Every 2-3 months at first. Then every 6-12 months.

12.6   Amaurosis Fugax

Symptoms   Monocular visual loss that usually last seconds to minutes, but may last up to 1-2 hours. Vision returns to normal.

Critical Signs   May see an embolus within an arteriole or the ocular examination may be normal.

Other Signs   Signs of the ocular ischemic syndrome (dilated veins, mid-peripheral dot/blot hemorrhages, neovascularization of the iris, disc, or retina), an old branch retinal artery occlusion (sheathed arteriole), or neurologic signs due to ischemia of a cerebral hemisphere (e.g., contralateral arm or leg weakness).

Etiology   Embolus from the carotid artery (most common), heart, or aorta; talc emboli from IV drug abuse; vascular insufficiency due to arteriosclerotic disease of vessels anywhere along the path from the aorta to the globe (and precipitated by a postural change or cardiac arrhythmia); hypercoagulable/hyperviscosity state.

Differential Diagnosis   All of the following may produce transient visual loss:
- Papilledema   (Optic-disc swelling is evident.)
- Giant-cell arteritis   (Patients are typically 55 years or older and have an elevated ESR, temporal headache, scalp tenderness, jaw claudication, or muscle pains.)
- Impending central retinal vein occlusion   (Dilated, tortuous retinal veins are observed on funduscopic examination.)
- Glaucoma   (Characteristic optic-nerve changes.)
- Retinal migraine   (Usually a diagnosis of exclusion. Typically <40 years old. May have recurrent episodes.)

Work-up

1. History: Monocular visual loss or homonymous hemianopsia? (Did the patient cover one eye to test vision?) Duration of visual loss? Previous episodes of amaurosis fugax or transient cerebral ischemia? Atherosclerotic risk factors? Use of birth control pills? Heart disease/operations? IV drug abuse?

2. Ocular examination, including a confrontational visual field examination and a dilated retinal evaluation. (Look for an embolus or signs of other disorders mentioned above.)
3. Medical examination (cardiac and carotid auscultation).
4. Consider a fluorescein angiogram (focal arterial staining at the site of the embolus may be seen).
5. Immediate ESR when giant-cell arteritis is suspected.
6. CBC with differential and platelet count, fasting blood sugar +/− glucose tolerance test, and lipid profile (rule out polycythemia, thrombocytosis, diabetes, hyperlipidemia).
7. Noninvasive carotid artery evaluation (e.g., Doppler, ultrasound, etc.).
8. Cardiac evaluation (including an echocardiogram).
9. Check the arms of young patients for signs of IV drug abuse.
10. Carotid arteriogram is reserved for patients in whom carotid surgery is to be performed.

Treatment

A. Carotid disease
   1. Consider aspirin 325 mg po q day.
   2. Consider carotid endarterectomy in the presence of a surgically accessible high grade carotid stenosis or occlusion *if* the potential benefit of the procedure outweighs the risks.
   3. Control hypertension and diabetes (follow-up with a medical internist).
   4. Stop smoking.
B. Cardiac disease
   1. Consider aspirin 325 mg po q day for mitral valve prolapse.
   2. Consider hospitalization and anticoagulation (e.g., heparin therapy) in the presence of a mural thrombus.
   3. Consider cardiac surgery as needed.
   4. Control arteriosclerotic risk factors as above.

Follow-up Patients with recurrent episodes of amaurosis fugax (especially if accompanied by signs of cerebral transient ischemic attacks) require immediate diagnostic and, sometimes, therapeutic attention.

12.7 Ocular Ischemic Syndrome

(Carotid Occlusive Disease)

Symptoms Decreased vision, ocular or periorbital pain, after-images or prolonged recovery of vision following exposure to bright light, may have a history of transient monocular visual loss (amaurosis fugax). Usually unilateral. Age typically 50-80 years.

Critical Signs   Dilated retinal veins that are irregular in caliber, narrowed retinal arterioles, mid-peripheral retinal hemorrhages, neovascularization of the iris, disc, and/or retina.

Other Signs   Episcleral injection, corneal edema, mild anterior uveitis, neovascular glaucoma, iris atrophy, cataract, retinal microaneurysms, cotton wool spots, and spontaneous pulsations of the central retinal artery. A central retinal artery occlusion may occur.

Etiology   Carotid disease (usually >90% stenosis).

Differential Diagnosis

- Central retinal vein occlusion (CRVO)   (Similar signs, but may have optociliary shunt vessels or edema of the disc and dilated retinal veins that are tortuous and regular in caliber. Decreased vision after exposure to light and orbital pain are not typically found. Ophthalmodynamometry may distinguish [see below].)
- Diabetes   (Bilateral, usually symmetric. Retinal hemorrhages usually concentrate in the posterior pole and hard exudates are often present.)
- Aortic arch disease (due to atherosclerosis, syphilis, or Takayasu's disease)   (Ocular ischemia producing an identical picture, usually bilaterally. Examination reveals absent arm and neck pulses, cold hands, and spasm of the arm muscles with exercise.)

Work-up

1. History: Previous episodes of transient monocular visual loss? Cold hands, spasm of arm muscles with exercise, etc.?
2. Complete ocular examination, searching carefully for neovascularization of the iris, disc, or retina.
3. Medical examination (arm pulses, cardiac and carotid auscultation).
4. Consider fluorescein angiography for diagnostic or therapeutic purposes.
5. Non-invasive carotid artery evaluation (e.g., ultrasound, Doppler, oculoplethysmography (OPG), etc.).
6. Consider ophthalmodynamometry if the diagnosis of a CRVO cannot be excluded (ophthalmic artery pressure is low in carotid disease, but normal to elevated in a CRVO).
7. Carotid arteriography is reserved for patients in whom surgery is to be performed.

8. Consider a cardiology consultation, as there is a high association with cardiac disease.

Treatment   Often unsuccessful.

1. Consider carotid surgery if indicated.
2. Consider panretinal photocoagulation in the presence of neovascularization.
3. Manage glaucoma if present (see "Neovascular Glaucoma," Section 10.13.)
4. Control hypertension and diabetes and reduce cholesterol level (follow-up with internist).
5. Stop smoking.

Follow-up   Depends upon the age and general health of the patient and the symptoms and signs of disease. Surgical candidates should be evaluated urgently.

12.8   Central Serous Choroidopathy

Symptoms   Blurred or dim vision, objects appear distorted and minified in size, colors are "washed out," or a blind spot is perceived in the central field of vision. Usually unilateral. Sometimes asymptomatic. Generally occurs in men age 25-50 years.

Critical Signs   Localized detachment of the sensory retina from the underlying pigment epithelium by clear serous fluid in the macular area. The margins of the detachment are sloping and merge gradually into attached retina. It is best seen with a fundus contact lens (e.g., Goldmann contact lens) using a slit-lamp. No blood is present.

Other Signs   Visual acuity generally ranges from 20/20-20/80, Amsler grid testing reveals distortion of straight lines often with a scotoma, a small afferent pupillary defect or a concomitant retinal pigment epithelial detachment may be present.

Differential Diagnosis   The entities below may produce a serous detachment of the sensory retina in the macular area.

- Age-related macular degeneration (ARMD) (Age generally >50 years, drusen, pigment epithelial alterations, may have a choroidal [subretinal] neovascular membrane, often bilateral.)

- Optic pit   (The optic disc has a small defect, a pit, in the nerve tissue. A serous retinal detachment may be present contiguous with the optic disc.)
- Macular detachment due to a rhegmatogenous retinal detachment   (A hole in the retina can be found.)
- Choroidal tumor   (A mass is visible by indirect ophthalmoscopy.)
- Pigment epithelial detachment   (The margins of a pigment epithelial detachment are more distinct. It may accompany central serous choroidopathy or ARMD.)

Work-up

1. Amsler grid test to document the area of field involved, see Appendix 3.
2. Slit-lamp examination of the macula with a fundus contact, Hruby, or a 60 or 90 diopter lens to rule out a concomitant choroidal neovascular membrane. Additionally, search for an optic pit of the disc.
3. Dilated retinal examination using indirect ophthalmoscopy to rule out a choroidal tumor and rhegmatogenous retinal detachment.
4. Obtain an intravenous fluorescein angiogram if the diagnosis is uncertain, a choroidal neovascular membrane is suspected, or laser treatment is to be instituted.

Treatment/Follow-up   Final visual outcome has not been shown to be improved or worsened by laser therapy, but it is restored more rapidly. Due to the small but significant risks of laser photocoagulation, however, the following recommendations have been made.

1. Follow most cases every 6-8 weeks until the condition spontaneously resolves or, if no resolution, for 4-6 months.
2. Laser photocoagulation may be considered under the following circumstances:
   a. Persistence of a serous detachment beyond 4-6 months.
   b. Recurrence of the condition in an eye which sustained a permanent visual deficit from a previous episode.
   c. Occurrence in the fellow eye after a permanent visual deficit resulted from a previous episode.
   d. Patient requires prompt restoration of vision (e.g., occupational requirement).

REFERENCE

Basic and Clinical Science Course. Section 4: Retina and vitreous. San Francisco: Am Academy of Ophthalmol, 1989.

12.9   Optic Pit

Symptoms   Asymptomatic if isolated. May notice distortion of straight lines or edges, blurred vision, a blind spot, or micropsia if a serous macular detachment develops.

Critical Sign   Small defect (usually hypopigmented or gray in appearance) in the nerve tissue of the optic disc, a pit.

Other Signs   May develop a localized detachment of the sensory retina extending from the disc to the macula, usually unilateral.

Differential Diagnosis

- Pseudopit   (Seen in patients with low-tension glaucoma or primary open-angle glaucoma, occasionally accompanied by flame hemorrhages.)
- Other causes of a serous macular detachment (see "Central Serous Choroidopathy," Section 12.8.)

Work-up

1. Optic-disc evaluation to detect the pit.
2. Slit-lamp examination of the macula with a fundus contact lens or 60 or 90 diopter lens to evaluate for a serous macular detachment (rule out a choroidal [subretinal] neovascular membrane).
3. Check the intraocular pressure.
4. Consider a fluorescein angiogram to help detect a pit and rule out a choroidal neovascular membrane in cases with a serous macular detachment.

Treatment

A. *Isolated optic pit:* No treatment required.
B. *Optic pit with a serous macular detachment:* Laser photocoagulation to the temporal margin of the optic disc is used in most cases. Surgery (vitrectomy) may be used in refractile cases.

Follow-up

A. *Isolated optic pits:* Yearly examination; sooner if symptomatic.
B. *Optic pits with serous macular detachment:* Reexamine every few weeks after treatment to watch for resorption of subretinal fluid. Watch for amblyopia in children.

12.10   Age-related Macular Degeneration

Two types: Nonexudative (dry form) and exudative (wet form). Both forms almost always occur in patients >50 years old.

A. Nonexudative

Symptoms   Gradual loss of central vision, may be asymptomatic.

Critical Sign   Drusen, almost always in the macular area of both eyes.

Other Signs   Pigment clumping and atrophic areas (geographic atrophy), absent foveal reflex, Amsler grid defect.

Differential Diagnosis

- Peripheral drusen   (Drusen are located outside of the macular area, not within it.)

Work-up

1. Amsler grid to document or detect a central or paracentral scotoma, see Appendix 3.
2. Macular examination with a 60 or 90 diopter or a fundus contact lens, looking for signs of the exudative form.

Treatment   No proven treatment is available. Low-vision aids may benefit patients with bilateral loss of macular function.

Follow-up   Every 6 months. Patients are given an Amsler grid to take home and use on a daily basis. They are instructed to return immediately if a change is noted on the Amsler grid.

B. Exudative

1. Choroidal (Subretinal) Neovascular Membrane without a Pigment Epithelial Detachment

Symptoms   Distortion of straight lines or edges, rapid onset of visual loss, blind spot in the central (or paracentral) visual field.

Critical Signs   Drusen accompanied by a choroidal neovascular membrane (dirty gray membrane beneath the retina).

Other Signs   Subretinal hemorrhages, subretinal exudates, subretinal pigment ring, disciform scar, retinal or vitreous hemorrhage. Nonexudative signs may be present.

Differential Diagnosis   All of the following are associated with a choroidal neovascular membrane.

- Ocular histoplasmosis syndrome   (Small atrophic chorioretinal scars, white-yellow in appearance, are seen in the mid-periphery and posterior pole along with chorioretinal scarring adjacent to the optic disc.)
- Angioid streaks   (Bilateral subretinal red-brown or gray bands of irregular contour which radiate from the optic disc.)
- High myopia   (Significant myopic refractive error, lacquer cracks in the posterior pole, myopic disc changes.)
- Traumatic choroidal rupture   (History of trauma, usually unilateral; a choroidal tear concentric to the optic disc is often noted.)
- Others   (Drusen of the optic nerve, choroidal tumors, photocoagulation scars, inflammatory chorioretinal lesions, and idiopathic.)

Work-up

1. Amsler grid testing to detect and document the degree of central field involved, see Appendix 3.
2. Macular slit-lamp examination with a 60 or 90 diopter or fundus contact lens to detect a choroidal neovascular membrane. Must examine *both* eyes.
3. Fluorescein angiography (FA) is performed as soon as possible if a choroidal neovascular membrane (CNVM) is suspected on clinical examination.

NOTE   FA is not indicated when there is no hope of preserving central vision such as in advanced stages of macular scarring (despite the presence of choroidal neovascularization).

Treatment   When a macular CNVM is identified by FA to be at least 200 microns from the center of the foveal avascular zone (FAZ)[1] and there is no hemorrhage nor exudate in the foveola, laser photocoagulation should be applied within 72 hours of the FA to reduce the risk of severe visual loss.

---

[1]The FAZ is an avascular area, about 500 microns in diameter, in the center of the fovea. It is easily observed with FA.

Follow-up

PATIENTS TREATED FOR A CNVM WITH LASER PHOTOCOAGULATION

Due to the high rate of neovascular activity following treatment (persistent and new CNVM), patients need to be followed closely, especially during the first post-treatment year:

1. Amsler grid to be used at home daily. The patient is instructed to return immediately if a change is noted.
2. Scheduled examinations at 2 weeks, 6 weeks, 3 months, and 6 months post-treatment, and then every 6 months. Careful macular examination is performed as described above.
3. FA is repeated 2 weeks following treatment and only again when renewed neovascular activity is suspected.
4. If a macular CNVM at least 200 microns from the center of the FAZ is detected, treatment by laser photocoagulation should be reinstituted within 72 hours.

2. Retinal Pigment Epithelial (RPE) Detachment

May have any of the symptoms or signs described above, but always has a well-defined elevated area of retina (and retinal pigment epithelium) with sharp borders. The work-up is the same as described above.

Treatment   Laser therapy is typically applied to a CNVM when one is located adjacent to the pigment epithelial detachment, but there is a risk of an RPE tear. If no CNVM is present, patients are usually observed.

Follow-up   Follow closely for the development of a treatable CNVM. Some pigment epithelial detachments may flatten or tear spontaneously. An Amsler grid should be used as described in Appendix 3.

12.11   Ocular Histoplasmosis Syndrome

Symptoms   May be asymptomatic or have decreased or distorted vision. Patients often have lived in or visited the Ohio-Mississippi River Valley area and are usually in the 20-50 year age range. A history of exposure to chickens, pigeons, or parakeets many years earlier may be elicited.

Critical Signs   (Classic triad.)

1. Yellow-white "punched-out" round spots usually less than 1 mm in diameter, deep to the retina in any fundus location ("histo-spots").
2. A macular choroidal (subretinal) neovascular membrane appearing as a gray-green patch beneath the retina associated with a detachment of the sensory retina, subretinal blood or exudate, or a pigment ring.
3. Atrophy or scarring adjacent to the optic disc sometimes with nodules or hemorrhage. There may be a rim of pigment separating the disc from the area of atrophy or scarring.

Other Signs   Linear streaks of chorioretinal atrophy in the peripheral fundus and a macular scar. The eye is uninflamed with minimal-to-no vitreous cells and no aqueous cell or flare.

Differential Diagnosis

- High myopia   (May have atrophic spots in the posterior pole and a myopic crescent on the temporal side of the disc. A choroidal neovascular membrane may develop. The atrophic spots are whiter than "histo-spots" and are not seen beyond the posterior pole. The myopic crescent has a rim of pigment on the outer [not inner] edge, separating the crescent from the retina. May have lacquer cracks. The disc is often tilted.)
- Age-related macular degeneration   (The macular changes may appear similar, but typically there are macular drusen and patients are greater than 50 years old. There are no atrophic round spots similar to histoplasmosis and no scarring or atrophy around the disc.)
- Toxoplasmosis   (White chorioretinal lesion associated with vitreous and sometimes aqueous cells.)
- Angioid streaks   ("Histo-like spots" may be seen in the mid-periphery and macular degeneration may occur. Jagged red, brown, or gray lines appearing deep to the retinal vessels and radiating from a point near the optic disc are also seen. Often associated with pseudoxanthoma elasticum, sickle-cell anemia, Paget's disease, and others.)
- Multifocal choroiditis with panuveitis   (Similar clinical findings, except anterior and/or vitreous inflammatory cells are additionally present.)

Work-up

1. History: Time spent in the Ohio-Mississippi River Valley area? Exposure to fowl?
2. Amsler grid test (see Appendix 3) to evaluate the central visual field of each eye.

3. Slit-lamp examination: Anterior-chamber cells and flare should not be present.
4. Dilated fundus examination concentrating on the macular area with a slit-lamp and fundus contact, Hruby, or 60 or 90 diopter lens. (Look for signs of a choroidal neovascular membrane and vitreous cells.)
5. Fluorescein angiography (to help detect or treat a choroidal neovascular membrane).

Treatment Laser photocoagulation is indicated when a choroidal neovascular membrane 200-2500 microns from the center of the fovea is discovered. Laser treatment is usually not indicated in the presence of foveal hemorrhage, exudate, or scarring in which central vision is irreparably lost. Prophylactic laser photocoagulation (i.e., in the absence of a neovascular membrane) is usually not recommended. Antifungal treatment is not helpful.

Follow-up Treatment should be instituted within 72 hours of confirming the presence of a choroidal neovascular membrane by fluorescein angiography. All patients (whether they will be, will not be, or have been treated) are taught how to use an Amsler grid and told to test themselves daily. Patients are instructed to return immediately if a change in vision is noted. Treated patients are seen at 2-3 weeks, 4-6 weeks, 3 months, and 6 months post-treatment and then every 6 months. A careful macular examination is performed at each visit. Fluorescein angiography is repeated at the 2 to 3-week post-treatment visit and whenever renewed neovascular activity is suspected.

- If a recurrent or new CNVM is detected 200-2500 microns from the center of the fovea, laser photocoagulation treatment is reinstituted within 72 hours.
- Patients without a CNVM are seen every 6 months when a macular "histo-spot" is present in one or both eyes, and yearly when one is not present in either eye.

REFERENCES

MACULAR PHOTOCOAGULATION STUDY GROUP. Argon laser photocoagulation for neovascular maculopathy: Three year results from randomized clinical trials. *Arch Ophthalmol* 104: 694, 1986.

MACULAR PHOTOCOAGULATION STUDY GROUP. Argon laser photocoagulation for ocular histoplasmosis: Results of a randomized clinical trial. *Arch Ophthalmol* 101: 1347, 1983.

12.12   High Myopia

Symptoms   Decreased vision.

Critical Signs   Myopic crescent (a crescent-shaped area of white sclera or choroidal vessels adjacent to the disc, separated from the normal-appearing fundus
by a hyperpigmented line; this crescent may enlarge with time), an oblique
(tilted) insertion of the optic disc, macular pigmentary abnormalities, a dark
spot in the macula (Fuchs' spot) and typically, but not always, a refractive
correction of more than -6.00 to -8.00 diopters.

Other Signs   Temporal optic-disc pallor, posterior staphyloma, entrance of the
retinal vessels into the nasal part of the cup, the retina and choroid may be
seen to extend over the nasal border of the disc, well-circumscribed areas of
atrophy, choroidal sclerosis, yellow subretinal streaks (lacquer cracks), peripheral retinal thinning, and lattice degeneration. A choroidal (subretinal)
neovascular membrane (CNVM) or retinal detachment may develop. Visual
field defects may be present.

Differential Diagnosis

- Age-related macular degeneration   (May develop a CNVM and a similar
  macular appearance, but typically drusen are present and the myopic features
  of the optic disc described above are absent.)
- Ocular histoplasmosis   (May also develop a CNVM and exhibit a peripapillary scar. A pigmented ring may separate the disc from the peripapillary
  atrophy—as opposed to a pigmented ring separating the atrophic area from
  the adjacent retina. Round choroidal scars [punched-out lesions] may also
  be seen scattered throughout the fundus.)
- Tilted discs   (Anomalous discs with a scleral crescent inferiorly, an irregular
  vascular pattern as the vessels emerge from the disc [situs inversus], and
  areas of fundus ectasia temporally. Many patients are myopic; however,
  they do not have chorioretinal degeneration nor lacquer cracks. Visual field
  defects may occur.)
- Gyrate atrophy   (Rare. Multiple sharply defined areas of chorioretinal atrophy beginning in the mid-periphery in childhood and then coalescing to
  involve a large portion of the fundus. Body fluid levels of ornithine are
  markedly elevated. Patients are often highly myopic. Autosomal recessive.)

Work-up

1. Manifest and/or cycloplegic refraction.
2. Intraocular pressure (IOP) measurement by applanation tonometry (Schiötz
   tonometry may underestimate the IOP in highly myopic eyes.)

3. Dilated retinal examination, using indirect ophthalmoscopy to search for retinal breaks or detachment. Scleral depression helps to see the far peripheral retina, but should not be performed over a staphyloma.
4. Slit-lamp and fundus contact, Hruby, or 60 or 90 diopter lens examination of the macula, searching for a CNVM (dirty-gray or green lesion beneath the retina, subretinal blood or exudate, or subretinal fluid).
5. Fluorescein angiography when a CNVM is suspected.
6. Formal visual field examinations (e.g., Humphrey or Octopus) to document field stability or change when glaucoma is suspected.

Treatment

1. Symptomatic retinal breaks are treated with laser photocoagulation, cryotherapy, or scleral buckling surgery. Treatment of asymptomatic retinal breaks should be considered when there is no surrounding demarcation line.
2. Macular choroidal neovascular membranes more than 200 microns from the center of the fovea may be considered for laser photocoagulation therapy within several days of obtaining a fluorescein angiogram. Laser treatment is usually not indicated in the presence of foveal hemorrhage, exudate, or scarring in which central vision is irreparably lost. The efficacy of this treatment has not been proven.
3. For glaucoma suspects, a single visual field often cannot distinguish myopic visual field loss from early glaucoma. Progression of visual field loss in the absence of progressive myopia, however, suggests the presence of glaucoma and the need for therapy (see "Primary Open-Angle Glaucoma," Section 10.1).

Follow-up In the absence of complications, reexamine every 6–12 months, watching for the related disorders discussed above. See "Primary Open-Angle Glaucoma" (Section 10.1), "Retinal Break" (Section 12.18), "Retinal Detachment" (Section 12.19), and "Age-related Macular Degeneration" (Section 12.10) (for treatment of choroidal neovascularization) for further information on these conditions.

12.13 Angioid Streaks

Symptoms Usually asymptomatic; decreased vision may result from choroidal (subretinal) neovascularization.

Critical Signs Bilateral reddish-brown or gray bands radiating in an irregular or spokelike pattern from the optic disc (similar to cracks in cement), located deep to the retina. Macular degeneration due to choroidal neovascularization is the complication of greatest concern.

Other Signs Mottled-background fundus appearance (''peau d'orange''), subretinal hemorrhages, retinal pigment epithelial atrophy, or small white pinpoint chorioretinal scars (''histo-like spots'') may be seen in the mid-periphery.

Etiology (50% are associated with systemic diseases, the remainder are idiopathic.)

- Pseudoxanthoma elasticum (Loose skin folds in the neck and on flexor aspects of joints, cardiovascular complications, increased risk of GI bleeds.)
- Paget's disease (Enlarged skull, bone pain, history of bone fractures, hearing loss, may have cardiovascular complications or may be asymptomatic. Increased serum alkaline phosphatase and urine calcium.)
- Sickle-cell disease (May be asymptomatic, may have decreased vision from fundus abnormalities [see ''Sickle-Cell Disease,'' Section 12.23], or may have a history of recurrent infections or painful crises. Positive sickle-cell prep and abnormal hemoglobin [Hgb] electrophoresis.)
- Ehlers-Danlos syndrome (Hyperelasticity of skin, loose jointedness.)
- Less common (Acromegaly, senile elastosis, lead poisoning, Marfan's syndrome.)

Differential Diagnosis

- Myopic chorioretinal degeneration (lacquer cracks) (High myopia, often with a tilted disc and peripapillary atrophy; may have macular degeneration.)
- Choroidal rupture (Subretinal streaks are usually concentric to the optic disc, yellow-white in color, and result from ocular trauma.)

Work-up

1. History: Any known systemic disorders? Previous ocular trauma?
2. Complete ocular examination, looking carefully at the macula with a slit lamp and a Hruby, 60 or 90 diopter, or a fundus contact lens to detect choroidal neovascularization.
3. Fluorescein angiogram if uncertain of the diagnosis or if choroidal neovascularization is suspected.
4. Physical examination, looking for clinical signs of etiologic diseases.
5. Serum alkaline phosphatase and urine calcium levels if suspect Paget's disease.
6. Sickle-cell prep and Hgb electrophoresis in black patients.

7. Skin biopsy if pseudoxanthoma elasticum is suspected.

Treatment

1. Focal laser treatment if choroidal neovascularization develops outside of the foveal avascular zone.
2. Management of any underlying systemic disease, if present, by a medical internist.

Follow-up   Fundus examination every 6 months, observing for choroidal neovascularization. An Amsler grid (see Appendix 3) is to be used at home on a daily basis. Patients are instructed to return immediately if a change is noted on the Amsler grid.

See ''Age-related Macular Degeneration,'' Section 12.10, for management of choroidal neovascularization.

12.14   Cystoid Macular Edema (CME)

Symptoms   Decreased vision.

Critical Signs   Irregularity and blurring of the foveal light reflex, macular thickening, tiny macular cysts.

Other Signs   Loss of the choroidal vascular pattern underlying the macula. Vitreous cells and optic nerve swelling can appear in severe cases. A macular hole causing permanent visual loss can develop.

Etiology

• After any type of ocular surgery (including laser photocoagulation and cryotherapy)   (The peak incidence after cataract surgery is about 6-10 weeks; the incidence increases with surgical complications including vitreous to the wound, iris prolapse, and vitreous loss.)
• Diabetic retinopathy.
• Central and branch retinal vein occlusions.
• Uveitis (particularly pars planitis and occasionally toxoplasmosis).
• Retinitis pigmentosa.
• Topical epinephrine (or dipivefrin) drops in postoperative cataract patients   (Often reversed by discontinuing the drops.)

- Retinal vasculitis (e.g., Eales' disease, Behçet's syndrome, sarcoidosis, necrotizing angiitis, multiple sclerosis, cytomegalovirus retinitis).
- Retinal telangiectasias (e.g., Coats' disease).
- Niacin (nicotinic acid) maculopathy   (Niacin is a component of some medications used to treat hypercholesterolemia.)
- Others   (e.g., intraocular tumors, systemic hypertension, collagen vascular disease, surface wrinkling retinopathy).

Work-up

1. History: Recent intraocular surgery? Diabetes? Previous uveitis or eye inflammation? Night blindness or family history of eye disease? Medications, including topical epinephrine or dipivefrin use?
2. Complete ocular examination, including a peripheral fundus evaluation (scleral depression inferiorly may be required to detect pars planitis). A macular examination is best performed with a slit-lamp and a fundus contact lens, a Hruby lens, or a 60 or 90 diopter lens.
3. Fluorescein angiography (Often shows early leakage of dye out of perifoveal capillaries and late macular staining, classically in a "flower petal" or "spoke-wheel" pattern. Fluorescein leakage does not occur in niacin maculopathy.)
4. Other diagnostic tests when indicated (e.g., fasting blood sugar or glucose tolerance test, electroretinogram, etc.)

NOTE   Subclinical CME commonly develops after cataract extraction and is noted on fluorescein angiography. These cases are not treated.

Treatment   Not well established for macular edema developing after ocular surgery. Most of these cases resolve spontaneously within 6 months.

1. Treat the underlying disorder if possible.
2. Discontinue topical epinephrine/dipivefrin drops and medications containing niacin (nicotinic acid).
3. Consider acetazolamide (e.g., Diamox) 250 mg po q day (especially for postoperative patients, but also those with retinitis pigmentosa and uveitis).
4. Other forms of therapy that have unproven efficacy, but are occasionally used:
   a. Nonsteroidal antiinflammatory drugs (e.g., indomethacin 25 mg po tid × 6 weeks).
   b. Topical steroids (e.g., prednisolone acetate 1% qid × 3 weeks, then taper over 3 weeks).
   c. Systemic steroids (e.g., prednisone 40 mg po q day × 5 days, then taper over 2 weeks).

- Diabetic macular edema may benefit from focal laser treatment, see "Diabetes Mellitus," Section 14.6.
- Macular edema persisting for 3-6 months after a branch retinal vein occlusion and reducing vision below 20/40 often improves with laser photocoagulation, see "Branch Retinal Vein Occlusion," Section 12.4.
- Macular edema in the presence of vitreous incarceration in a surgical wound may be improved by anterior vitrectomy or YAG laser lysis of the vitreous strand.
- Macular edema from pars planitis is often treated with steroids when vision is reduced below 20/40, see "Pars Planitis," Section 13.5.

Follow-up   Postsurgical CME is not an urgent condition. Other forms of macular edema may require an etiologic work-up and may benefit from early treatment (e.g., elimination of niacin-containing medications).

12.15   Macular Hole

Symptoms   Decreased vision, typically around the 20/200 level for a full thickness hole, better for a partial thickness hole; sometimes distortion of vision. More commonly middle-aged to elderly women are affected.

Critical Signs   A round red spot in the center of the macula, usually from ⅓-⅔ of a disc diameter in size, with a gray halo (marginal retinal detachment) surrounding it.

Other Signs   Small yellow deposits within the hole, deep to the retina; retinal cysts at the margin of the hole, and/or a small operculum above the hole (anterior to the retina).

NOTE   A partial thickness (lamellar) hole is not as red in color, and the surrounding gray halo is usually not present.

Etiology   May be due to vitreous or epiretinal membrane traction on the macula, trauma, or cystoid macular edema.

Differential Diagnosis

- Macular pucker with a pseudohole   (A condensation of a membrane on the surface of the retina may simulate a macular hole.)
- Solar retinopathy   (Small, round, red or yellow lesion at the center of the fovea, with surrounding fine gray pigment in a sun gazer or eclipse watcher.)

Work-up

1. History: Previous trauma? Previous eye surgery? Sun gazer?
2. Complete ocular examination, including a macular examination with a slit lamp and 60 or 90 diopter, Hruby, or fundus contact lens.

Treatment   No effective treatment is known. Visual loss is irreversible and the risk of retinal detachment is very small. Symptoms of a retinal detachment (e.g., sudden increase in flashes and floaters, abundant ''cobwebs'' in the vision, or a curtain coming across the field of vision), however, are explained to patients, particularly those with high myopia. It is in this latter group that the macular hole sometimes leads to a retinal detachment. Retinal detachment requires repair.

Follow-up   High myopes are seen every 6 months, other patients may be seen yearly. All patients are seen sooner if retinal detachment symptoms develop. There is a small risk that the condition may develop in the fellow eye.

12.16   Macular Pucker

(Surface Wrinkling Retinopathy)

Symptoms   Decreased and/or distorted vision. Occasionally bilateral. Typically middle-aged to elderly patients.

Critical Signs   Spectrum ranges from a fine glistening membrane (cellophane retinopathy) to a thick gray-white membrane (macular pucker) present on the surface of the retina in the macular area.

NOTE   When the preretinal membrane is thin, it is often best appreciated with an indirect ophthalmoscope by moving the lens up and down in your hand. A glistening sparkle, much like cellophane, may be observed in the macular area.

Other Signs   Retinal folds radiating out from the membrane, displacement or straightening of the macular retinal vessels, macular edema or detachment, signs of other ocular disease. A round, dark condensation of the epiretinal membrane in the macula may simulate a macular hole.

Etiology   Idiopathic, retinal break, rhegmatogenous retinal detachment, following retinal cryotherapy or photocoagulation, following intraocular surgery, trauma, uveitis, retinal vascular disease, and others.

Differential Diagnosis

• Diabetic retinopathy   (May produce preretinal fibrovascular tissue which may displace retinal vessels or detach the macula. Macular edema may be present. Hemorrhages and microaneurysms are usually found in addition, and the changes are commonly bilateral.)

Work-up

1. History: Previous eye surgery or eye disease? Diabetes?
2. Complete ocular examination, particularly a thorough dilated fundus evaluation. The macula is often best seen with a slit lamp and a 60 or 90 diopter, Hruby, or fundus contact lens.

Treatment   Treat the underlying disorder. Surgical peeling of the membrane can be performed when it reduces the vision to 20/80-20/100 or worse.

Follow-up   This is not an urgent condition, and treatment may be instituted at any time. Some membranes separate from the retina and vision may improve spontaneously. A small percentage of preretinal membranes recur after surgical removal.

12.17   Posterior Vitreous Detachment (PVD)

Symptoms   Floaters (''cobwebs'' or ''flies'' which move with eye movement) and/or flashes of light which are more common in dim illumination.

Critical Signs   One or more discrete pigmented vitreous opacities, often in the shape of a ring, suspended over the optic disc. The opacities float within the vitreous as the eye moves from side to side.

Other Signs   Vitreous hemorrhage, peripheral retinal and disc margin hemorrhages, pigmented cells in the anterior vitreous, retinal break or detachment.

NOTE   The presence of pigmented cells in the anterior vitreous or vitreous hemorrhage in association with an acute PVD indicates a high probability of a coexisting retinal break, see Section 12.18.

Differential Diagnosis

- Vitritis   (It may be difficult to distinguish a PVD with pigmented anterior vitreous cells from vitreous inflammatory cells. In vitritis, the vitreous cells may be found in both the posterior and anterior vitreous, the condition may be bilateral, and the cells are not typically pigmented. A history of uveitis may be elicited.)
- Migraine   (Patients complain of flashing lights that last approximately 20 minutes. A headache may or may not follow. No vitreous or retinal abnormalities are found on examination.)

The following may occur with or without a PVD, producing similar symptoms:

- Retinal break
- Vitreous hemorrhage
- Retinal detachment

Work-up

1. History: Distinguish between the flashing lights of migraine which typically occur in a "zig-zag" pattern, obstruct vision, and last approximately 20 minutes from the light sparks of a PVD, which are commonly accompanied by floaters. Determine the duration of the symptoms.
2. Complete ocular examination, particularly a dilated retinal examination using indirect ophthalmoscopy and scleral depression to rule out a retinal break and detachment. A slit-lamp examination of the anterior vitreous looking for pigmented cells is often performed, see Appendix 9.
3. A PVD may be visualized by focusing in the vitreous, above the disc, using:
   a. Indirect ophthalmoscopy
   b. Direct ophthalmoscopy (The ophthalmoscope is initially focused on the cornea, the lens wheel is moved from a higher black number toward a lower black number, and the patient is asked to move his eye from left to right. The PVD is seen to float by.)
   c. A slit lamp and a 60 or 90 diopter or Hruby lens. (Pull the slit lamp back toward you once you have focused on the disc. A black strand may be seen in the vitreous.)

Treatment   No treatment is indicated for a PVD. If a retinal break is found the patient should receive laser or cryotherapy within 24-72 hours to avoid the development of a retinal detachment, see Section 12.18.

NOTE   A retinal break surrounded by pigment is old and usually does not require treatment.

Follow-up   The patient should be given a list of retinal detachment symptoms (an increase in floaters or flashing lights, or the appearance of a curtain or shadow anywhere in the field of vision), and told to return immediately if these symptoms develop.

- If no retinal break nor hemorrhage is found, the patient should be scheduled for repeat examination with scleral depression in 2-3 weeks, 2-3 months, and 6 months after the symptoms first developed.
- If no retinal break is found, but mild vitreous hemorrhage or peripheral punctate retinal hemorrhages are present, repeat examinations are performed 1-2 weeks, 4 weeks, 3 months, and 6 months after the event.
- If a vitreous hemorrhage which is dense enough to obscure the entire retina is found, ultrasonography is indicated to rule out a retinal detachment or tumor. Bed rest, with the head of the bed elevated, often with bilateral patches, is employed to hasten settling of the blood, see Section 12.22.

12.18   Retinal Break

Symptoms

Acute retinal break   Flashes of light and floaters ("cobwebs" or "flies" which move with eye movement).
Chronic retinal break or an atrophic retinal hole   Usually asymptomatic.

Critical Sign   A full-thickness retinal defect.

Other Signs

Acute retinal break   Pigmented cells in the anterior vitreous, vitreous hemorrhage, posterior vitreous detachment, retinal flap, or an operculum (a free-floating piece of retina) suspended in the vitreous cavity above the retinal hole.

Chronic retinal break A ring of pigmentation surrounds the break, a demarcation line between attached and detached retina, and signs (but not symptoms) of an acute retinal break.

Predisposing Lesions Lattice degeneration, senile retinoschisis, vitreoretinal tufts, and meridional folds.

Work-up Complete ocular examination, particularly a dilated fundus examination of both eyes using indirect ophthalmoscopy and scleral depression. Scleral depression is generally *not* performed until 3-4 weeks following a traumaic hyphema or microhyphema. A slit-lamp examination with a fundus contact lens is often quite helpful in evaluating retinal breaks.

Treatment In general, laser, cryotherapy, or scleral buckling surgery is required within 24-72 hours for acute retinal breaks, and only rarely for chronic breaks. While each case must be individualized, we follow these general guidelines:

A. Treatment recommended
    1. Acute symptomatic break (e.g., a horseshoe or operculated tear).
    2. Acute traumatic break (including a dialysis).
B. Treatment to be considered
    1. Asymptomatic retinal break which is large (e.g., >1.5 mm) and/or above the horizontal meridian.
    2. Asymptomatic retinal break in an aphakic or pseudophakic eye, an eye in which the involved eye or the fellow eye has had a retinal detachment, or in a highly myopic eye.

Follow-up Patients with predisposing lesions or retinal breaks which do not require treatment are followed every 6-12 months. Patients treated for a retinal break are reexamined in one week, 1 month, 3 months, and then every 6-12 months. Retinal detachment symptoms (an increase in floaters or flashing lights or the appearance of a curtain or shadow anywhere in the field of vision) are explained to all patients, and patients are told to return immediately if these symptoms develop.

12.19 Retinal Detachment

There are three distinct types of retinal detachment (RD). All three forms show an elevation of the retina, the thin transparent tissue containing the retinal vessels.

A. Rhegmatogenous (RRD)

Symptoms Flashes of light, floaters, a curtain or shadow moving over the field of vision, peripheral and/or central visual loss.

Critical Sign Elevation of the retina along with a flap tear or break in the retina.

Other Signs Pigmented cells in the anterior vitreous, vitreous hemorrhage, posterior vitreous detachment, lower intraocular pressure in the affected eye than the fellow eye, clear subretinal fluid that does not shift with body position, and sometimes fixed folds. The detached retina moves with eye motion and is corrugated in appearance. An afferent pupillary defect (APD) may be present.

NOTE A chronic RRD often shows a pigmented demarcation line at the posterior extent of the RD, intraretinal cysts, fixed folds, or white dots underneath the retina.

B. Exudative (ERD)

Symptoms Minimal-to-severe visual loss or a visual field defect.

Critical Sign Serous elevation of the retina with shifting subretinal fluid (SRF). (The area of detached retina changes when the patient changes position: while sitting, the SRF accumulates inferiorly, detaching the retina inferiorly; while in the supine position, the fluid accumulates in the posterior pole, detaching the macula.)

Other Signs The detached retina is smooth and may become so elevated that it reaches the lens. A mild APD may be present.

Etiology

- Neoplastic (e.g., choroidal malignant melanoma, metastasis, choroidal hemangioma).
- Inflammatory disease (e.g., Vogt-Koyanagi-Harada syndrome, posterior scleritis, other chronic inflammatory processes).
- Congenital abnormalities (e.g., optic pit, morning glory syndrome, choroidal coloboma, Coats' disease).
- Nanophthalmos (Small eyes with a small cornea and a shallow anterior chamber, but a large lens and a thick sclera.)

- The uveal effusion syndrome   (Bilateral detachments of the peripheral choroid, ciliary body, and retina; leopard-spot retinal pigment epithelial changes; cells in the vitreous; dilated episcleral vessels.)

C. Tractional (TRD)

Symptoms   Visual loss or visual field defect, may be asymptomatic.

Critical Signs   The detached retina appears concave in shape with a smooth surface; vitreous membranes pulling the retina are present.

Other Signs   The retina is immobile, and the detachment rarely extends to the ora serrata. A mild APD may be present.

Etiology   Fibrous bands in the vitreous (resulting from proliferative diabetic retinopathy, sickle-cell retinopathy, retinopathy of prematurity, toxocariasis, etc.) contract and pull the retina off the retinal pigment epithelium.

Differential Diagnosis for All Three Types of Retinal Detachment

- Senile retinoschisis   (Commonly bilateral, usually temporal, no pigmented cells or hemorrhage is present in the vitreous, the retinal vessels over the schisis are often sheathed, white"snowflakes" are often seen on the inner layer of the schisis near the ora serrata, and the patient is asymptomatic. An absolute scotoma—as opposed to a relative scotoma as seen with a RRD—is found on visual field testing. A demarcation line is generally not present unless an RD develops from the schisis.)
- Juvenile retinoschisis   (Cystoid foveal changes are present, x-linked recessive, bilateral, the retinoschisis does not extend to the ora serrata.)
- Choroidal detachment   (Orange-brown in color, more solid in appearance than a RD, the ora serrata can usually be seen without scleral depression, and the detachment often extends 360 degrees around the globe. Hypotony is generally present.)

Treatment/Follow-up

1. Patients with acute RRD which *involve* or *threaten* the macula or those with TRD, which *involve* the macula should be admitted to the hospital immediately and placed at bedrest until surgical repair can be performed.
2. All other RRD which do not threaten the macula are repaired at the earliest convenience, preferably within 1-2 days.
3. Chronic retinal detachments are treated within 1 week.

4. For ERD, successful treatment of the underlying condition often leads to resolution of the detachment.

12.20 Retinoschisis

Retinoschisis, a splitting of the retina, occurs in juvenile and senile forms.

A. Juvenile Retinoschisis

Symptoms Decreased vision (often due to vitreous hemorrhage) or asymptomatic. The condition is congenital, but may not be detected until years later. A positive family history may or may not be elicited.

Critical Signs Cystoid foveal changes with retinal folds which radiate from the center of the foveal configuration. Unlike the cysts of cystoid macular edema, they do not stain on fluorescein angiography.

Other Signs Separation of the inner retinal layers from the outer retinal layers in the retinal periphery with the development of inner-layer retinal breaks; this peripheral retinoschisis occurs most commonly in the inferotemporal quadrant of the fundus and is bilateral. The retinoschisis does not extend to the ora serrata. Retinal detachment, vitreous hemorrhage, and a pigmentary degeneration similar to retinitis pigmentosa may also occur.

Inheritance X-linked recessive.

Differential Diagnosis
- Senile retinoschisis (See below.)
- Rhegmatogenous retinal detachment   (Usually unilateral and acquired. It extends to the ora serrata and lacks the foveal changes described above. Anterior-chamber cells and flare and pigment in the vitreous are often seen.)

Work-up
1. Family history.
2. Dilated retinal examination with scleral depression to rule out an outer-layer retinal break or detachment.

Treatment   Surgical repair of a retinal detachment should be performed if present. Superimposed amblyopia should always be considered in children <9-11 years of age when one eye is more severely affected, and a trial of patching should be considered, see Section 9.5.

Follow-up   Every 6 months; sooner if treating amblyopia.

B. Senile Retinoschisis

Symptoms   Usually none, may have decreased vision.

Critical Signs   The retinal split is usually bilateral and may show sheathing of retinal vessels, ''snow flakes,'' or ''frosting'' on the elevated inner wall of the schisis cavity. The schisis cavity is dome-shaped with a smooth surface and is usually located temporally, especially inferotemporally.

Other Signs   Prominent cystoid degeneration near the ora serrata, an absolute scotoma is found on visual field testing, hyperopia is common, and there are no pigment cells nor hemorrhage in the vitreous. A rhegmatogenous retinal detachment may develop.

Differential Diagnosis

* Rhegmatogenous retinal detachment   (The surface is not smooth, but corrugated in appearance and can be seen to move more with eye movements than schisis does; retinal vessels are not sheathed and no ''snow flakes'' nor ''frosting'' can be seen on the retinal elevation; one or more full-thickness holes are present, and pigmented cells or hemorrhage may be present in the vitreous. A long-standing retinal detachment may resemble retinoschisis, but intraretinal cysts, demarcation lines between attached and detached retina, and white retroretinal dots may be seen. A relative scotoma is found on visual field testing.)
* Juvenile retinoschisis (see above.)

Work-up

1. Slit-lamp evaluation to rule out the presence of anterior-chamber inflammation or pigmented anterior-vitreous cells (both of which should not be present in isolated retinoschisis).
2. Dilated retinal examination with scleral depression to rule out a concomitant retinal detachment or an outer-layer retinal hole which may lead to a retinal detachment.

3. A fundus contact lens evaluation of the retina as needed to aid in recognizing outer-layer retinal breaks.

Treatment Surgery is indicated when a clinically significant retinal detachment develops. A small retinal detachment walled off by a demarcation line is generally not treated.

Follow-up Every 6 months. Retinal detachment symptoms (an increase in floaters or flashing lights or the appearance of a curtain or shadow anywhere in the field of vision) are explained to all patients, and patients are told to return immediately if these symptoms develop.

12.21 Choroidal Detachment

Symptoms Decreased vision or asymptomatic in a serous choroidal detachment. Severe pain, decreased vision, and red eye in a hemorrhagic choroidal detachment.

Critical Signs Smooth, bullous elevation of the retina and choroid, orange-brown in color, usually extending 360 degrees around the periphery in a lobular configuration. The ora serrata can be seen without scleral depression.

Other Signs

A. *Serous choroidal detachment:* Low intraocular pressure (IOP) (often less than 6 mm Hg), shallow anterior chamber with mild cell and flare, positive transillumination.
B. *Hemorrhagic choroidal detachment:* High IOP, shallow anterior chamber with mild cell and flare, no transillumination.

Etiology

A. SEROUS

- Postsurgical (Wound leak, perforation of the sclera from a superior rectus bridle suture, iritis, cyclodialysis cleft, leakage or excess filtration from a filtering bleb, or following laser photocoagulation or cryotherapy. May occur days to weeks after the surgery.)
- Traumatic (Often associated with a ruptured globe.)
- Inflammatory (e.g., scleritis, Vogt-Koyanagi-Harada [VKH] syndrome)
- Tumor (Primary or metastasis.)

- Rhegmatogenous retinal detachment or after scleral buckling repair of a detachment.
- Others   (Nanophthalmos, uveal effusion syndrome, carotid-cavernous fistula.)

B. HEMORRHAGIC

- Postsurgical   (From anterior displacement of the ocular contents and rupture of the short posterior ciliary arteries.)
- Spontaneous (e.g., after perforation of a corneal ulcer).
- Rupture of a choroidal neovascular membrane in a patient on anticoagulants.

Differential Diagnosis

- Ring melanoma of the ciliary body   (Not typically multilobular nor symmetrical in each quadrant of the globe. Pigmented melanomas do not transilluminate. B-scan ultrasound may help to differentiate between the two.)
- Rhegmatogenous retinal detachment   (Appears white in color and undulates with eye movements. A break is usually seen in the retina, and pigment cells are present in the vitreous.)

Work-up

1. History: Recent ocular surgery or trauma? Known eye or medical problem?
2. Slit-lamp examination: Check for the presence of a filtering bleb and perform a Seidel test to rule out a wound leak, see Appendix 4.
3. Gonioscopy of the anterior-chamber angle: Look for a cyclodialysis cleft.
4. Dilated retinal examination: Determine whether there is subretinal fluid, indicating a concomitant retinal detachment, and whether an underlying choroidal disease or tumor is present. Examination of the fellow eye may be helpful in diagnosis.
5. In cases suspicious for melanoma, B-scan ultrasonography and transillumination of the globe are helpful.
6. Check the skin for vitiligo and the head for alopecia (VKH).

Treatment

A. General treatment
  1. Cycloplegic (e.g., atropine 1% tid).
  2. Topical steroid (e.g., prednisolone acetate 1% 4-6×/day).
  3. Surgical drainage of the suprachoroidal fluid may be indicated for a flat or progressively shallow anterior chamber, particularly in the presence of inflammation (due to the risk of peripheral anterior synechiae),

corneal decompensation secondary to lens-cornea touch, or ''kissing'' choroidals (apposition of two lobules of detached choroid).

B. Specific treatment: Repair the underlying problem.

SEROUS

- Wound leak or leaky filtering bleb: Patch × 24 hours, suture the site, use cyanoacrylate glue, and/or place a bandage contact lens on the eye.
- Cyclodialysis cleft: Laser, diathermy, cryotherapy, or suture the cleft to close it.
- Uveitis: Topical cycloplegic and steroid as above.
- Inflammatory disease (See the specific entity elsewhere in this book.)
- Retinal detachment: Surgical repair.

HEMORRHAGIC

An anterior vitrectomy and drainage of the choroidal detachment is performed for severe cases with vitreous to the wound. Otherwise treat as in (A).

Follow-up   In accordance with the underlying problem.

12.22   Vitreous Hemorrhage

Symptoms   Sudden painless loss of vision or sudden appearance of black spots with flashing lights.

Critical Signs   In a severe vitreous hemorrhage the red fundus reflex may be absent and there may be no fundus view on ophthalmoscopy. Red blood cells can sometimes be appreciated when a slit lamp is focused posterior to the lens. In a mild vitreous hemorrhage, blood may be seen to obscure part of the retina and retinal vessels.

Other Signs   A mild afferent pupillary defect. Depending on the etiology, there may be other fundus abnormalities.

Etiology

- Diabetic retinopathy   (Almost always have a known history of diabetes and usually one of diabetic retinopathy. Diabetic retinopathy is usually evident in the fellow eye.)
- Retinal break   (Commonly superior in cases of dense vitreous hemorrhage.)

- Retinal detachment (May be diagnosed by ultrasound if the retina cannot be viewed on clinical examination.)
- Retinal vein occlusion (usually a branch retinal vein occlusion) (Commonly in older patients with a history of high blood pressure. May have a history of a vein occlusion or sudden visual loss in the eye months to years previously.)
- Posterior vitreous detachment (Common in middle-aged to elderly patients. Usually patients note floaters and flashing lights.)
- Age-related macular degeneration (ARMD) (Patients often acknowledge poor vision prior to the vitreous hemorrhage due to their underlying disease. Macular drusen and/or other findings of ARMD are found in the fellow eye.)
- Sickle-cell disease (particularly SC disease) (Black patients. May have peripheral retinal neovascularization in the fellow eye, typically in a "sea-fan" configuration.)
- Trauma (By history)
- Intraocular tumor (May be visible on ophthalmoscopy or B-scan ultrasonography.)
- Subarachnoid or subdural hemorrhage (Terson's syndrome) (Frequently bilateral preretinal or vitreous hemorrhages may occur. A severe headache usually precedes the fundus findings. Coma may occur.)
- Eales' disease (A disease usually of men 20-30 years of age with peripheral retinal ischemia and neovascularization of unknown etiology. Decreased vision due to vitreous hemorrhage is frequently the presenting sign. The disease is often bilateral and is a diagnosis of exclusion.)
- Others (Coats' disease, retinopathy of prematurity, retinal angiomas of von Hippel-Lindau, congenital prepapillary vascular loop, hypertension, radiation retinopathy, anterior segment hemorrhage due to an intraocular lens, bleeding diathesis, etc.)

Differential Diagnosis

- Vitritis (*white* blood cells in the vitreous) (The onset is rarely as sudden; anterior or posterior uveitis may also be present. No red blood cells and no hemorrhage in the vitreous are present.)
- Retinal detachment (May occur without a vitreous hemorrhage, yet the symptoms may be identical. The fundus view may be difficult in a highly elevated detachment; however, the retina can usually be viewed with an indirect ophthalmoscope. In cases of highly elevated detachments, slit-lamp examination may show the retina behind the lens.)

Work-up

1. History: Any ocular or systemic diseases, specifically the ones mentioned above? Trauma?

2. Complete ocular examination, including a slit-lamp examination to check for iris neovascularization, an intraocular pressure measurement, and a dilated fundus examination of *both eyes* using indirect ophthalmoscopy. In cases of spontaneous vitreous hemorrhage, scleral depression is performed if a retinal view can be obtained (we do not generally depress eyes until 3-4 weeks after traumatic hemorrhages.)
3. When no retinal view can be obtained, a B-scan ultrasound is performed to detect an associated retinal detachment or intraocular tumor.
4. A fluorescein angiogram may aid in defining the etiology (although the quality of the angiogram may depend on the density of the hemorrhage).

Treatment

1. If the etiology of the vitreous hemorrhage is not known and a retinal break and/or a retinal detachment cannot be ruled out (e.g., there is no known history of one of the diseases mentioned above, there are no changes in the fellow eye, and the fundus is obscured by a total vitreous hemorrhage), the patient is admitted to the hospital. Others are treated as outpatients.
2. Bed rest with the head of the bed elevated (and sometimes bilateral patching) for 2-3 days (this reduces the chance of recurrent bleeding and allows the blood to settle inferiorly, permitting a view of the superior peripheral fundus, a common site for responsible retinal breaks).
3. Eliminate aspirin, nonsteroidal antiinflammatory drugs, and other anti-clotting agents unless they are medically necessary.
4. The underlying etiology is treated as soon as possible—e.g., retinal breaks are sealed with cryotherapy or laser photocoagulation, detached retinas are repaired, and proliferative retinal vascular diseases are treated with laser photocoagulation (or cryotherapy when there is no retinal view).
5. Surgical removal of the blood (vitrectomy) is usually performed for:
   a. Vitreous hemorrhage accompanied by retinal detachment.
   b. Chronic vitreous hemorrhage (greater than 6 months' duration).
   c. Vitreous hemorrhage with neovascularization of the iris.
   d. Hemolytic glaucoma.

NOTE Vitrectomy for isolated vitreous hemorrhage (e.g., without retinal detachment) may be considered earlier than 6 months for diabetics or those patients with bilateral vitreous hemorrhage.

Follow-up

Inpatient The patient is evaluated daily for the first 2-3 days. If a total vitreous hemorrhage persists and the etiology remains unknown, the patient is discharged and followed with a B-scan ultrasound every 1-3 weeks to rule out a retinal detachment.

Outpatient   Follow-up in 1-3 days. Monitor the treatment of the underlying problem.

12.23   Sickle-Cell Disease

(Sickle-Cell Hemoglobin C Disease, Sickle-Cell Thalassemia, Sickle-Cell Anemia, and Sickle-Cell Trait)

Symptoms   Usually without ocular symptoms. May have floaters, flashing lights, or loss of vision with advanced disease. Systemically, patients with sickle-cell anemia often have painful crises with severe abdominal or musculoskeletal discomfort. Patients are black or of Mediterranean extraction in most cases.

Critical Signs   Peripheral retinal neovascularization in the shape of a fan ("sea-fan" sign), sclerosed peripheral retinal vessels, or an abnormal dull gray peripheral fundus background color (due to peripheral arteriolar occlusions and ischemia).

Other Signs   Tortuosity of retinal veins, black mid-peripheral fundus lesions with spiculated borders (black sunbursts), intraretinal and subretinal hemorrhages ("salmon patch"), refractile (iridescent) deposits, angioid streaks, "comma-shaped" capillaries of the conjunctiva (especially along the inferior fornix). Vitreous hemorrhage and traction bands, retinal detachment, central retinal artery occlusion, and macular arteriolar occlusions may develop.

NOTE   Proliferative sickle cell retinopathy is thought to progress from peripheral arteriolar occlusions (stage 1) to peripheral arteriovenous anastomoses (stage 2) to retinal neovascularization (stage 3). The retinal neovascularization may spontaneously regress or may produce vitreous hemorrhage (stage 4) or traction retinal detachment (stage 5).

Differential Diagnosis   (Other causes of peripheral retinal neovascularization.)

- Sarcoidosis   (May also produce peripheral "sea-fan" neovascularization in young black individuals. However, granulomatous uveitis, vitritis with vitreous opacities, and sheathing of retinal vessels are often present.)
- Diabetes   (Tends to have a more posterior retinal location, dot/blot hemorrhages, and an elevated blood sugar.)

- Branch retinal vein occlusion   (Flame-shaped hemorrhages involving a sector or half of the retina—the inferior or superior half; the hemorrhages do not cross the horizontal raphé. May only see a sclerosed, arteriole in late cases.)
- Embolic (e.g., talc) retinopathy   (History of intravenous drug abuse. May see refractile talc particles in the macular arterioles.)
- Eales' disease   (Peripheral retinal vascular occlusion of unknown etiology; a diagnosis of exclusion.)
- Others   (Retinopathy of prematurity, familial exudative vitreoretinopathy, chronic myelogenous leukemia, radiation retinopathy, pars planitis, carotid-cavernous fistula, and collagen vascular disease)

Work-up

1. Past medical history and family history: Sickle-cell disease, diabetes, or known medical problem? Intravenous drug abuse?
2. Dilated fundus examination using indirect ophthalmoscopy.
3. Sickle-cell prep and hemoglobin electrophoresis (patients with sickle-cell trait, as well as hemoglobin C disease, may have a negative sickle-cell prep).
4. Consider fluorescein angiography to aid in diagnostic and therapeutic considerations.

Treatment   There are no well-established indications or guidelines for treatment at this time. The presence of vitreous hemorrhage or retinal detachment, however, typically warrants treatment. Laser photocoagulation or retinal surgery is usually used.

Follow-up

- No retinal pathology present: Repeat dilated fundus examination yearly.
- Retinal pathology present: Repeat dilated fundus examination every 1-6 months, depending upon the degree of pathology.

12.24   Retinitis Pigmentosa (RP)

Symptoms   Difficulty with night vision (often night blindness) and loss of peripheral vision are most common. Rarely, poor central vision or difficulty with color vision occur. Often relatives have the same problem.

Critical Signs   Classically, clumps of pigment dispersed throughout the peripheral retina in a perivascular pattern, often assuming a "bone spicule" arrangement, areas of depigmentation or atrophy of the retinal pigment epithelium (RPE), narrowing of arterioles, vitreous cells and, later, optic-disc pallor. The diagnosis is confirmed by finding an abnormal or nonrecordable electroretinogram (ERG) and progressive visual field loss (initially the visual field defect is in the form of a ring scotoma).

Other Signs   "Salt and pepper" appearance to the retina, focal or sectorial pigment clumping, visual deterioration, cystoid macular edema, epiretinal membrane, posterior subcapsular cataract.

Inheritance   May be autosomal recessive, autosomal dominant, x-linked recessive, or simplex (only one affected member in the pedigree).

Systemic Diseases Associated with Hereditary Retinal Degeneration   There are many systemic diseases and syndromes associated with RP. The following is a short list of conditions which should be considered when evaluating an RP patient, as treatment may be beneficial.

- Refsum's disease   (Autosomal recessive RP+ increased serum phytanic acid level. May have ataxia, progressive weakness of distal extremities, deafness, dry skin, anosmia, or progressive restriction of ocular motility.)
- Hereditary abetalipoproteinemia (Bassen-Kornzweig syndrome)   (RP + fat intolerance, diarrhea, crenated erythrocytes [acanthocytes], ataxia, progressive restriction of ocular motility and other neurologic symptoms due to deficiency in lipoproteins and malabsorption of the fat-soluble vitamins A, D, E, and K.)
- Kearns-Sayre syndrome   (Autosomal recessive pigmentary degeneration of the retina [often "salt and pepper" in appearance] with normal arterioles, progressive limitation of ocular movement, ptosis, and later heart block. Ocular signs generally appear before age 20 years.)

Differential Diagnosis

A. *Disorders which produce a fundus picture similar to RP (pseudoretinitis pigmentosa)*
   - Phenothiazine toxicity   (Especially in patients taking greater than 800 mg/day of thioridazine.)
   - Syphilis   (Positive FTA-ABS, asymmetric visual fields, abnormal fundus appearance, may have a history of recurrent uveitis, no family history of RP; the ERG is generally preserved to some degree.)
   - Congenital rubella   (A "salt and pepper" fundus appearance may be accompanied by microphthalmos, cataract, deafness, a congenital heart

abnormality, or another systemic abnormality. The ERG is usually normal.)
- Following resolution of an exudative retinal detachment, often from toxemia of pregnancy or Harada's disease (The history is diagnostic.)
- Pigmented paravenous retinochoroidal atrophy (Paravenous localization of RPE degeneration and pigment deposition. No definite hereditary pattern. Variable visual fields and ERG. May be nonprogressive, but long-term follow-up is not available.)

B. *Disorders which produce night blindness*
- Gyrate atrophy (The fundus shows well-demarcated, scalloped areas of full thickness atrophy [white-yellow in appearance] with thin margins of pigment outlining the areas of atrophy; the changes extend from the periphery toward the macula. Patients have hyperornithinemia in their blood [often ten times normal levels], urine, aqueous humor, and cerebrospinal fluid. Abnormal or nonrecordable ERG, visual field defects, high myopia and cataracts are common. Autosomal recessive.)
- Choroideremia (Choroidal atrophy accompanies scattered small pigment granules, sparing the macula. "Bone spicules" are not seen. X-linked recessive.)
- Vitamin A deficiency (Usually acquired from malnutrition or surgical resection of the bowel, but may be inherited [familial carotinemia]. There is marked night blindness, numerous small, yellow-white, well-demarcated spots deep in the retina seen peripherally, dry eye and/or Bitot's spots [white lesions] on the conjunctiva.)
- Congenital stationary night blindness (Night blindness from birth, normal visual fields, may have a normal or abnormal fundus, not progressive.)

Work-up
1. Medical and ocular history pertaining to the diseases discussed above.
2. Drug history.
3. Family history (for diagnostic and counseling purposes).
4. Ophthalmoscopic examination.
5. Formal visual field testing (e.g., Goldmann).
6. ERG (may help distinguish stationary rod-cone dysfunction from RP, a progressive disease) and dark adaptation studies.
7. Fundus photographs.
8. FTA-ABS if the diagnosis is uncertain.
9. If the patient is a male and the type of inheritance is unknown, examine his mother and perform an ERG on her (women carriers of X-linked disease often have abnormal pigmentation in the mid-periphery and have abnormal dark adapted ERGs.)

10. If neurological abnormalities such as ataxia, polyneuropathy, deafness, or anosmia are present, obtain a fasting (at least 14 hours) serum phytanic acid level (rule out Refsum's disease).
11. If hereditary abetalipoproteinemia is suspected, obtain a serum cholesterol and triglyceride level (levels are low), a serum protein and lipoprotein electrophoresis (lipoprotein deficiency is detected), and peripheral blood smears (acanthocytosis is seen).
12. If Kearns-Sayre syndrome is suspected, the patient must be followed by a cardiologist with sequential electrocardiograms checking for a cardiac conduction abnormality.

Treatment/Follow-up   See ''Acquired Syphilis'' (Section 14.2), ''Gyrate Atrophy'' (Section 12.26), ''Choroideremia'' (Section 12.25), and ''Vitamin A Deficiency'' (Section 14.10) if these conditions are suspected. No effective treatment for retinitis pigmentosa is currently known. However, there may be an effective treatment of some of the systemic conditions mentioned above. All patients will benefit from genetic counseling and instruction on how to deal with their visual handicap. In advanced cases, low-vision aids and vocational rehabilitation are helpful.

REFSUM'S DISEASE

1. Place on a low–phytanic acid, low-phytol diet (minimize the amount of milk products, animal fats, and green leafy vegetables in the patient's diet).
2. Follow serum phytanic acid levels every 6 months.

HEREDITARY ABETALIPOPROTEINEMIA

1. Water-miscible vitamin A 10,000-15,000 IU po q day.
2. Vitamin E 200-300 IU/kg po q day.
3. Vitamin K 5 mg po every week.
4. Restrict dietary fat to 15 percent of caloric intake.
5. Biannual serum levels of vitamin A and E; yearly ERG, dark adaptometry, and prothrombin time; periodic nerve conduction studies.
6. Consider supplementing the patient's diet with zinc.

KEARNS-SAYRE SYNDROME

Refer the patient to a cardiologist for yearly electrocardiograms. Patients may need a pacemaker.

12.25 Choroideremia

Symptoms   Night blindness in males ages 4-30 years followed by insidious loss of peripheral vision. Decreased central vision occurs late in the disease. Females are carriers and asymptomatic.

Critical Signs

Males   Dispersed pigment granules throughout the fundus accompanied by atrophy of the choroid, sparing the macula. The choroidal vasculature is not well seen despite a light fundus background.

Females   Small scattered, square intraretinal pigment granules overlying choroidal atrophy, most marked in the mid-periphery.

Other Signs   Retinal arteriolar narrowing and optic atrophy can occur late in the process, constriction of visual fields, normal color vision, abnormal electroretinogram (ERG).

Inheritance   X-linked recessive.

Differential Diagnosis

- Retinitis pigmentosa   (No choroidal atrophy, may see "bone spicules" of pigment.)
- Gyrate atrophy   (Scalloped retinal pigment epithelial [RPE] and choriocapillaris atrophy, posterior subcapsular cataract, high myopia with astigmatism, hyperornithinemia. Autosomal recessive.)
- Albinism   (Blond fundus without RPE clumping; the choroidal vasculature is easily seen. Iris transillumination defects are present and the foveal reflex is absent.)
- Thioridazine (e.g., Mellaril) retinopathy   (Patients taking >800 mg/day of thioridazine.)

Work-up

1. History: Family history? Medications?
2. Dilated fundus examination of the patient and family members if possible.
3. Formal visual fields (e.g., Octopus or Humphrey).
4. ERG +/− dark adaptation studies.
5. Fluorescein angiogram (may be diagnostic).

Treatment   No effective treatment for this condition is currently available. The following may be helpful in management.

1. Darkly tinted sunglasses may ameliorate symptoms.
2. Genetic counseling.

12.26   Gyrate Atrophy

Symptoms   Decreased vision, night blindness.

Critical Signs   Multiple sharply defined areas of chorioretinal atrophy separated from each other by thin margins of pigment. The lesions begin in the mid-periphery in childhood and then coalesce to involve the entire fundus, sparing the fovea until late in the disease, usually in midlife. Ornithine levels are markedly elevated in all body fluids.

Other Signs   Posterior subcapsular cataract, high myopia, and astigmatism; optic-disc pallor, and narrowing of the retinal vessels appear later in the disease. Constriction of visual fields, and abnormal-to-nonrecordable electro-retinogram (ERG), electro-oculogram, and dark adaptation studies occur. Color vision typically remains relatively intact until late in the course. Carriers have normal fundi, but may have mild elevation of ornithine levels.

Inheritance   Autosomal recessive.

Differential Diagnosis   All of the following can be distinguished by the presence of normal ornithine levels.

- Paving stone degeneration   (Patches of chorioretinal atrophy limited to the retinal periphery, usually inferiorly.)
- Choroideremia   (Diffuse retinal pigment epithelial and choroidal atrophy spread throughout the fundus. X-linked recessive.)
- High myopia   (Chorioretinal atrophy most marked in the posterior pole, often with a staphyloma.)
- Thioridazine retinopathy   (Patient taking >800 mg/day of thioridazine.)

Work-up

1. Family history: Check for night blindness or severely decreased vision.
2. Dilated fundus examination.
3. Plasma ornithine and amino acid levels (expect ornithine to be 6-10 times its normal level).
4. Consider an ERG and fluorescein angiogram if the ornithine level is not markedly elevated.

Treatment

1. Supplemental vitamin B-6 (pyridoxine) (the dose is not currently established—can try 20 mg/day po initially and increase up to 500 mg/day po if there is no response).

NOTE   Only a small percentage of patients are vitamin B-6 responders.

2. Reduce dietary protein consumption and substitute artificially flavored solutions of essential amino acids without arginine.

Follow-up

- Frequent serum ornithine levels are obtained initially to determine the amount of supplemental vitamin B-6 and the degree to which dietary protein needs to be restricted. Serum ornithine levels between 0.15-0.20 mM are optimal. The frequency of blood tests may be reduced after the ornithine levels stabilize in this range.
- Serum ammonia levels are followed in patients restricting dietary arginine.

12.27   Cone Dystrophies

Symptoms   Slowly progressive bilateral visual loss, photophobia, and poor color vision. Vision is worse during the day than at night.

Critical Signs

   Early   Essentially a normal fundus examination (even with poor visual acuity). Abnormal cone function on the electroretinogram (ERG) (i.e., a reduced single-flash photopic response and a reduced flicker response).
   Late   "Bull's eye" macular appearance.

Other Signs   Nystagmus, temporal pallor of the optic disc, spotty pigment clumping in the macular area. Rarely, rod degeneration may ensue leading to a retinitis pigmentosa-like picture (i.e., a cone-rod degeneration, which may have an autosomal dominant inheritance pattern).

Differential Diagnosis

- Stargardt's disease/fundus flavimaculatus   (Bilateral visual loss in the first or second decades of life often precedes the fundus findings, normal night vision and peripheral visual fields, macular atrophy with accompanying yellow flecks may develop. A normal ERG is usually present in the early stage. Primarily autosomal recessive.)
- Chloroquine retinopathy   (May produce a "bull's eye" macular appearance and poor color vision. History of chloroquine/hydroxychloroquine use, no family history of cone degeneration, no nystagmus.)

- Congenital color blindness   (Normal visual acuity, onset at birth, not progressive.)
- Retinitis pigmentosa   (Night blindness and peripheral visual field loss are the first symptoms. Often peripheral retinal "bone spicules" are seen. Can be distinguished by dark-adaptation testing and an ERG.)
- Nonphysiologic visual loss   (Normal ophthalmoscopic examination, fluorescein angiogram, ERG, and electro-oculogram. Patients can often be tricked into seeing better by special testing).

Work-up

1. Family history.
2. Complete ophthalmic examination, including color plates and formal color testing (e.g., Farnsworth-Munsell 100 hue test).
3. Formal visual field test (e.g., Humphrey or Octopus).
4. ERG.
5. Fluorescein angiogram to help detect the "bull's eye" macular pattern.

Treatment   There is no proven cure for this disease. The following measures may be palliative:

1. Heavily tinted glasses or contact lenses may help maximize vision.
2. Miotic drops (e.g., pilocarpine ½-1% qid during the day) are occasionally tried to improve vision and reduce photophobia.
3. Genetic counseling.
4. Low-vision aids as needed.

Follow-up   Yearly.

12.28   Stargardt's Disease

(Fundus Flavimaculatus)

Symptoms   Usually bilateral decreased vision in childhood or young adulthood. In the early stages the decrease in vision is often out of proportion to the clinical ophthalmoscopic appearance.

Critical Signs   Any of the following may be present.

A. A relatively normal-appearing fundus except for a heavily pigmented retinal pigment epithelium (RPE).
B. Yellow or yellow-white flecklike deposits at the level of the RPE.
C. Atrophic macular degeneration: May have a "bull's eye" appearance due to atrophy of the RPE around a normal central core of RPE, a "beaten-metal appearance," pigment clumping, or marked geographic atrophy.

Other Signs Atrophy of the RPE just outside of the macula or in the mid-peripheral fundus, normal peripheral visual fields in most cases, and rarely an accompanying cone or rod dystrophy. The electroretinogram (ERG) is typically normal in the early stages, but may become abnormal late in the disease. The electro-oculogram (EOG) is usually normal.

Inheritance Usually autosomal recessive, rarely autosomal dominant.

Differential Diagnosis

• Fundus albipunctatus (Diffuse small, white, discrete dots most prominent in the mid-peripheral fundus and rarely present in the fovea, nonprogressive congenital night blindness, no atrophic macular degeneration nor pigmentary changes. Visual acuity and visual fields remain normal.)
• Retinitis punctata albescens (Similar clinical appearance to fundus albipunctatus, but visual acuity, visual field, and night blindness progressively worsen. A markedly abnormal ERG develops.)
• Drusen (Small yellow-white spots deep to the retina, sometimes calcified, and usually developing later in life. Fluorescein angiography helps distinguish: All drusen hyperfluoresce; whereas, some lesions of fundus flavimaculatus do and some lesions do not hyperfluoresce [and some areas without flecks show hyperfluorescence].)
• Cone or cone-rod dystrophy (May have a "bull's eye" macula, but have a significant color vision deficit and a characteristic ERG.)
• Chloroquine/hydroxychloroquine maculopathy (History of use of this medication. Dose-related.)
• Nonphysiologic visual loss (Normal ophthalmoscopic examination, fluorescein angiogram, ERG, and EOG. Patients can often be tricked into seeing better by special testing.)

Work-up Indicated when the diagnosis is uncertain or needs to be confirmed.

1. History: Age at onset, medications, family history?
2. Dilated retinal examination.
3. Fluorescein angiogram (often shows blockage of choroidal fluorescence producing a "silent choroid" or "midnight fundus").
4. ERG and EOG.

5. Formal visual field examination (e.g., Octopus or Humphrey).

Treatment   No known medical or surgical therapy is beneficial. The patient may benefit from low-vision aids, services dedicated to helping the visually handicapped, and genetic counseling.

12.29   Phenothiazine Toxicity

A. Thioridazine (e.g., Mellaril)

Symptoms   Blurred vision, brownish vision, difficulty with night vision.

Signs   Pigment clumps between the posterior pole and the equator, areas of retinal depigmentation, retinal edema, visual field abnormalities (central scotoma and general constriction), depressed or extinguished electroretinogram (ERG).

NOTE   Symptoms and signs may occur within weeks of starting phenothiazine therapy, particularly if very large doses (e.g., >2000 mg/day) are taken.

Dosage Generally Required to Produce Toxicity   800 mg/day chronically.

Differential Diagnosis   (Pigment clumps in the retina.)

• Retinitis pigmentosa   (Positive family history, pale optic disc, narrowed arterioles.)
• Old syphilitic chorioretinopathy   (Positive FTA-ABS, may have a history of an acute visual problem.)
• Viral chorioretinitis   (Often associated with an anterior-chamber reaction, vitreous cells, and other ocular signs.)
• Trauma   (Usually unilateral, history of trauma.)

Treatment   Discontinue the medication.

Baseline Work-up   (For patients in whom long-term treatment is anticipated.)

1. Visual acuity.
2. Complete ophthalmoscopic examination.
3. Fundus photographs.
4. Visual field (preferably automated, e.g., Humphrey or Octopus).
5. Consider an ERG.

6. Color vision testing (preferably with a Farnsworth-Munsell 100 hue test).

Follow-up Every 6 months.

B. Chlorpromazine (e.g., Thorazine)

Symptoms Abnormal ocular and skin pigmentation as described in "signs" below.

Signs Abnormal pigmentation of the eyelids, cornea, conjunctiva (especially within the palpebral fissure), and anterior-lens capsule; anterior and posterior subcapsular cataract; rarely a pigmentary retinopathy with the visual field and ERG changes described for thioridazine.

Dosage Generally Required to Produce Toxicity 1200-2400 mg/day for over 12 months.

Treatment Discontinue the medication.

Baseline Work-up Same as for thioridazine.

Follow-up Every 6 months.

12.30 Chloroquine/Hydroxychloroquine Toxicity

Symptoms Decreased vision, abnormal color vision, difficulty adjusting to darkness.

Critical Signs "Bull's eye" macula (a ring of depigmentation surrounded by a ring of increased pigmentation), loss of the foveal reflex.

Other Signs Increased pigmentation in the macula, arteriolar narrowing, vascular sheathing, peripheral pigmentation, decreased color vision, visual field abnormalities (central, paracentral, or peripheral scotoma), abnormal electroretinogram (ERG) and electro-oculogram (EOG), and normal dark adaptation. Whorl-like corneal changes may also be observed.

Dosage Generally Required to Produce Toxicity

Chloroquine: >300 g total cumulative dose.
Hydroxychloroquine: >750 mg/day taken over months to years.
   (Some feel retinopathy will not develop if the daily dose is kept <4.4 mg/kg/day of chloroquine and 7.7 mg/kg/day of hydroxychloroquine.)

Differential Diagnosis   The following can produce a "bull's eye" macula.

- Cone dystrophy   (Positive family history, generally <30 years old, severe photophobia, abnormal to nonrecordable photopic ERG.)
- Stargardt's disease/fundus flavimaculatus   (Positive family history, generally <25 years old, may have white-yellow flecks in the posterior pole and mid-periphery.)
- Age-related macular degeneration   (Drusen, +/− pigment clumping and atrophy, +/− detachment of the retinal pigment epithelium or sensory retina.)
- Spielmeyer-Vogt syndrome   (Retinitis pigmentosa, seizures, ataxia, and progressive dementia.)

Treatment   Discontinue the medication if signs of toxicity develop.

Baseline Work-up   (For patients in whom long-term treatment is anticipated.)

1. Visual acuity.
2. Ophthalmoscopic examination.
3. Posterior pole fundus photographs.
4. Visual field, preferably automated (e.g., Humphrey or Octopus).
5. Color vision testing (preferably Farnsworth-Munsell 100 hue test).

Follow-up   Every 6 months.

NOTE   Once ocular toxicity develops, it usually does not regress even if the drug is withdrawn. In fact, new toxic effects may develop and old ones may progress even after the chloroquine/hydroxychloroquine has been discontinued.

12.31   Best's Disease

(Vitelliform Macular Dystrophy)

Symptoms   Decreased vision or asymptomatic. Onset in childhood, but may not be detected until years later.

Critical Signs Yellow, round, subretinal lesion(s) likened to an "egg yolk." Typically bilateral and located in the fovea, measuring approximately one to two disc areas in size. Normal electroretinogram (ERG); abnormal electro-oculogram (EOG).

Other Signs The lesions may degenerate and macular choroidal (subretinal) neovascularization, hemorrhage, and scarring may develop. In the scar stage it may be indistinguishable from age-related macular degeneration.

Inheritance Autosomal dominant with variable penetrance and expressivity. Carriers may have normal fundi, but have an abnormal EOG.

Work-up
1. Family history (often helpful to examine family members).
2. Complete ocular examination, including a dilated retinal examination, carefully inspecting the macula with a slit lamp and a fundus contact, Hruby, or 60 or 90 diopter lens.
3. EOG to confirm the diagnosis or to detect the carrier state of the disease.
4. Consider a fluorescein angiogram to confirm the presence of or delineate a choroidal neovascular membrane.

Treatment There is no effective treatment for the underlying disease. Choroidal neovascularization may need to be treated by laser photocoagulation.

Follow-up Patients with treatable choroidal neovascular membranes should be attended to promptly. Otherwise there is no urgency in seeing patients with this disease. Patients are given an Amsler grid (see Appendix 3), instructed on its use, and told to return immediately if a change is noted.

NOTE An adult form of vitelliform macular dystrophy (a "pattern dystrophy") has been described. The "egg yolk" lesions usually appear from age 30-50 years, the disease is dominantly inherited, and the EOG may or may not be abnormal. There is also no effective treatment for this entity.

13

Uveitis

13.1 Anterior Uveitis

(Iritis / Iridocyclitis)

Symptoms

> *Acute*   Pain, red eye, photophobia, mild decreased vision, tearing.
> *Chronic*   Recurrent episodes, fewer or none of the above symptoms.

Critical Signs   Cells and flare in the anterior chamber.

Differentiating Signs

> *Nongranulomatous*   Fine keratic precipitates (KP) (white cells on the corneal endothelium).
> *Granulomatous*   Large "mutton-fat" KP, Koeppe nodules (clusters of cells on the pupillary border), Busacca nodules (clusters of cells on the anterior iris surface).

Other Signs   Cells in the anterior vitreous (spillover), posterior synechiae (adhesions of the iris to the lens), miosis, low intraocular pressure (IOP) (but occasionally elevated), injection of the perilimbal blood vessels, hypopyon (layering of white cells in the anterior chamber) if severe, cystoid macular edema if chronic, occasionally a cataract.

NOTE Patients will often complain of increased pain in the involved eye when light is shined in the uninvolved eye.

Etiology

ACUTE, NONGRANULOMATOUS

- Trauma (see "Traumatic Iritis," Section 3.7.)
- Ankylosing spondylitis (Young adult males, often with low back pain, abnormal sacroiliac spine x-rays, elevated ESR, [+] HLA B27.)
- Inflammatory bowel disease (Chronic intermittent diarrhea often alternating with constipation.)
- Reiter's syndrome (Young adult males, conjunctivitis, urethritis, polyarthritis, occasionally keratitis, elevated ESR, [+] HLA B27, may have recurrent episodes.)
- Psoriatic arthritis (Iritis is not associated with psoriasis without arthritis.)
- Glaucomatocyclitic crisis (Recurrent episodes of acute [IOP] rise, open angle on gonioscopy, corneal edema, fine KP, fixed mid-dilated pupil and mild iritis.)
- Lens-induced uveitis (Often after incomplete extracapsular cataract extraction or trauma damaging the lens capsule; may also be secondary to a hypermature cataract.)
- Herpes simplex/herpes zoster/varicella (Usually with a dendritic keratitis, occasionally skin vesicles, glaucoma, iris atrophy.)
- Postoperative iritis (An anterior-chamber reaction is expected after intraocular surgery. Severe reactions with excessive pain, however, must make one consider endophthalmitis. See "Postoperative Uveitis," Section 13.9.)
- UGH syndrome (uveitis-glaucoma-hyphema) (Usually secondary to irritation from an intraocular lens.)
- Behçet's disease (Young adults, acute hypopyon iritis, aphthous mouth ulcers, genital ulcerations, erythema nodosum, [+] Behçet's skin puncture test if active systemic disease is present, occasionally retinal vasculitis and hemorrhages, may have recurrent episodes.)
- Lyme disease (Often a history of a tick bite. May have a skin rash and/ or arthritis.)
- Mumps, influenza, adenovirus, measles, chlamydia (Rare causes of transient anterior uveitis.)
- Other rare causes of anterior uveitis (e.g., tight contact lens, Leptosporosis, Kawasaki's disease, rickettsial disease.)

CHRONIC, USUALLY NONGRANULOMATOUS

- Juvenile rheumatoid arthritis (JRA)   (Usually young girls, eye may be white and without pain, often bilateral, iritis can occur before the arthritis, pauciarticular arthritis [fewer than 5 joints involved], [+] ANA, [−] rheumatoid factor, elevated ESR, occasionally fever and lymphadenopathy.)
- Chronic iridocyclitis of children   (Usually young girls, same as JRA except no arthritis.)
- Fuchs' heterochromic iridocyclitis   (Usually unilateral, few symptoms, diffuse iris stromal atrophy often causing a lighter colored iris, iris transillumination defects, blunting of the iris architecture, fine KP over the *entire* corneal endothelium, mild anterior-chamber reaction, few if any posterior synechiae. Vitreous opacities, glaucoma, and cataracts are common.)

CHRONIC, USUALLY GRANULOMATOUS

- Sarcoidosis   (Usually blacks, usually bilateral, may have dense posterior synechiae, conjunctival nodules, or signs of posterior uveitis [see Section 13.2]. Mild-to-moderate anergy, an abnormal chest x-ray, a [+] gallium scan, and an elevated serum angiotensin converting enzyme [ACE] are common.)
- Syphilis   (May have a maculopapular rash [often on the palms and soles], iris roseola [vascular papules on the iris], and interstitial keratitis with ghost vessels in late stages. A [+] VDRL or RPR and [+] FTA-ABS are usually present.)
- Tuberculosis   ([+]PPD, typical chest x-ray, occasionally phlyctenular keratitis and sometimes signs of posterior uveitis [see Section 13.2].)
- Others   (Rare, e.g., leprosy, brucellosis.)

Differential Diagnosis   The following may be associated with an anterior-chamber reaction.

- Rhegmatogenous retinal detachment   (Elevated retina with a retinal break, pigment cells in the vitreous or anterior chamber.)
- Posterior segment tumor (e.g., retinoblastoma or leukemia in children, malignant melanoma in adults)
- Juvenile xanthogranuloma   (Age <15 years, often with a spontaneous hyphema, yellow-gray poorly demarcated iris nodules, and slightly raised orange skin lesions.)
- Intraocular foreign body
- Sclerouveitis   (Uveitis secondary to scleritis.)

Work-up

1. Obtain a history attempting to define the etiology.

2. Complete ocular examination, including an IOP check and a dilated fundus examination. The vitreous should be evaluated for cells (see Appendix 9 for the technique).

If a unilateral, nongranulomatous uveitis develops for the first time *and* the history and examination are unremarkable, no further work-up is pursued.

If the uveitis is bilateral, granulomatous, *or* recurrent and the history and examination are unremarkable then a nonspecific initial work-up is conducted:

3. CBC
4. ESR
5. ANA
6. RPR or VDRL
7. FTA-ABS or MHA-TP
8. PPD and anergy panel
9. Chest x-ray (especially ruling out sarcoidosis and tuberculosis)
10. In endemic areas, a Lyme titer is recommended (see below)

If the history, symptoms, and/or signs point strongly to a certain etiology then the work-up should be tailored accordingly:

- Ankylosing spondylitis: Sacroiliac spine x-rays (show sclerosis and narrowing of the joint spaces), ESR, and sometimes an HLA B27.
- Inflammatory bowel disease: Medicine or GI consult, consider an HLA B27.
- Reiter's syndrome: Conjunctival, urethral, and prostatic cultures if indicated; joint x-rays if arthritis is present; a medicine or rheumatology consult; consider an HLA B27.
- Psoriatic arthritis: A rheumatology or dermatology consult, consider an HLA B27.
- Glaucomatocyclitic crisis: Diagnosed clinically.
- Lens-induced uveitis: Diagnosed clinically. See "Phacoanaphylactic Endophthalmitis" (Section 13.14), "Phacolytic Glaucoma" (Section 10.8), and "Lens-Particle Glaucoma" (Section 10.9).
- Herpes: Diagnosed clinically.
- UGH: Diagnosed clinically.
- Behçet's disease: Behçet's skin puncture test (if a blister develops minutes to hours after puncturing the skin intradermally with a sterile 25- to 30-gauge needle, a positive test is noted), a medicine or rheumatology consult, consider an HLA B27 or HLA B5.
- Lyme disease: Lyme immunofluorescent assay or enzyme-linked immunosorbent assay.

- JRA: ANA, rheumatoid factor, x-rays of arthritic joints (if no arthritic symptoms are present then x-rays of the knees are obtained), and a pediatric or rheumatology consult.
- Chronic iridocyclitis of children: Same as JRA.
- Fuchs' heterochromic iridocyclitis: Diagnosed clinically.
- Sarcoidosis: Chest x-ray, angiotensin converting enzyme (ACE), $+/-$ scrum lysozyme, PPD and anergy panel, and gallium scan of the head and neck; consider a biopsy of any skin or conjunctival nodule for pathological diagnosis—see "Sarcoidosis," Section 13.4. (NOTE The ACE and gallium scan may give false negative results if the patient is on systemic steroids.)
- Syphilis: RPR or VDRL, FTA-ABS or MHA-TP.
- Tuberculosis: PPD and anergy panel, chest x-ray, referral to a medical specialist.

Treatment

1. Cycloplegic (e.g., cyclopentolate 1-2% tid for mild-to-moderate inflammation; scopolamine ¼% or atropine 1% tid for moderate-to-severe inflammation).
2. Topical steroid (e.g., prednisolone acetate 1% q 1-6 hours depending on the severity).

    If the anterior uveitis is severe and not responding well to frequent topical steroids, then consider periocular repository steroids (e.g., methylprednisolone 40-80 mg subtenons). Before injecting depot steroids periocularly, it is wise to use topical steroids at full strength for 6 weeks to make certain that the patient is not a steroid responder, i.e., develops a significant IOP rise secondary to steroids. See Appendix 8 describing the technique of a subtenons injection.

    If there is no improvement on maximal topical and repository steroids then consider systemic steroids or lastly systemic immunosuppressive agents. A medicine or rheumatology consult is often advisable when systemic therapy is to be instituted. See Appendix 5 for a systemic steroid work-up.

3. Treat secondary glaucoma. Glaucoma may result from:
    a. A severe inflammatory reaction with cellular blockage of the trabecular meshwork. See "Inflammatory Open-Angle Glaucoma," Section 10.4.
    b. Synechiae formation giving rise to secondary angle-closure. See "Acute Angle-Closure Glaucoma," Section 10.10.
    c. Neovascularization of the iris producing blockage of the trabecular meshwork or closure of the angle. See "Neovascular Glaucoma," Section 10.13.

d. A response to steroids. See "Steroid Response/Glaucoma," Section 10.5.
4. If an exact etiology for the anterior uveitis is determined then the specific management outlined below should be added to the above treatment:

Ankylosing spondylitis   Often requires systemic antiinflammatory agents (e.g., aspirin, indomethacin etc.). Consider consulting cardiology (there is a high incidence of heart block and aortic insufficiency), rheumatology, and physical therapy.

Inflammatory bowel disease   Often benefits from systemic steroids and/or sulfadiazine and supplemental vitamin A. Consider a medicine or GI consult.

Reiter's syndrome   If urethritis is present then the patient and sexual partners are treated (e.g., tetracycline 250-500 mg qid, doxycycline 100 mg bid, or erythromycin 250-500 mg qid for 3-4 weeks). Consult medicine, rheumatology and/or physical therapy.

Psoriatic arthritis   Consider a rheumatology consult.

Glaucomatocyclitic crisis   See Section 10.12.

Lens-induced uveitis   Usually requires removal of lens material, see "Phacoanaphylactic Endophthalmitis" (Section 13.14), "Phacolytic Glaucoma" (Section 10.8), and "Lens-Particle Glaucoma" (Section 10.9).

Herpes uveitis   See "Herpes Simplex Virus" (Section 4.15) or "Herpes Zoster Virus" (Section 4.16).

UGH   See "Postoperative Glaucoma," Section 10.15.

Behçet's disease   Often needs systemic steroids or immunosuppressive agents (responds well to chlorambucil); consider a medicine or rheumatology consult.

Lyme disease   See Section 14.4.

JRA   The steroid dosage is adjusted according to the degree of cells, not flare, present in the anterior chamber; chronic cycloplegic therapy (e.g., tropicamide 0.5% qhs) may be required. A rheumatology or pediatric consult for possible aspirin or systemic steroid therapy is usually obtained. NOTE   There is a high complication rate with cataract surgery.

Chronic iridocyclitis of children   Same as JRA.

Fuchs' heterochromic iridocyclitis   Usually does not respond to nor require steroids (a trial of steroids may be attempted, but they should be tapered quickly if there is no response); cycloplegics are rarely necessary. NOTE   Patients usually do well with cataract surgery.

Sarcoidosis   Often needs periocular and systemic steroids; a medicine or pulmonary consult is advisable for systemic evaluation, see Section 13.4.

Syphilis   See "Acquired Syphilis" (Section 14.2) or "Congenital Syphilis" (Section 14.3).

Tuberculosis   Referral to an internist for consideration of systemic antituberculous treatment.

Follow-up Every 1-7 days in the acute phase depending on the severity; every 1-6 months chronically when stable. At each visit, the anterior-chamber reaction and IOP should be evaluated. A vitreous and fundus examination should be performed for all flare-ups, when vision is affected, or every 3-6 months. If the anterior-chamber reaction is improving then the steroid drops can be slowly tapered (usually 1 drop per day every 3-7 days, e.g., qid for 1 week, then tid for 1 week, then bid for 1 week, etc.) Steroids are usually stopped once all cells have disappeared from the anterior chamber (flare is often still present). Rarely, chronic low-dose steroids every day or every other day are required to keep the inflammation from recurring. The cycloplegic agents can also be tapered as the anterior-chamber reaction improves. Slow tapering is advised for granulomatous reactions due to a higher tendency to form posterior synechiae. Cycloplegics should be used at least qhs until the anterior chamber is free of cells.

NOTE   As with most ocular and systemic diseases requiring steroid therapy, the steroid (be it topical or systemic) should never be stopped abruptly. Sudden discontinuation of steroids can lead to severe rebound inflammation.

13.2   Posterior Uveitis

Symptoms   Blurred vision, floaters, occasionally redness, pain, and photophobia.

Critical Signs   White blood cells and opacities in the vitreous (vitritis), retinal or choroidal infiltrates, edema, or vascular sheathing.

Other Signs   Disc swelling, retinal hemorrhages or exudates, or signs of anterior-segment inflammation (e.g., aqueous cells and flare, posterior synechiae) may be present. Glaucoma, cataract, choroidal (subretinal) neovascularization, or retinal detachment may develop.

Etiology

A. More common
   • Toxoplasmosis   (A yellow-white fuzzy retinal lesion, commonly in the posterior pole. It may be difficult to view due to a severe accompanying vitritis. A chorioretinal scar is frequently seen adjacent to the acute active lesion. A negative antitoxoplasma antibody titer [undiluted] in an immunocompetent host usually rules out toxoplasmosis.)

- Sarcoidosis   (White-yellow exudates or sheathing around retinal veins, retinal or vitreous white nodules, and other retinal or choroidal abnormalities may be present. Vitritis and granulomatous uveitis are common. Patients are typically black and often have pulmonary, skin, CNS, or other systemic involvement. An elevated angiotensin converting enzyme [ACE] level is often present.)
- Syphilis   (Produces an acute chorioretinitis and vitritis which may mimic almost any other condition. A concomitant skin rash on the palms and/ or soles may be present. Retinal pigment clumping, sometimes similar to retinitis pigmentosa, may later occur. Congenital syphilis typically produces a ''salt and pepper''-appearing fundus. [+] FTA-ABS.)
- Pars planitis   (Considered an ''intermediate uveitis.'' Usually a bilateral vitritis in patients age 15-40 years with white exudative material covering the inferior ora serrata and pars plana. Cellular clumps in the vitreous [appearing as ''snowballs''] and peripheral vascular sheathing may be present.)
- Ocular histoplasmosis   (Common in the Ohio-Mississippi River Valley area. Yellow-white choroidal spots, usually less than 1 mm in diameter, macular degenerative changes, sometimes with choroidal neovascularization, and peripapillary atrophy or scarring is seen. Minimal-to-no vitreous nor aqueous cells are seen.)

B. Following surgery or trauma: See ''Postoperative Uveitis'' (Section 13.9), ''Postoperative Endophthalmitis'' (Section 13.10), ''Traumatic Endophthalmitis'' (Section 13.11), and ''Sympathetic Ophthalmia'' (Section 13.15).

C. Immunocompromised host (e.g., AIDS, patients being treated with chemotherapy, etc.)
- Cytomegalovirus (CMV)   (Yellow-white patches of necrotic retina are mixed with retinal hemorrhage. Also seen in neonates. See ''Acquired Immune Deficiency Syndrome,'' Section 14.1.)
- Candida   (Seen also in hospitalized patients being treated with prolonged antibiotic therapy, IV drug abusers, and patients with long-standing catheters. Yellow-white fluffy retinal or preretinal lesions are found initially. Later, associated ''cotton balls'' in the vitreous develop. Candida may be cultured from the blood, urine, or an IV site.)
- Endogenous endophthalmitis   (Patients are typically septic, and many have an anterior-chamber reaction or hypopyon in addition to the vitritis.)
- Others (e.g., herpes simplex, varicella-zoster, fungi, mycobacteria)

D. Less common
- Acute posterior multifocal placoid pigment epitheliopathy (AMPPE) (Acute visual loss, typically in young adults, sometimes following a viral illness. Multiple creamy white subretinal lesions with indistinct margins approximately ½ disc diameter in size are usually found in the posterior pole of both eyes. Vitreous cells, disc edema, serous retinal detachment, and rarely CNS signs may be present. Vision usually returns to normal in 2-6 weeks.)

- Acute retinal necrosis (Unilateral or bilateral multiple opaque white patches of thickened retina with vascular sheathing, usually in the retinal periphery. The patches of necrotic retina gradually enlarge and coalesce. Vitreous cells are abundant. May have a retinal detachment.)
- Acute retinal pigment epitheliitis (Krill's disease) (Young adults with sudden visual loss. Gray spots are seen at the level of the retinal pigment epithelium in the macula, each of which is surrounded by a lighter-colored halo. The spots occur in 2-4 distinct clusters. The condition may be unilateral or bilateral. It resolves in 6-12 weeks without treatment.)
- Behçet's disease (Usually a bilateral ocular disease of young adult males. Retinal and optic-disc edema, vascular sheathing, and occasionally hemorrhages or exudate may accompany a vitritis and anterior uveitis, sometimes with a hypopyon. The eye is typically not red. Recurrent oral and/or genital ulcers, erythema nodosum, or arthritis may be noted. See "Anterior Uveitis," Section 13.1.)
- Birdshot (vitiliginous) retinochoroidopathy (Usually middle-aged adults with bilateral multiple creamy-yellow spots deep to the retina, approximately 1 mm in diameter, scattered around the equator of the fundus. With time, the spots coalesce and spread to the macula. Vitreous cells are more abundant than aqueous cells. Retinal and/or optic nerve edema may be present. [+] HLA A29 in most patients. Visual loss appears to be irreversible.)
- Diffuse unilateral subacute neuroretinitis (Unilateral visual loss in children and young adults, thought to be due to a nematode. Optic-nerve swelling, vitreous cells, and deep gray-white retinal lesions are present initially. Later, optic atrophy, narrowing of retinal vessels, and atrophic pigment epithelial changes develop. Vision and visual fields deteriorate with time.)
- Embolic retinitis (Sudden onset of decreased vision in a systemically ill patient. Retinal edema, vascular sheathing, and hemorrhages with white centers [Roth spots] may be accompanied by vitreous cells. Diseased heart valves are common sources.)
- Lyme disease (Produces varied forms of posterior uveitis. More common in the New England and Middle Atlantic states, particularly in patients who spend time camping outdoors. A history of a tick bite, skin rash, Bell's palsy, or arthritis may be elicited.)
- Multiple evanescent white-dot syndrome (Acute unilateral visual loss, often following a viral illness usually in young women. Multiple creamy white-colored lesions at the level of the retinal pigment epithelium are accompanied by a granularity of the fovea. There are few vitreous cells and occasional sheathing of retinal vessels. There is often an enlarged blind spot on formal visual field testing. Vision typically returns to normal within weeks without treatment.)
- Recurrent multifocal choroiditis (multifocal choroiditis with panuveitis) (Unilateral visual loss in young women [who often have bilateral fundus involvement]. Multiple, small, round, pale inflammatory lesions

at the level of the pigment epithelium and choriocapillaris are found
[similar to "histo-spots"], sometimes associated with choroidal neovascularization. Vitreous cells, mild disc edema, and, less commonly,
anterior-chamber cells and flare may be present. The lesions are predominantly in the macular area, frequently respond to oral or periocular
steroids, but typically recur. Myopia is common. Laser photocoagulation
may be considered in the presence of a choroidal neovascular membrane.)
- Rubella   (Usually seen in infants whose mother developed rubella during the pregnancy. "Salt and pepper" pigmentation of the retina is
typical. A small eye, cataract, or iris transillumination defects may be
present. The optic nerve may be pale. An elevated antirubella antibody
titer can usually be demonstrated.)
- Serpiginous choroidopathy   (Typically bilateral, recurrent chorioretinitis characterized by acute lesions [yellow-white subretinal patches with
indistinct margins] bordering old atrophic scars. The chorioretinal changes
usually extend from the optic disc outward. Patients are typically 30-60
years old. A choroidal neovascular membrane may develop, requiring
laser photocoagulation to prevent visual loss.)
- Toxocariasis   (Usually occurs in children, affecting only one eye. An
elevated white retinal lesion may be seen in the posterior pole or peripheral fundus. The peripheral lesion may be associated with a fibrous
band extending to the optic disc, sometimes dragging the macular vessels
away from their normal course. A severe vitritis and anterior uveitis
may be present. A negative undiluted toxocara titer in an immunocompetent host usually rules out this disease.)
- Tuberculosis   (Produces varied clinical manifestations. The diagnosis
is usually made by ancillary laboratory tests. Miliary tuberculosis may
produce multifocal small yellow-white choroidal lesions. Most patients
have concomitant anterior [granulomatous or nongranulomatous] uveitis.
A 2-week therapeutic trial of isoniazid 300 mg po q day + pyridoxine
[vitamin B-6] 10 mg/day may be given. If the uveitis is due to tuberculosis, it should improve significantly on this regimen.)
- Vogt-Koyanagi-Harada syndrome   (Exudative retinal detachment with
vitreous cells, a swollen optic disc, or atrophic patches at the level of
the retinal pigment epithelium may accompany an anterior-chamber reaction. Patients are darkly pigmented, typically of Asian or American
Indian ancestry, and have or develop systemic signs including meningeal
signs, vitiligo, alopecia, and poliosis.)
- Whipple's disease   (Rare. Small white vitreous opacities, retinal hemorrhages and exudates, or exudative material over the pars plana in a
patient with diarrhea, arthralgia, and weight loss. The diagnosis is made
by intestinal biopsy or, less commonly, pars plana vitrectomy.)
- Others   (Nocardia, Coccidioides, Aspergillus, Cryptococcus, menin-
gococcus, ophthalmomyiasis, onchocerciasis and cysticercosis [seen in
Africa, Central and South America], measles, Eales' disease, Crohn's

disease, multiple sclerosis, subacute sclerosing panencephalitis, and age-related vitritis.)

Differential Diagnosis (masquerade syndromes)

- Reticulum-cell sarcoma (large-cell lymphoma) (Persistent vitreous cells in patients greater than 50 years of age which usually do not respond completely to systemic steroids. Yellow-white subretinal infiltrates, retinal edema and hemorrhage, anterior-chamber inflammation, or neurologic signs may be present.)
- Malignant melanoma (A retinal detachment and associated vitritis may obscure the underlying tumor. B-scan ultrasound will usually detect the tumor in cases not detectable by indirect ophthalmoscopy.)
- Retinitis pigmentosa (Vitreous cells and macular edema may accompany "bone spicule" pigmentary changes and attenuated retinal vessels. Drusen of the optic disc may be mistaken for disc swelling. Electroretinography aids in diagnosis.)
- Rhegmatogenous retinal detachment (A small number of pigmented anterior vitreous cells and a mild anterior uveitis frequently accompany a rhegmatogenous retinal detachment.)
- Retained intraocular foreign body (Persistent inflammation following a penetrating ocular injury. May have iris heterochromia. Diagnosed by indirect ophthalmoscopy, B-scan ultrasound, or CT scan of the globe.)
- Posterior scleritis (May or may not have an accompanying anterior scleritis. Vitritis is accompanied by a subretinal mass and often an exudative retinal detachment. Chorioretinal folds may be seen. Fluorescein angiography and B-scan ultrasonography are helpful in diagnosis.)
- Retinoblastoma (Almost always occurs in young children. May present with a "pseudohypopyon" and vitreous cells. One or more elevated white retinal lesions is usually, but not always, present. A retinal detachment and/or iris neovascularization may be found. Fluorescein angiography, CT scan, and B-scan ultrasonography may aid in diagnosis.)
- Leukemia (Unilateral retinitis and vitritis may occur in patients already known to have leukemia.)
- Amyloidosis (Rare. Vitreous "globules" or "membranes" without any signs of anterior-segment inflammation. A serum protein electrophoresis and diagnostic vitrectomy confirm the diagnosis.)
- Asteroid hyalosis (Small white refractile particles adherent to and floating in the vitreous. Usually asymptomatic and of no clinical significance.)

Work-up

1. History: Systemic disease or infection, skin rash, IV drug abuse, indwelling catheter, risk factors for AIDS? Recent eye trauma or surgery? Travel to the Ohio-Mississippi River Valley, New England, or Middle Atlantic area? Tick bite?

2. Complete ocular examination, including an intraocular pressure measurement and careful ophthalmoscopic examination. Indirect ophthalmoscopy with scleral depression of the inferior ora seratta is essential.
3. Consider fluorescein angiography to help in diagnosis or plan for therapy.
4. Blood tests (any of the following are obtained, depending on the suspected diagnosis): Toxoplasma titer, ACE level, FTA-ABS, RPR, ESR, ANA, HLA B5 (Behçet's), HLA A29 (Birdshot), Toxocara titer, Lyme immunofluorescent assay or enzyme-linked immunosorbent assay, and in neonates or immunocompromised patients, titers for CMV, herpes simplex, varicella-zoster, or rubella virus. Cultures of blood (and IV sites) may be helpful when infectious etiologies are suspected.
5. PPD with anergy panel.
6. Chest x-ray.
7. Urine for CMV in immunocompromised patients.
8. CT scan of the brain and lumbar puncture when reticulum-cell sarcoma is suspected.
9. Diagnostic vitrectomy when appropriate (see individual sections).

See the individual sections for more specific guidelines for work-up and treatment.

13.3   Toxoplasmosis

Symptoms   Blurred vision, floaters, may have pain.

Critical Signs   Unilateral white-yellow retinal lesion associated with a hazy vitreous (due to vitreous cells). An old chorioretinal scar can often be seen adjacent to the new white-yellow lesion, but is not always present.

Other Signs   Vitreous precipitates on the posterior surface of the detached vitreous, vitreous debris, optic-disc swelling, mild granulomatous iritis, localized vasculitis, or retinal artery or vein occlusion in the area of the inflammation. Chorioretinal scars are occasionally found in the uninvolved eye. Large visual field loss may result from peripapillary toxoplasmosis. A choroidal (subretinal) neovascular membrane develops on rare occasions.

NOTE   Toxoplasmosis can also develop in the deep retina, in which case few to no vitreous cells may be present.

Differential Diagnosis   See "Posterior Uveitis," Section 13.2, for a complete list. The following may closely simulate toxoplasmosis.

- Syphilis (Positive FTA-ABS.)
- Tuberculosis (Positive PPD +/− chest x-ray. Rare.)
- Toxocariasis (Usually affects children. A fibrous band may be seen radiating from a white retinal mass. Old chorioretinal scars are not typically seen. May have a history of exposure to puppies or eating dirt. Positive Toxocara enzyme-linked immunosorbent assay [ELISA].)

Work-up See "Posterior Uveitis," Section 13.2, for a nonspecific work-up when the diagnosis is in doubt.

1. History: Does the patient eat raw meat or has he been exposed to cats (sources of acquired infection)? Inquire about risk factors for AIDS in atypical cases (e.g., several active lesions without old chorioretinal scars).
2. Complete ocular examination, including a dilated fundus evaluation.
3. Serum antitoxoplasma antibody titer. Should have a positive titer from current or previous infection (the dilution is unimportant). NOTE Ask the lab to do a 1:1 dilution, as you are only looking for a positive result.
4. FTA-ABS, PPD with anergy panel, chest x-ray, and a toxocara ELISA when the diagnosis is uncertain.
5. Fluorescein angiogram if a choroidal neovascular membrane is suspected.
6. Consider an HIV test in atypical cases or when the patient is a high risk candidate for AIDS.

Treatment

A. Small peripheral retinochoroiditis (not affecting or threatening vision): If an anterior-chamber reaction is present, a topical cycloplegic (e.g., cyclopentolate 2% tid) +/− a topical steroid (e.g., prednisolone acetate 1%) qid is given. No additional treatment is indicated. The drops are tapered as the anterior-chamber reaction resolves.
B. Active lesions which are within 2-3 millimeters of the disc or fovea and threaten or are affecting vision, or extramacular lesions accompanied by severe vitritis:
   1. Sulfadiazine 2-4 g po load, then 1 g po qid × 6 weeks.
   2. Clindamycin[1] 300 mg po qid × 4-6 weeks (warn the patient about the risk of pseudomembranous colitis, and discontinue the drug if the patient develops greater than 4 bowel movements/day).
   3. Consider prednisone 60-100 mg po q day × 7-14 days and then taper over 2-3 weeks. Periocular steroids are not given.

   NOTE Systemic steroids should never be given without antimicrobial treatment, should not be given to immunocompromised patients or

---

[1]Clindamycin has not been approved for use in toxoplasmosis by the Federal Drug Administration.

patients with tuberculosis, and should be avoided in patients with systemic infection. Diabetics may have difficulty controlling their blood sugar. See Appendix 5 for a systemic steroid work-up.

4. Topical cycloplegic (e.g., cyclopentolate 2% tid) +/− a topical steroid (e.g., prednisolone acetate 1% qid) if an anterior-chamber reaction is present.
5. If a monocular patient who is reliable enough to return for blood tests has a parafoveal lesion, then pyrimethamine 75 mg po load, followed by 25 mg po q day × 6 weeks, plus folinic acid 3 mg im 3×/week or 5 mg po q day is given in addition to the above therapy.

If a patient is placed on pyrimethamine, a platelet count and CBC are obtained once or twice per week to check for a low platelet count and a low red or white blood cell count (pyrimethamine can depress the bone marrow). If the platelet count falls below 100,000 then reduce the dosage of pyrimethamine and increase the folinic acid.
Patients on pyrimethamine should not take vitamins which contain folic acid.

Follow-up   In 3-7 days for blood tests and/or ocular assessment, then every 2 weeks on therapy. Patients taking pyrimethamine are followed more closely.

NOTES

1. If a patient cannot use or must discontinue clindamycin, tetracycline 2 g load po followed by 250 mg po qid is used alternatively. Do not give tetracycline to children or pregnant or breast-feeding women.
2. Pyrimethamine should be given with meals to reduce anorexia.
3. Pyrimethamine should not be given to pregnant or breast-feeding women.
4. Only women who develop toxoplasmosis *during* pregnancy can transmit it to their fetus. A woman cannot transmit congenital toxoplasmosis.

See "AIDS" for additional information.

13.4   Sarcoidosis

Symptoms   Pain, photophobia, decreased vision. Typically affects blacks in the 20- to 50-year age group.

Critical Ocular Signs   Granulomatous iritis with large "mutton-fat" keratic precipitates on the corneal endothelium (or less commonly a nongranulomatous iritis), vitritis with white fluffy opacities in the inferior vitreous or yellow-white nodules or exudates ("candle wax drippings") and sheathing along peripheral retinal veins.

Other Ocular Signs Iris and/or choroidal nodules, retinal hemorrhage, conjunctival granuloma, band keratopathy, posterior synechiae, glaucoma, cataract, lacrimal-gland enlargement, dry eye, optic-disc swelling, optic-nerve granuloma, optic neuritis, extraocular muscle palsy, and proptosis. Retinal neovascularization and cystoid macular edema may occur.

Systemic Signs Facial-nerve palsy, salivary-gland enlargement, bilateral hilar adenopathy on chest x-ray, erythema nodosum (erythematous, tender nodules beneath the skin, often in the anterior tibial area), arthritis, lymphadenopathy, hepatosplenomegaly, and other skin, central nervous system, and bone changes may be found.

Differential Diagnosis

- Sickle-cell disease (May also produce peripheral retinal neovascularization in young black individuals, but it is more commonly "sea-fan" in appearance. The aqueous and vitreous have few to no cells and a hemoglobin electrophoresis is abnormal in sickle-cell disease.)
- Tuberculosis (TB) (Rare. May appear identical to sarcoidosis. Positive PPD +/− chest x-ray in most cases.)
- Idiopathic pars planitis (White fluffy vitreous opacities and cells along with white exudative material accumulating along the ora serrata and pars plana, typically inferiorly.)
- Others (See "Anterior Uveitis," Section 13.1 and "Posterior Uveitis," Section 13.2.)

Work-up Below are listed the tests which are obtained when sarcoidosis is suspected clinically (see "Anterior Uveitis," Section 13.1, and "Posterior Uveitis," Section 13.2, for nonspecific uveitis work-ups).

1. Chest x-ray.
2. Serum angiotensin converting enzyme (ACE): Usually, but not always elevated in active systemic sarcoidosis. May also be elevated in tuberculosis, diabetes, leprosy, histoplasmosis, and other conditions which do *not* produce uveitis. Normal ACE values vary with age, requiring comparison with age-matched controls. Steroids usually suppress the ACE level soon after starting treatment.
3. PPD with anergy panel: Used to distinguish TB (induration of 10 mm or more in most cases) from sarcoidosis (anergy in 50% of cases).

4. Biopsy of any conjunctival granuloma or the palpebral lobe of the lacrimal gland when it is enlarged. (An acid-fast stain and a methenamine-silver stain should be performed at the time of biopsy to rule out TB and fungal infection.)

If the above work-up is inconclusive, yet sarcoidosis is still suspected, the following tests may be obtained:

5. Gallium scan of the head, neck, and mediastinum (it often shows increased uptake in patients with active systemic sarcoidosis).
6. Serum lysozyme (may be elevated) and serum protein electrophoresis (may show hypergammaglobulinemia).
7. Skin, lymph node, or lung biopsy by a qualified physician.
8. Blind conjunctival biopsy (unilateral or bilateral).
9. Kveim skin test (rarely available).

Serum calcium levels are sometimes obtained in patients diagnosed with sarcoidosis to ascertain that the blood calcium is not dangerously high.

Treatment   All patients are referred to an internist for medical management.

A. Uveitis
  1. Cycloplegic (e.g., cyclopentolate 2% or scopolamine ¼% tid).
  2. Topical steroid (e.g., prednisolone acetate 1% q 1-6 hours, depending on the degree of inflammation).
  3. Periocular steroids (e.g., triamcinolone 40 mg subtenons q 3-4 weeks) may be required when the uveitis does not respond to q 1 hour topical steroids. See Appendix 8 for the technique.
  4. Systemic steroids are often required in the presence of posterior uveitis (including optic neuritis) (e.g., prednisone 60-100 mg po q day) + an H_2 blocker (e.g., ranitidine 150 mg po bid). See Appendix 5 when considering systemic steroids.
B. Cystoid macular edema: See Section 12.14.
C. Glaucoma: See "Inflammatory Open-Angle Glaucoma" (Section 10.4), "Acute Angle-Closure Glaucoma" (Section 10.10), "Neovascular Glaucoma" (Section 10.13), or "Steroid Response/Glaucoma" (Section 10.5), depending on the etiology of the glaucoma.
D. Retinal neovascularization: May require panretinal photocoagulation.
E. Orbital disease is managed with systemic steroids as above.
F. Seventh-nerve palsy, central nervous system disease, pulmonary disease, and renal disease all require systemic steroids and management by an internist. Hypercalcemia may also require medical treatment.

Follow-up   Patients are reexamined in 3-7 days. The steroids are adjusted in accordance with the response to treatment. As the inflammation subsides, the steroids and cycloplegic agent are tapered slowly. Intraocular pressure is monitored and fundus reevaluation is performed periodically. Asymptomatic patients with quiet eyes are seen every 6 months. Patients being treated with steroids need to be followed more closely (e.g., every 1-3 months). Children with sarcoidosis are reexamined every 3 months due to the frequent occurrence of asymptomatic but damaging uveitis.

13.5   Pars Planitis

Symptoms   Floaters and cloudy vision, rarely red eye, pain, or photophobia. Usually age 15-40 years and bilateral.

Critical Signs   "Snowbanking" (white exudative material over the inferior ora serrata and pars plana) and vitreous cells.

NOTE   "Snowbanking" can often only be seen with indirect ophthalmoscopy and scleral depression.

Other Signs   Cellular aggregates in the vitreous, especially inferiorly ("snowball" opacities), peripheral retinal vascular sheathing, anterior-chamber inflammation, cystoid macular edema (CME), posterior subcapsular cataract, secondary glaucoma, posterior vitreous detachment, vitreous hemorrhage, retinal detachment, retinal tears, or peripapillary edema may develop.

Differential Diagnosis   See "Posterior Uveitis," Section 13.2.

Work-up   See "Posterior Uveitis," Section 13.2.

Treatment   No treatment is necessary for a visual acuity of 20/40 or better. For patients with a visual acuity worse than 20/40 due to CME, any or all of the following may be tried (although (2) and (3) are not generally given simultaneously).

1. Topical prednisolone acetate 1% (e.g., Pred Forte) q 1-2 hours may serve a dual purpose, relieving discomfort from an anterior-chamber reaction, and sometimes improving the CME.
2. Periocular repository steroids (e.g., methylprednisolone 40 mg subtenons). Repeat the injections every 1-2 months until the vision and CME are no longer improving and then slowly taper the frequency of injections. (See Appendix 8 for the technique).

NOTE   Sometimes methylprednisolone 20 mg retrobulbar (one dose) is given.

3. If there is no improvement after the first three subtenons injections then consider systemic steroids (e.g., prednisone 60 mg po q day × 4-6 weeks, tapering gradually according to the response) or other immunosuppressive agents.

In bilateral cases, systemic steroid therapy is often preferred over bilateral periocular injections.

NOTES

1. Some physicians delay periocular repository steroid therapy for several weeks in order to observe whether the patient is a steroid responder (i.e., develops a significant intraocular pressure rise secondary to the topical steroids). If a steroid response is found then the periocular steroid may need to be withheld.
2. Acetazolamide (e.g., Diamox) 250 mg po q day may be tried in refractory cases.

Follow-up   In the acute phase, patients are reevaluated every 1 to 4 weeks depending on the severity of the condition. In the chronic phase, reexamination is performed every 3 to 6 months.

13.6   Acute Retinal Necrosis (ARN)

Symptoms   Blurred vision, ocular pain, and photophobia, sometimes developing bilaterally. Most patients are in good systemic health, but underlying AIDS should be considered.

Critical Signs   Multiple white opaque patches of thickened retina, usually in the periphery, which gradually enlarge and coalesce. There is a sharp demarcation line between the involved and normal retina. Vitreous cells are often abundant.

Other Signs   Sheathed retinal arterioles and sometimes venules, predominantly in the periphery, retinal hemorrhages, optic-disc edema, an anterior-chamber reaction, increased intraocular pressure (IOP), or retinal detachment may occur. An optic neuropathy (an afferent pupillary defect, decreased color vision, and a central scotoma) sometimes develops.

Etiology Unknown. Varicella-zoster, herpes simplex, and cytomegalovirus (CMV) viruses have been implicated.

Differential Diagnosis See "Posterior Uveitis," Section 13.2.

Work-up See "Posterior Uveitis," Section 13.2, for a nonspecific uveitis work-up.

1. History: Risk factors for AIDS? Immunocompromised? If yes, CMV retinitis may be more likely.
2. Complete ocular examination, evaluating the anterior chamber and the vitreous for cells, measuring the IOP, and performing a dilated retinal examination using indirect ophthalmoscopy and scleral depression.
3. Consider a CBC with differential, FTA-ABS, RPR, ESR, toxoplasmosis titers, PPD with anergy panel, chest x-ray, and urine for CMV to rule out other causes of retinitis.
4. Consider serum titers for herpes simplex, varicella-zoster, and cytomegalovirus virus.
5. An orbital CT scan or B-scan ultrasound is usually obtained, looking for an enlarged optic nerve.
6. Consider a fluorescein angiogram.

Treatment

1. Admit to the hospital.
2. Acyclovir[2] 1500 mg/m^2 of body surface area/day iv in 3 divided doses × 10 days.

   NOTE Knowing a patient's height and weight, a conversion table or logarithmic formula can be used to determine the patients body surface area in square meters. This table is available in hospital pharmacies. The vast majority of people have a body surface area of 1-2.5 m^2.

3. Topical cycloplegic (e.g., atropine 1% tid) and topical steroid (e.g., prednisolone acetate 1% q 2-6 hours) in the presence of anterior-segment inflammation.
4. Consider anticoagulation (e.g., heparin then warfarin for a total of 2-3 weeks).
5. Systemic steroids (controversial): Some physicians administer steroids aggressively at the time of diagnosis (e.g., methylprednisolone 250 mg iv qid × 3 days followed by prednisone 60 mg po bid × 1-2 weeks), particularly when the optic nerve is thought to be involved. Most delay

---

[2]The dosage of acyclovir needs to be reduced in patients with renal insufficiency. BUN and creatinine levels are followed closely.

steroid therapy for one or more weeks until the retinitis begins to clear (e.g., prednisone 60-100 mg po q day).

6. Consider laser photocoagulation to the areas of necrotic retina to strengthen retinal adherence and possibly avoid detachment.
7. See "Inflammatory Open-Angle Glaucoma," Section 10.4, for treatment of elevated IOP.
8. Optic-nerve sheath decompression surgery has been used for ARN when the optic nerve is enlarged and the patient's condition worsens or does not improve with medical therapy.

Follow-up   Patients are seen daily in the hospital and are then followed every few weeks to months for the following year. A careful fundus evaluation with scleral depression is performed at each visit to rule out retinal holes which may lead to a detachment. If the retinitis crosses the margin of prior laser treatment, consider applying additional laser. A pupillary examination should always be performed and an optic neuropathy considered if the retinopathy does not explain the amount of visual loss.

13.7   Vogt-Koyanagi-Harada (VKH) Syndrome

Symptoms   Bilaterally decreased vision, photophobia, pain, and red eyes, accompanied by or preceded by a headache, stiff neck, nausea, vomiting, fever, and malaise. Hearing loss and tinnitus frequently occur.

Critical Signs   Bilateral serous retinal detachments with underlying choroidal infiltrates, posterior vitreous cells and opacities, retinal hemorrhages, optic-disc edema, anterior-chamber flare and cells, and keratic precipitates. Perilimbal vitiligo is common. Alopecia, vitiligo, and poliosis may develop later.

Other Signs   May see mottling of the retinal pigment epithelium after the serous retinal detachment resolves, hyphema, iris nodules, peripheral anterior and posterior synechiae, scleritis, hypotony, venous engorgement, retinal vasculitis, or choroidal neovascularization. Neurologic signs including loss of consciousness, paralysis, and seizures may occur. Typically patients are 20-50 years old and are of a darkly pigmented heritage such as Asian or American Indian.

Differential Diagnosis   See "Posterior Uveitis," Section 13.2, for a complete list. In particular consider the following:

- Sympathetic ophthalmia (Prior history of trauma or surgery to the other eye. Generally no CNS, skin, nor hair manifestations.)
- Acute posterior multifocal placoid pigment epitheliopathy (AMPPE) (Ophthalmoscopic and fluorescein angiographic features may be very similar, but there is less vitreous inflammation and no anterior-segment involvement.)
- Other granulomatous panuveitides (e.g., syphilis, sarcoidosis, tuberculosis)

Work-up See "Posterior Uveitis," Section 13.2, for a nonspecific uveitis work-up.

1. History: Neurologic symptoms, hearing loss, or hair loss? Previous eye surgery or trauma?
2. Complete ocular examination, including a dilated retinal evaluation.
3. CBC, RPR, FTA-ABS, $+/-$ chest x-ray, angiotension converting enzyme (ACE), and PPD with anergy panel to rule out similar-appearing disorders.
4. Consider a CT scan with and without contrast or MRI of the brain during attacks with neurologic signs to rule out a CNS disorder.
5. Lumbar puncture during attacks with meningeal symptoms for cell count and differential, protein, glucose, VDRL, Gram's and methenamine-silver stains, and culture. (Lymphocytosis is often seen in VKH and AMPPE.)
6. Fluorescein angiogram may help in the diagnosis.

Treatment Inflammation is controlled with steroids, the dose depending upon the severity of the inflammation. In moderate-to-severe cases, the following regimen can be used initially. Steroids are tapered slowly as the condition improves.

1. Topical steroids (e.g., prednisolone acetate 1% q 1 hour).
2. Systemic steroids (e.g., prednisone 60-80 mg po q day) plus an H_2 blocker (e.g., ranitidine 150 mg po bid). See Appendix 5 for a systemic steroid work-up.
3. Topical cycloplegic (e.g., scopolamine ¼% tid).
4. Treatment of any specific neurologic disorders (e.g., seizures or coma).

Follow-up Initial management may require hospitalization. Weekly then monthly reexamination is performed, watching for recurrent inflammation and increased intraocular pressure. The steroids are tapered slowly. Inflammation may recur up to 9 months after the steroids have been discontinued. If that should occur, the above treatment regimen should be reinstituted.

13.8 Reticulum-Cell Sarcoma

(Large-Cell Lymphoma)

Symptoms Painless decrease in vision, floaters. Usually no history of prior uveitis.

Critical Signs Large amount of vitreous cells and debris in a patient older than 40 years (typically >50 years) which do not respond well to systemic steroids. Usually bilateral.

Other Signs May see patches of yellow-white chorioretinal or subretinal pigment epithelial infiltrates, retinal edema and hemorrhages, or a mild anterior-chamber reaction with fine keratic precipitates. Neurologic manifestations may be present.

Differential Diagnosis See "Posterior Uveitis," Section 13.2.

Work-up See "Posterior Uveitis," Section 13.2, for a nonspecific uveitis work-up.

1. History: Previous uveitis? Recent intraocular surgery? Immunocompromised or risk group for AIDS? Concomitant systemic symptoms or signs (e.g., skin rash, difficulty breathing, or diarrhea)? If yes, see "Posterior Uveitis," Section 13.2.
2. Complete ocular examination.
3. CT scan (axial and coronal views) with and without contrast or MRI of the orbit and head (and a body CT scan if indicated).
4. Lumbar puncture (cell count, cytology, VDRL, protein, glucose, culture, Gram's and methenamine-silver stains).
5. Consider a diagnostic vitrectomy with cytologic and immunohistologic studies.
6. Biopsy suspicious lymph nodes as needed.
7. Bone marrow biopsy if indicated.

Treatment In cooperation with an oncologist and radiation therapist.

1. Ocular and brain radiation therapy.
2. Intravenous chemotherapy.
3. Systemic radiation therapy (if there is visceral involvement).
4. Intrathecal chemotherapy if indicated.

Follow-up   In conjunction with the oncologist and radiation therapist.

13.9   Postoperative Uveitis

Postoperative inflammation is typically mild-to-moderate, usually resolving within six weeks. This section presents several etiologies of postoperative uveitis and a work-up that may be considered when postoperative inflammation is atypical.

Etiology
  A. Severe intraocular inflammation in the early postoperative course
   • Infectious endophthalmitis   (Progressive and often severe ocular pain [but not always], deteriorating vision, corneal edema, eyelid swelling, chemosis, sometimes a hypopyon, and commonly vitreous inflammation and blunting of the red reflex.)
   • Phacoanaphylactic endophthalmitis   (A severe granulomatous inflammation with mutton-fat keratic precipitates, resulting from an autoimmune reaction to lens protein exposed during surgery.)
   • Aseptic endophthalmitis   (A severe sterile postoperative uveitis due to excess tissue manipulation, especially vitreous manipulation, during surgery. A hypopyon and a mild vitreous cellular reaction may develop. Generally *not* characterized by profound or progressive pain or visual loss. Eyelid swelling and chemosis are atypical. Usually resolves with topical steroid therapy.)
  B. Persistent postoperative inflammation (e.g., beyond 6 weeks)
   • Patient noncompliance with steroid drops (e.g., not taking or not shaking the drops properly).
   • Steroid drops tapered too abruptly.
   • Iris or vitreous incarceration in the wound.
   • Uveitis-glaucoma-hyphema (UGH) syndrome   (Irritation of the iris or ciliary body by an intraocular lens. Increased intraocular pressure [IOP] and red blood cells in the anterior chamber accompany the anterior-segment inflammation.)
   • Retinal detachment   (Often produces a low-grade anterior-chamber reaction.)
   • Low-grade endophthalmitis (e.g., Proprionibacterium acnes, fungal, or partially treated bacterial endophthalmitis)
   • Inflammatory reaction to contaminants on the intraocular lens (e.g., polishing substances or substances used to sterilize the lens) or to the viscoelastic substance.

- Epithelial downgrowth or fibrous ingrowth   (Corneal epithelium or fibrous tissue grows into the eye through a corneal wound, and may be seen on the posterior corneal surface. The iris may appear flattened due to the spread of the membrane over the anterior-chamber angle onto the iris. Large cells may be seen in the anterior chamber and glaucoma may be present. The diagnosis can be confirmed by observing the immediate appearance of white spots after argon laser treatment [medium power] to the areas of iris covered by the membrane.)
  - Preexisting uveitis (see "Anterior Uveitis," Section 13.1.)
  C. Sympathetic ophthalmia   (Diffuse granulomatous inflammation in *both* eyes following trauma or surgery to one eye.)

Work-up

1. History: Is the patient taking and shaking the steroid drops properly? Did the patient stop the steroid drops abruptly? Was there a postoperative wound leak allowing for epithelial downgrowth or fibrous ingrowth? Previous history of uveitis?
2. Complete ocular examination of both eyes, including a slit-lamp assessment of the anterior-chamber reaction, a determination of whether vitreous or residual lens material is present in the anterior chamber, and an inspection of the posterior lens capsule looking for posterior capsular opacities (as is seen in some cases of P. acnes). Gonioscopy (checking for iris or vitreous to the wound), an IOP measurement, a dilated indirect ophthalmoscopic examination (to rule out a retinal detachment or signs of chorioretinitis), and a posterior vitreous evaluation with a slit-lamp and a 60 diopter or Hruby lens looking for inflammatory cells should be performed.
3. Obtain a B-scan ultrasound when the fundus view is obscured.
4. A diagnostic surgical vitrectomy is usually performed for smears and cultures when infectious endophthalmitis is suspected. Anaerobic cultures, using both solid media and broth, should be obtained to isolate P. acnes (routine cultures are also obtained, see "Postoperative Endophthalmitis," Section 13.10). The anaerobic cultures should be incubated in an anaerobic environment as rapidly as possible and allowed to grow for at least two weeks.
5. Consider an anterior-chamber paracentesis for diagnostic smears and cultures.
6. Consider diagnostic argon laser treatment (medium power) to the areas of iris thought to be covered by epithelial downgrowth or fibrous ingrowth.

If the above work-up is negative, no underlying etiology can be elicited, and a trial of steroids only transiently reduces the inflammation, surgical removal of the capsular bag and intraocular lens should be considered in an effort to isolate P. acnes.

See "Postoperative Endophthalmitis" (Section 13.10), "Phacoanaphylactic Endophthalmitis" (Section 13.14), "Anterior Uveitis" (Section 13.1), "Posterior Uveitis" (Section 13.2), and "Sympathetic Ophthalmia" (Section 13.15) for more specific information on diagnosis and treatment.

13.10   Postoperative Endophthalmitis

Acute (One to several days after surgery.)

Symptoms   Sudden onset of progressively decreasing vision, redness, and increasing eye pain.

Critical Signs   More ocular inflammation than would be expected after the ocular procedure performed. Intense flare and cell in the anterior chamber and vitreous, $+/-$ hypopyon, eyelid edema, chemosis, and a reduced red reflex.

NOTE   Pain and a hypopyon do not have to be present.

Other Signs   Corneal edema, iris hyperemia, purulent discharge.

Organisms

   Most common   Staph. epidermidis.
   Common   Staph. aureus, streptococcal species (except Pneumococcus, which is not a common cause).
   Less common   Gram negative bacteria (Pseudomonas, Aerobacter, Proteus, H. influenza, Klebsiella, E. coli, Bacillus, Enterobacter) and anaerobes.

Differential Diagnosis   See "Postoperative Uveitis," Section 13.9.

Work-up

  1. Complete ocular history and examination.
  2. Consider a B-scan ultrasound (may confirm the clinical suspicion by revealing marked vitreous cells, and establishes a baseline against which the success of therapy can be measured).
  3. A diagnostic (and therapeutic) vitrectomy is often performed. Cultures (blood, chocolate, Sabouraud's, thioglycolate) and smears (Gram's and Giemsa stains) are obtained, and intravitreal antibiotics are given as described below. An anterior-chamber paracentesis should be considered.
  4. CBC with differential and serum electrolytes.

Treatment

1. Hospitalization.
2. Topical fortified antibiotics (e.g., fortified cefazolin q 1 hour + fortified gentamicin or tobramycin q 1 hour alternating every ½ hour) (See Appendix 10 describing fortified drop preparation.)
3. Subconjunctival antibiotics (e.g., gentamicin 40 mg + vancomycin 25-50 mg [or clindamycin 40 mg]); can be repeated daily if bacteria are isolated. See Appendix 8 for the technique.
4. Systemic antibiotics (e.g., cefazolin 500-1000 mg iv q 6 hours + gentamicin 1.75 mg/kg iv load followed by 1 mg/kg q 8 hours).[3]
5. Intravitreal antibiotics (e.g., gentamicin 0.1-0.4 mg in 0.1 ml + vancomycin 1.0 mg in 0.1 ml; clindamycin 1 mg in 0.1-0.2 ml may be used in place of vancomycin) at the time of vitrectomy.
6. Topical cycloplegic (e.g., atropine 1%) 3-4×/day.

Steroids are usually started topically, subconjunctivally, and intravitreally since fungus is not usually suspected in acute onset postoperative endophthalmitis.

7. Topical steroid (e.g., prednisolone acetate 1%) 6×/day.
8. Subconjunctival steroid (e.g., triamcinolone 40 mg) at the time of vitrectomy and sometimes daily (Appendix 8 explains the technique).
9. Intravitreal steroid (e.g., dexamethasone 0.4 mg) at the time of vitrectomy.

NOTE Antibiotic and steroid therapy is usually withheld until *after* the vitrectomy is performed unless a prolonged delay before surgery is expected.

Follow-up

1. Monitor the clinical course every 4-8 hours.
2. The antibiotic regimen is refined according to the patient's response to treatment and to the culture and sensitivity results. If a patient is getting worse or an identified organism is found resistant to the intravitreal antibiotics injected, an additional intravitreal injection of one antibiotic can be given 48 hours after the initial injection.
3. If the patient is responding well to treatment, topical fortified antibiotics may be slowly tapered after 48 hours and then switched to regular strength. Intravenous antibiotics are maintained for 6-10 days, depending on the ocular status, and then comparable oral antibiotics are substituted for a

---

[3]Systemic antibiotic doses may need to be reduced in patients with renal disease. Check gentamicin peak and trough levels ½ hour before and after the fifth dose and follow the BUN and creatinine every other day. Adjust the doses accordingly.

total 14-day course. Patients are usually discharged from the hospital after intravenous antibiotics are discontinued. Close outpatient follow-up is warranted.

NOTE   Some physicians administer a systemic steroid (e.g., prednisone 60-100 mg po q day) once the responsible organism has been treated appropriately for 24 hours. This is maintained for 7-10 days and then tapered. We do not generally do this.

Delayed-Onset (A week to a month or more after surgery.)

Symptoms   Insidious decreased vision, increasing redness and pain.

Critical Signs   Reduced visual acuity, anterior-chamber and vitreous inflammation, vitreous abscesses, hypopyon, or clumps of exudate in the anterior chamber, on the iris surface, or along the pupillary border.

Other Signs   Corneal infiltrate and edema, may have a surgical bleb.

Etiology/Organisms

- Fungi (Aspergillus, Candida, Cephalosporium, Penicillium, others)
- Proprionibacterium acnes   (Recurrent, granulomatous anterior uveitis often with a hypopyon, but minimal conjunctival injection and pain. A white plaque or opacities on the posterior lens capsule may be evident. There is only a transient response to steroids.)
- Other bacteria   (Related to a filtering bleb [often streptococci], vitreous wick, or partial suppression with antibiotics during or after surgery.)

Differential Diagnosis   See Postoperative Uveitis, Section 13.9.

Work-up

1. Complete ocular history and examination.
2. Vitrectomy for smears (Gram's, Giemsa, and methenamine-silver) and cultures (blood, chocolate, Sabouraud's, thioglycolate, and a solid media for anaerobic culture [e.g., Brucella or blood agar]; P. acnes will be missed unless proper anaerobic cultures are obtained). Intravitreal antibiotics are given as described below.
3. CBC with differential, serum electrolytes, liver function studies.

Treatment

1. Initially treat as acute postoperative endophthalmitis as described above, but do *not* start steroids.
2. If a fungal infection is suspected or an intraoperative smear is consistent with fungus, administer intravitreal amphotericin B, 5-10 micrograms at the time of vitrectomy.
3. Broad-spectrum antifungal therapy is delayed until a fungus is positively identified in a direct smear or culture. Antifungal therapy consists of:
   a. Topical natamycin (5% suspension) q 1 hour.
   b. Flucytosine 37.5 mg/kg po q 6 hours.
   c. Amphotericin B 0.25 to 0.3 mg/kg/day iv initially (in test doses of 1 mg), then increase the dose slowly to 0.75 to 1.0 mg/kg/day iv in divided doses.
   d. Consider miconazole 10 mg in 1.0 ml subconjunctivally.
   e. A therapeutic vitrectomy should be performed if it was not done with the initial cultures.

   Antifungal therapy is modified in accordance with sensitivity testing, clinical course, and tolerance to antifungal agents.
4. Removal of the lens and capsular remnants may be required for diagnosis and treatment of P. acnes. P. acnes may be sensitive to intravitreal penicillin, cefoxitin, or clindamycin.

Follow-up   Dependent upon the organism. In general follow-up is as described above for acute postoperative endophthalmitis. Repeat CBC, serum electrolytes, and liver function tests 2×/week during treatment for fungal endophthalmitis.

13.11   Traumatic Endophthalmitis

This condition constitutes an emergency. If suspected, prompt action is required.

Symptoms and Signs   Same as ''Acute Postoperative Endophthalmitis,'' Section 13.10.

   NOTE   Patients with Bacillus endophthalmitis may develop a high fever, leukocytosis, proptosis, a corneal abscess in the form of a ring, and rapid visual deterioration.

Organisms   Bacillus species, staph. epidermidis, gram negative species, fungi, streptococcus species, and others. A mixed flora may be present.

Differential Diagnosis

- Sterile inflammatory response from a retained intraocular foreign body or blood in the vitreous.
- Sterile inflammation due to surgical complications.
- Phacoanaphylactic endophthalmitis   (A sterile autoimmune inflammatory reaction due to exposed lens protein. See Section 13.14.)

Work-up   Same as for ''Acute Postoperative Endophthalmitis,'' Section 13.10. An orbital CT scan (axial and coronal views) and ultrasound are also performed to rule out an intraocular foreign body.

Treatment

1. Hospitalization.
2. Management for a ruptured globe/penetrating ocular injury if present, see Section 3.15.
3. Topical fortified gentamicin or tobramycin q 1 hour + fortified cefazolin q 1 hour, alternating q ½ hour (see Appendix 10 describing fortified drop preparation.)
4. Subconjunctival gentamicin 40 mg and subconjunctival clindamycin 34 mg. Can be repeated daily as needed. (See Appendix 8 for the technique.)
5. Systemic antibiotics (e.g., gentamicin 1.75 mg/kg iv load followed by 1.0 mg/kg iv q 8 hour + clindamycin 300 mg iv q 6 hours +/− cefazolin 500-1000 mg iv q 8 hour).[4]
6. Intravitreal antibiotics (gentamicin 0.1-0.4 mg in 0.1 ml + clindamycin 1.0 mg in 0.1 ml; vancomycin 1.0 mg in 0.1 ml may be used in place of clindamycin)—these may be repeated every 48-72 hours as needed.
7. A surgical vitrectomy is performed once the condition is highly suspected.

NOTES

1. Antibiotics are usually withheld until after the vitrectomy is performed unless a prolonged delay until surgery is expected.
2. Steroids should *not* be given initially since a fungal etiology cannot be ruled out. If cultures are negative for fungi, topical, subconjunctival,

---

[4]The drug doses may need to be reduced in children and those with renal disease. Check gentamicin peak and trough levels ½ hour before and after the fifth dose and follow the BUN and creatinine.

+/− systemic steroids may be started (e.g., topical prednisolone acetate 1% 6×/day + subconjunctival dexamethasone 4 mg +/− prednisone 40-80 mg po q day).

Follow-up Same as for "Postoperative Endophthalmitis," Section 13.10. The specific antibiotics and the frequency of their administration should be modified in accordance with the response to treatment as well as the culture and sensitivity results.

13.12 Endogenous Bacterial Endophthalmitis

Symptoms Decreased vision in an acutely ill (e.g., septic) patient, an immunocompromised host, or an IV drug abuser. No history of recent intraocular surgery.

Critical Signs Vitreous cells and debris, anterior-chamber cell and flare, or a hypopyon in a high-risk patient.

Other Signs Iris microabscess, absent red fundus reflex, retinal inflammatory infiltrates, flame-shaped retinal hemorrhages with or without white centers, corneal edema, eyelid edema, chemosis, and conjunctival injection. Panophthalmitis (orbital involvement [proptosis, restricted ocular motility] + endophthalmitis) may develop.

Etiology Bacillus cereus (especially in IV drug abusers), streptococci, Neisseria meningidis, Staphylococcus aureus, Hemophilus influenza, others).

Differential Diagnosis
- Endogenous fungal endophthalmitis (May see fluffy white vitreous opacities. Fungi grow out on cultures. See "Candida Retinitis/Uveitis/Endophthalmitis," Section 13.13.)
- Retinochoroidal infection (e.g., toxoplasmosis and toxocariasis) (Yellow or white retinochoroidal lesion present.)
- Noninfectious posterior uveitis (e.g., sarcoidosis, pars planitis) (May have a known history of uveitis. Unlikely to coincidentally get the first episode during sepsis.)
- Neoplastic conditions (e.g., reticulum-cell sarcoma [usually beyond 50-55 years of age], retinoblastoma [usually in first few years of life].)

Work-up

1. History: Duration of symptoms? Underlying disease or infections? IV drug abuse? Immunocompromised?
2. Complete ocular examination including a dilated fundus examination.
3. B-scan ultrasound to determine the extent of posterior segment ocular involvement if it cannot be determined on clinical examination.
4. Complete medical work-up by an infectious disease expert.
5. Cultures of the blood, urine, and all indwelling catheters and IV lines (as well as Gram's stain of any discharge). A lumbar puncture is indicated when meningeal signs are present.
6. Vitrectomy with intraocular antibiotics (e.g., gentamicin 0.1-0.4 mg in 0.1 ml, + vancomycin 1.0 mg in 0.1 ml; clindamycin 1.0 mg in 0.1 ml may be used in place of vancomycin): The timing of this procedure is controversial. We perform it as soon as possible. (Other physicians initially perform aqueous and vitreous aspirations when the systemic cultures are negative and the organism remains unknown.)

Treatment   (In conjunction with a medical internist.)

1. Hospitalize.
2. Broad-spectrum antibiotics are started after appropriate smears and cultures are obtained. Antibiotic choices vary according to the suspected source of septic infection (e.g., GI tract, GU tract, etc.) and are determined by an infectious disease expert. Dosages recommended for meningitis and severe infections are used.

   NOTE   IV drug abusers are given an aminoglycoside plus clindamycin to cover Bacillus cereus.

3. Topical cycloplegic (e.g., atropine 1% tid).
4. Topical steroid (e.g., prednisolone acetate 1% q 1-6 hours, depending on the degree of anterior-segment inflammation).
5. Periocular antibiotics (e.g., subconjunctival or subtenons injections) are sometimes used (see Appendix 8 for injection techniques).

Follow-up   Daily in the hospital. Peak and trough levels for many antibiotic agents are followed every few days. BUN and creatinine levels are monitored during aminoglycoside therapy. The antibiotic regimen is guided by the culture and sensitivity results as well as the clinical response to treatment. IV antibiotics are maintained for at least 2 weeks and until the condition has resolved.

13.13 Candida Retinitis / Uveitis / Endophthalmitis

Symptoms Decreased vision, floaters, pain, often bilateral. Patients typically are IV drug abusers, immunocompromised hosts (e.g., due to cancer, immunosuppressive agents, AIDS, long-term antibiotics, or systemic steroids) or possess a long-term indwelling catheter (e.g., for hyperalimentation or hemodialysis).

Critical Signs Multifocal, yellow-white fluffy retinal lesions from one to several disc diameters in size. With time, the lesions increase in size, spread into the vitreous, and appear as "cotton-balls."

Other Signs Vitreous cells and haze, vitreous abscesses, retinal hemorrhages with or without pale centers (pale centers = Roth spots), aqueous cells and flare, or a hypopyon. Retinal detachment may develop.

Differential Diagnosis The following should be considered in immunocompromised hosts.

- Cytomegalovirus (CMV) retinitis   (Minimal-to-mild vitreous reaction, more retinal hemorrhage, tends to concentrate along vessels, consider strongly in AIDS patients.)
- Toxoplasmosis   (Yellow-white lesion confined to the retina. An adjacent chorioretinal scar may or may not be present. Vitreous cells and debris are common, but not vitreous abscesses or "cotton-balls.")
- Others (e.g., herpes simplex, Mycobacterium avium-intracellulare, Nocardia, Aspergillus, cryptococcus, coccidiomycosis)

Work-up

1. History: Medications? Medical problems? IV drug abuse? Other risk factors for AIDS?
2. Search the skin for scars from IV drug injection.
3. Complete ocular examination, including a dilated retinal evaluation.
4. Blood, urine, and catheter site (if present) cultures for Candida; often need to be repeated several times (may be negative despite ocular candidiasis).
5. Diagnostic (and therapeutic) vitrectomy is indicated when a significant amount of vitreous involvement is present. Cultures and smears are taken at the time of vitrectomy to confirm the diagnosis and to evaluate the organisms sensitivity to antifungal agents. Amphotericin B-5 micrograms is injected into the central vitreous cavity at the conclusion of the procedure.

6. Baseline CBC, BUN, creatinine, and liver function tests (LFTs).

Treatment

1. Hospitalize all unreliable patients, systemically ill patients, or those with moderate-to-severe vitreous involvement.
2. An infectious disease specialist or internist familiar with antifungal therapy should be consulted.
3. Ketoconazole 200-400 mg po q day.
4. Flucytosine[5] 150 mg/kg po q day divided into 4 doses × 3 weeks.
5. In resistant cases, amphotericin B may be administered. For the first few days, amphotericin B 1 mg iv is given 5×/day and then larger doses totaling 20 mg/day are administered. Therapy is discontinued when a total dose of 200 mg has been given. Patients with endophthalmitis can be given up to 1 mg/kg/day for several weeks, not to exceed a total dose of 2 grams.
6. Topical mydriatic/cycloplegic agent (e.g., atropine 1% tid).
7. See "Inflammatory Open-Angle Glaucoma," Section 10.4, for intraocular pressure (IOP) control. Note, however, that steroids are generally contraindicated in candidiasis.

Follow-up   Patients are seen daily. Visual acuity, IOP, and the degree of anterior-chamber and vitreous inflammation are assessed. Serum BUN, creatinine, and CBC are repeated a few times per week. LFTs are repeated periodically. Serum levels of antifungal agents are followed and dosages are adjusted accordingly.

REFERENCE

KANSKI JJ. Uveitis: a colour manual of diagnosis and treatment. London: Butterworth and Co., 64, 1987.

13.14   Phacoanaphylactic Endophthalmitis

Definition   A sterile autoimmune inflammatory reaction to exposed lens protein. It usually occurs one day to a few weeks following surgical, traumatic, or spontaneous disruption of the lens capsule.

---
[5]The dosage of flucytosine should be reduced in patients with renal insufficiency.

Symptoms Pain, photophobia, redness, decreased vision.

Critical Signs A greater anterior-chamber inflammatory reaction than is typically seen after a surgical procedure (more cells and flare and sometimes a hypopyon and "mutton-fat" keratic precipitates). Lens material may be seen in the anterior chamber.

Other Signs Eyelid edema, chemosis, increased intraocular pressure (IOP), posterior synechiae.

Differential Diagnosis See "Postoperative Uveitis," Section 13.9.

Work-up See "Postoperative Uveitis," Section 13.9, for a generalized uveitis work-up in a postoperative patient.

1. History: Recent ocular surgery or trauma?
2. Complete ocular examination, looking for lens particles in the anterior chamber, measuring the IOP, and searching for any inflammatory reaction in the vitreous. The red fundus reflex should be assessed during a dilated retinal examination.
3. If infectious endophthalmitis cannot be ruled out, cultures are obtained and antibiotics started (see "Postoperative Endophthalmitis," Section 13.10).
4. B-scan ultrasound to help in diagnosis and follow-up.

Treatment

1. Topical steroids (e.g., prednisolone acetate 1%) q 1-2 hours.
2. Subconjunctival steroids (e.g., methylprednisolone 40 mg) (see Appendix 8 for the technique).
3. If the IOP is elevated, see "Inflammatory Open-Angle Glaucoma," Section 10.4 and "Steroid Response/Glaucoma," Section 10.5, for management.

If severe:

4. Systemic steroids (e.g., prednisone 80-100 mg po q day) + an antacid or H_2-blocker (e.g., ranitidine 150 mg po bid). (See Appendix 5 for a steroid work-up.)
5. After the inflammation has subsided, surgery may be indicated to remove residual lens material and capsule.

Follow-up Every 1-7 days, depending on the severity of the condition (some patients may need to be hospitalized).

• Check the IOP, watching for glaucoma.

- Assess the degree of inflammation. Taper the steroids slowly as the inflammation subsides.

13.15 Sympathetic Ophthalmia

Symptoms Bilateral eye pain, photophobia, decreased vision (near vision is often affected before distance vision), and red eye. A history of penetrating trauma or intraocular surgery to one eye (usually 4-8 weeks prior, but the range is from 10 days to 50 years) may be elicited.

Critical Signs Bilateral severe anterior-chamber reaction with large "mutton-fat" keratic precipitates, small depigmented nodules at the level of the retinal pigment epithelium (Dalen-Fuchs' nodules), and thickening of the uveal tract. Signs of previous injury or surgery in one eye are usually present.

Other Signs Nodular infiltration of the iris, peripheral anterior synechiae, neovascularization of the iris, occlusion and seclusion of the pupil, cataract, exudative retinal detachment, papillitis. The earliest sign may be loss of accommodation or a mild anterior or posterior uveitis in the uninjured eye.

Differential Diagnosis

- Vogt-Koyanagi-Harada (VKH) syndrome (Similar signs, but often no history of ocular trauma or surgery. Other symptoms and signs may include headache, nausea, vomiting, fever, malaise, vertigo, bizarre behavior, focal neurologic symptoms, alopecia, vitiligo, or poliosis. Darkly pigmented persons—especially Asians—are more commonly affected.)
- Phacoanaphylactic endophthalmitis (Severe anterior-chamber reaction from injury to the lens capsule, usually from trauma or surgery. No posterior uveitis is present.)
- Sarcoidosis (May cause a granulomatous panuveitis with exudates over retinal veins or white clumps in the anterior vitreous inferiorly. Concomitant pulmonary disease is common.)
- Syphilis (Granulomatous panuveitis may be accompanied by interstitial keratitis, dilated capillary nests on the iris, or a diffuse pigmentary retinopathy. Positive FTA-ABS.)

Work-up

1. History: Any prior eye surgery or injury? Venereal disease? Difficulty breathing?

2. Complete ophthalmic examination, including a dilated retinal examination.
3. CBC, RPR, FTA-ABS, +/− angiotensin converting enzyme level if sarcoidosis is a serious consideration.
4. Chest x-ray (rule out sarcoidosis).
5. Fluorescein angiography and/or B-scan ultrasonography to help confirm the diagnosis.

Treatment

1. Prevention: Enucleation of a blind, traumatized eye before a sympathetic reaction can develop—usually considered within 7-14 days of the trauma. If sympathetic ophthalmia develops, enucleation may still be beneficial, regardless of the time period since the trauma.

Inflammation is controlled with steroids, the dose depending upon the severity of the inflammation. In moderate-to-severe cases the following regimen can be used initially. Steroids are tapered slowly as the condition improves.

2. Topical steroids (e.g., prednisolone acetate 1% q 1-2 hours)
3. Periocular steroids (e.g., subconjunctival dexamethasone 4-5 mg, 2-3 ×/week). See Appendix 8 for the administration technique.
4. Systemic steroids (e.g., prednisone 60-80 mg po q day + an antacid or H_2 blocker [e.g., ranitidine 150 mg po bid]. See Appendix 5 for a systemic steroid work-up).
5. Cycloplegic (e.g., scopolamine ¼% tid).
6. If steroids are ineffective or contraindicated, an immunosuppressive agent (e.g., methotrexate 45 mg po q 4 days, tapering to 15 mg q 4 days) may be tried, usually in conjunction with a medical consultant.

Follow-up Every 1-7 days at first to monitor the effectiveness of therapy. As the condition improves, the follow-up interval may be extended to every 3-4 weeks. Intraocular pressure must be monitored closely. Steroids should be maintained for 3-6 months after all signs of inflammation have cleared. Due to the possibility of recurrence, periodic checkups are important.

14

Systemic Disorders

14.1 Acquired Immune Deficiency Syndrome (AIDS)

Risk Groups

Homosexual or bisexual men, IV drug abusers, hemophiliacs and transfusion recipients, sexual partners of persons with AIDS or at risk for AIDS, prostitutes and their sexual partners, infants born to mothers with AIDS.

Laboratory Diagnosis

1. Serum ELISA (enzyme-linked immunosorbent assay) for human immunodeficiency virus (HIV) antibody (sensitive, but not very specific).
2. Western blot if ELISA is positive (very rarely is the Western blot falsely positive).

OCULAR COMPLICATIONS

External Disease

Herpes Zoster Ophthalmicus

May be the initial clinical manifestation of HIV infection. Seen in both AIDS-related complex (ARC) and AIDS.

Signs Vesicular lesions of the face in a trigeminal nerve distribution; may be associated with almost any eye abnormality (See "Herpes Zoster Virus," Section 4.16).

Treatment

1. Acyclovir 30 mg/kg/day iv in 3 divided doses × 7-10 days. (For patients with a creatinine > 2 mg/dl, the dosage is reduced to 20 mg/kg/day in 2 divided doses.) A maintenance dose may be required to prevent reactivation of infection.
2. When intraocular inflammation is present, a topical cycloplegic (e.g., scopolamine ¼% tid) and a topical steroid (e.g., prednisolone acetate 1% q 1-2 hours) are given.

- Cimetidine 400 mg po bid is controversial in prophylaxis against postherpetic neuralgia. We generally do not give this.
- Patients probably should not receive oral steroids for fear of further immunosuppression and extension of the infection.

Kaposi's Sarcoma

Signs Bright-red subconjunctival lesion most commonly located in the inferior cul-de-sac. It may be mistaken for a subconjunctival hemorrhage. Eyelid lesions are purple-red, nontender nodules and can have associated edema, trichiasis, or entropion formation. Orbital lesions with associated periorbital edema occur rarely.

Treatment

1. Vinblastine and vincristine have each had some success in causing remission of Kaposi's sarcoma.
2. Local treatment by excision, cryotherapy, or irradiation may be performed for single lesions.

Retinal Vascular Disease

Noninfectious Retinopathy

The following are common retinal abnormalities seen in patients with AIDS. They are nonspecific and not diagnostic of AIDS: Cotton-wool spots, flame hemorrhages, dot hemorrhages, Roth spots (white-centered hemorrhages), microaneurysms and microvascular abnormalities, perivasculitis with sheathing, and ischemic maculopathy (decreased visual acuity, retinal edema, and macular star formation).

Treatment   The guidelines are not well established. There may be a role for focal laser therapy in the presence of macular edema.

Cytomegalovirus (CMV) Retinopathy

Most common ocular infection in AIDS.

Symptoms   Painless, decreased vision in one or both eyes.

Critical Signs   Multiple distinct areas of white, granular retinal opacification with irregular feathered borders, often mixed with retinal hemorrhages. The necrotic areas usually initiate along the major vascular arcades in the posterior pole, and enlarge and coalesce with time.

Other Signs   The eye is typically white and quiet with little to no aqueous or vitreous cells. Atrophy and pigment dispersion result once the active process resolves. Optic neuritis, retinal detachment, or cystoid macular edema may develop.

Work-up

1. History and complete ocular examination, including dilated fundus examination.
2. Fluorescein angiography may be helpful in the fundus evaluation.
3. Referral to an internist for a systemic CMV work-up (e.g., urine for CMV and repeat complement fixation and neutralization titers).

Treatment   Ganciclovir (9-[1,3-dihydroxy-2-propoxymethyl] guanine) 2.5 mg/ kg iv q 8 hours or 5.0 mg/kg iv q 12 hours $\times$ 10-20 days in the hospital; then 6 mg/kg/day iv, 5 of 7 days as an outpatient (given through an indwelling catheter) indefinitely.

NOTES ON GANCICLOVIR

1. The dosage may need to be reduced in the presence of renal disease.
2. Patients should not be on systemic azidothymidine (AZT) at the same time.
3. This suppresses CMV and does not cure the retinitis. With discontinuation of the drug, the disease progresses.
4. A CBC needs to be repeated several ×/week during the initial therapy and less frequently during maintenance therapy.
5. Ganciclovir use requires approval by the Food and Drug Administration; treatment criteria are now being established.

Toxoplasmosis

Symptoms   Decreased vision, floaters, photophobia, pain, red eye.

Critical Signs   Hazy yellow-white retinochoroidal lesions accompanied by vitreous cells and debris. Hemorrhage is minimal. The infection is often newly acquired, and an old retinochoroidal scar is typically not observed. The lesions may be bilateral and/or multifocal.

Work-up

1. Complete ocular examination with special emphasis on the neuro-ophthalmic aspects.
2. Referral to an internist for a complete medical work-up (emphasize the need to watch for CNS toxoplasmosis).

NOTE   Toxoplasmosis antibody titers may be unreliable.

Treatment   Not well established. See "Toxoplasmosis," Section 13.3 for drug dosages.

1. Pyrimethamine plus (a) clindamycin (first choice) or (b) sulfadiazine or (c) tetracycline (or an equivalent).
2. Topical steroid (e.g., prednisolone acetate 1% q 1-6 hours, the dosage depending on the degree of anterior-segment inflammation).
3. Topical cycloplegic (e.g., scopolamine ¼% tid) in the presence of anterior-segment inflammation.

NOTES

1. Maintenance therapy may be required to prevent recurrence of the disease. Clindamycin should probably not be used for this purpose.

2. Systemic steroids may allow for advancement of infection, and their role in ocular toxoplasmosis in AIDS is uncertain.

Candida Retinitis: See Section 13.13.

Others

Herpes simplex virus, Mycobacterium tuberculosis or avium-intracellulare, Cryptococcus neoformans, Histoplasma capsulatum, herpes zoster, Aspergillus, and Nocardia are all rarely seen.

Neuro-ophthalmic Manifestations

Cranial-nerve palsies, pupillary abnormalities, visual field defects, and visual hallucinations may occur as a result of CNS infection (e.g., toxoplasmosis) or tumor. There is an increased incidence of neurosyphilis in the AIDS population, suggesting the need for lumbar puncture in all patients with syphilis and a (+) HIV titer. (See "Acquired Syphilis," Section 14.2.)

TREATMENT FOR AIDS

Azidothymidine (AZT) has demonstrated short-term improvement in many AIDS and ARC patients. Management is by an internist.

REFERENCES

HOLLAND GN, ENGSTROM RE JR., GLASGOW BJ, et al. Ocular toxoplasmosis in patients with the Acquired Immunodeficiency Syndrome. *Am J Ophthalmol* 106:653, 1988.

JABS DA, NEWMAN C, DE BUSTROS S, POLD BF. Treatment of cytomegalovirus retinitis with ganciclovir. *Ophthalmology* 94:824, 1987.

SEIFF SR, MARGOLIS T, GRAHAM SH, O'DONNELL JJ. Use of intravenous acyclovir for treatment of herpes zoster ophthalmicus in patients at risk for AIDS. *Ann Ophthalmol* 20:480, 1988.

SHEPP DH, DANDLIKER RN, MYERS JD. Treatment of varicella-zoster virus infection in severely immunocompromised patients: A randomized comparison of acyclovir and vidarabine. *N Engl J Med* 314:208-212, 1986.

14.2   Acquired Syphilis

Systemic Signs

STAGES

Primary   Chancre (ulcerated, painless lesion), regional lymphadenopathy.

Secondary   Skin/mucous membrane lesions, generalized lymphadenopathy, constitutional symptoms (e.g., sore throat, fever, etc.), and other less common, but more severe abnormalities, including symptomatic or asymptomatic meningitis.

Latent   No clinical manifestations.

Tertiary   Cardiovascular disease (e.g., aortitis), central nervous system disease (meningovascular disease, general paresis, tabes dorsalis).

Ocular Signs

Primary   A chancre may occur on the eyelid or conjunctiva.

Secondary   Uveitis, optic neuritis, active chorioretinitis, retinitis, retinal vasculitis, conjunctivitis, dacryoadenitis, dacryocystitis, episcleritis, scleritis, interstitial keratitis (monocular), others.

Tertiary   Optic atrophy, old chorioretinitis, interstitial keratitis, chronic iritis, Argyll Robertson pupil (will not react to light, but will accommodate; see Section 11.3), and other signs seen in secondary disease.

NOTE   Patchy hyperemia of the iris with the development of fleshy, pink nodules near the iris sphincter is pathognomonic of syphilis.

Differential Diagnosis   See "Anterior Uveitis" (Section 13.1) and "Posterior Uveitis" (Section 13.2).

Work-up   (See Sections 13.1 and 13.2 for a nonspecific uveitis work-up.)

1. Complete ophthalmic examination, including a pupillary evaluation, a slit-lamp examination, and a dilated fundus examination.
2. VDRL or RPR: Reflects the activity of the disease and is important in following the response to treatment. Used for screening, but many false negatives can occur in early primary, latent, or late syphilis. Not as specific as (3).
3. FTA-ABS or MHA-TP: Very sensitive and specific in all stages of syphilis. Once reactive, it does not revert back to normal and, therefore, cannot be used to assess the response to treatment.

4. Human immunodeficiency virus (HIV) serology: Should be offered to patients with sexually transmitted diseases.
5. Lumbar puncture (LP). The indications are controversial. We consider an LP in the following:
   a. (+) FTA-ABS and neurologic or neuro-ophthalmologic signs, papillitis, active chorioretinitis, or posterior uveitis.
   b. Patients who are HIV (+) as well as FTA-ABS (+).
   c. Treatment failures.
   d. Patients to be treated with a nonpenicillin regimen (as a baseline).
   e. Patients with untreated syphilis of unknown duration or greater than 1-year duration.

Treatment Indications

A. *(−) FTA-ABS:* No treatment indicated. Patient probably does not have syphilis.
B. *(+) FTA-ABS and (−) VDRL*
   If appropriate past treatment *cannot* be documented, treatment is indicated.
   If appropriate past treatment *can* be documented, treatment is not indicated.
C. *(+) FTA-ABS and (+) VDRL:* A VDRL titer of 1:8 or greater (e.g., 1:64) is expected to decline at least fourfold within one year of appropriate treatment, and should revert to negative (or at least to 1:4 or less) within 1 year in primary syphilis, 2 years in secondary syphilis, and 5 years in tertiary syphilis. A VDRL of less than 1:8 (e.g., 1:4) often does *not* drop fourfold. The following recommendations, therefore, are made:

   - If appropriate past treatment *cannot* be documented, treatment is indicated.
   - If appropriate past treatment *can* be documented and . . .

   A previous VDRL titer greater than or equal to fourfold the current titer can be documented, no treatment is indicated (unless 5 years have passed and the titer is still greater than 1:4).

   A previous VDRL titer was greater than or equal to 1:8 and did not drop fourfold, treatment is indicated.

   The previous VDRL titer was less than 1:8, treatment is not indicated unless the current titer has *risen* fourfold.

   A previous VDRL is unavailable, treatment is not required unless treatment was more than several years prior and the VDRL is still greater than 1:4.

NOTE   If active syphilitic signs (e.g., active chorioretinitis or papillitis) are present despite appropriate past treatment (regardless of the VDRL titer), LP and treatment may be needed.

Treatment

A. *Neurosyphilis* ([+] FTA-ABS in the serum and either cell count >5 WBC/mm^3, protein > 45 mg/dl, or [+] cerebrospinal fluid [CSF] VDRL on LP): IV aqueous crystalline penicillin (PCN) G 2-4 million units q 4 hours × 10-14 days followed by benzathine PCN 2.4 million units im q week × 3 weeks (1.2 million units to each buttock).

B. *Syphilis with abnormal ocular, but normal CSF findings:* Benzathine PCN 2.4 million units im q week × 3 weeks.

NOTES

1. The therapy for PCN allergic patients is not well established. Tetracycline 500 mg po qid × 30 days is used by some for both late and neurosyphilis, but better CSF penetration may be obtained with doxycycline or a third-generation cephalosporin.

2. If anterior-segment inflammation is present, treatment with a cycloplegic (e.g., cyclopentolate 2% tid) and topical steroid (e.g., prednisolone acetate 1% qid) may be beneficial.

Follow-up

A. *Neurosyphilis:* Repeat the LP every 6 months for 2 years, shorten if the cell count returns to normal sooner. The cell count should fall to a normal level within this time period and the CSF VDRL titer should drop fourfold (these changes typically occur within 6-12 months). An elevated CSF protein falls more slowly. If these indices do not fall as expected, retreatment may be indicated.

B. *Other forms of syphilis:* Repeat the VDRL titer at 3 and 6 months after treatment.

If a VDRL titer of 1:8 or more does not decline fourfold within 6 months, if the VDRL titer rises fourfold at any point, or if clinical symptoms or signs of syphilis persist or recur, Lp and retreatment are indicated.

If a pretreatment VDRL titer is less than 1:8, retreatment is only indicated when the titer rises during follow-up or symptoms or signs of syphilis recur.

See "Congenital Syphilis," Section 14.3, for additional information.

14.3 Congenital Syphilis

Presenting Ocular Signs Any of the following may be present.

1. *Interstitial keratitis (IK)* Usually presents acutely in the first or second decade of life with cellular infiltration and superficial and deep vascularization of the cornea (corneal "salmon patch"). Both eyes eventually become affected. As the inflammation resolves, the cornea may thin, opacify, or exhibit blood vessels containing no blood within their lumens (ghost vessels).
2. *Anterior uveitis* Cells and flare in the anterior chamber.
3. *Chorioretinitis* Typically appears as a "salt and pepper" fundus (pigmented areas interspersed among atrophic white areas).
4. *Optic atrophy* A pale optic nerve.

Systemic Signs Widely spaced, peg-shaped teeth (Hutchinson's teeth), frontal bossing, depressed nasal bridge (saddle nose), nerve deafness, recurrent arthropathy, linear scars at the angles of the mouth, mental retardation, and others.

Differential Diagnosis

- Other congenital infections (toxoplasmosis, rubella, cytomegalovirus, herpes simplex or zoster virus, or rubeola [measles]) (Specific serological titers will usually be positive; RPR and FTA-ABS will usually be negative.)

Work-up

1. History: Maternal syphilis? Medical problems since birth (persistent runny nose, rash, deafness, scars on the skin, others)? Previous treatment for syphilis?
2. Complete ocular examination, including a pupillary assessment, a slit-lamp examination if possible, and a dilated fundus examination (in interstitial keratitis, the fundus may not be well visualized).
3. B-scan ultrasound should be considered when no fundus view is obtained to rule out a retinal detachment and mass lesion.
4. Blood tests: RPR (or VDRL) and FTA-ABS (or MHA-TP)[1]; consider viral and toxoplasma titers when the diagnosis is uncertain.

---

[1] Both the RPR (or VDRL) and FTA-ABS (or MHA-TP) can be positive in a syphilis-free infant born to a mother with the disease. The RPR usually converts back to negative by 3 months of age in a disease-free child; the FTA-ABS is usually found to be negative by 6 months of age. A positive IgM-FTA-ABS in an infant suggests active disease in the infant.

5. Consider darkfield examination of scrapings from skin lesions (if available).
6. Lumbar puncture (LP) (for routine studies including a VDRL) is indicated in all cases of active disease or in cases of inactive disease not previously treated.

Treatment See "Acquired Syphilis," Section 14.2, for treatment indications.

1. Systemic antibiotic (one of the following):
    a. Aqueous crystalline penicillin G 50,000 units/kg/day im or iv in 2 divided doses × 10-14 days
    b. Aqueous procaine penicillin G 50,000 units/kg im daily × 10-14 days
    c. For penicillin allergic patients: Erythromycin 50 mg/kg/day po in 4 divided doses × 2 weeks
2. In the presence of acute interstitial keratitis or anterior-chamber inflammation, a topical steroid (prednisolone acetate 1% 4-8×/day) and a cycloplegic (e.g., scopolamine ¼% tid) should be used.
3. Intraocular pressure control (e.g., if >30 mm Hg, consider levobunolol ½% bid or timolol ¼-½% bid and/or acetazolamide 5 mg/kg po q 6 hours).

Follow-up Patients are seen daily until their systemic therapy is completed and then in 1-2 weeks. When the LP is abnormal (e.g., positive cerebrospinal fluid [CSF] VDRL, white blood cell count >5 WBC/mm^3 or protein >45 mg/dl), follow-up is as described for neurosyphilis (see "Acquired Syphilis," Section 14.2). Otherwise, follow-up is as described for other forms of acquired syphilis (see Section 14.2). Remember, the FTA-ABS typically remains reactive despite treatment.

REFERENCE

RAKEL RE, ed. Conn's Current Therapy. 39th ed. Philadelphia: WB Saunders Company, 594, 1987.

14.4 Lyme Disease

Symptoms Decreased vision, double vision, pain, photophobia, facial weakness. Patients may also complain of headache, malaise, fatigue, fever, chills, palpitations, or muscle or joint pains. A history of a tick bite within the previous few months can often be elicited.

Ocular Signs Optic neuritis, vitritis, iritis, choroiditis, exudative retinal detachment, cranial-nerve palsy (III, IV, or VI), bilateral optic-nerve swelling, conjunctivitis, episcleritis, exposure keratopathy, or other rare abnormalities, including orbital inflammatory pseudotumor.

Critical Systemic Signs One or more flat erythematous or "bull's eye" skin lesions which enlarge in all directions (erythema chronica migrans), unilateral or bilateral facial-nerve palsies, and arthritis. The skin lesions and arthritis may be transient and migratory. These findings may not be present at the time the ocular signs develop. A high serum antibody titer against the causative agent, Borrelia burgdorferi, is often, but not always present.

Other Systemic Signs Meningitis, peripheral radiculoneuropathy, synovitis, joint effusions, cardiac abnormalities, and/or a low false positive FTA-ABS titer.

Differential Diagnosis

• Syphilis   (High positive FTA-ABS titer, may produce a low false positive antibody titer against B. burgdorferi. No history of a tick bite. May have interstitial keratitis, patchy iris hyperemia, a "salt and pepper" chorioretinitis, or pigmented "bone spicules" on fundus examination.)
• Others   (Rickettsial infections, acute rheumatic fever, juvenile rheumatoid arthritis.)

Work-up

1. History: Prior tick bite, skin rash, Bell's palsy, joint or muscle pains, flu-like illness? Meningeal symptoms?
2. Complete systemic (especially neurological) and ocular examinations.
3. Serum antibody levels against B. burgdorferi, using an immunofluorescence assay or an enzyme-linked immunosorbent assay. (These tests are sometimes negative despite the presence of Lyme disease.)
4. Serum RPR and FTA-ABS.
5. Consider a lumbar puncture when meningitis is suspected or neurologic signs or symptoms are present.

Treatment Current recommendations vary, but include one of the following:

ADULTS

First choice Tetracycline 250 mg po qid or doxycycline 100 mg po bid × 10-20 days.
Second choice Penicillin VK 500 mg po qid × 10-20 days.
Third choice Erythromycin 250 mg po qid × 10-20 days.

CHILDREN

First choice   Penicillin 50 mg/kg/day po in 4 divided doses (not <1 g/day or >2 g/day) for 15-20 days.

Second choice   Erythromycin 30 mg/kg/day po in 3-4 divided doses for 15-20 days.

PATIENTS WITH NEURO-OPHTHALMIC SIGNS OR RECURRENT OR RESISTANT INFECTION

Ceftriaxone 2 g iv q 12 hours for 14 days.
Aqueous crystalline penicillin G 2-4 million units iv q 4 hours for 10 days.

Follow-up   Daily until improvement is demonstrated.

REFERENCES

BERTUCH AW, ROCCO E, SCHWARTZ, EG. Lyme Disease: Ocular manifestations. *Annals of Ophthalmol* 20:376, 1988.
FINKEL MF. Lyme disease and its neurological complications. *Arch Neurol* 45:99, 1988.
MACDONALD, AB. Lyme disease. *J Clin Neuro-ophthalmol* 7(4):1850, 1987.

14.5   Chicken Pox

Symptoms   Facial rash, red eye, foreign-body sensation.

Ocular Signs

Early   Acute conjunctivitis with vesicles or papules at the limbus, eyelid margin, or on the conjunctiva. Pseudodendritic corneal epithelial lesions, stromal keratitis, anterior uveitis, optic neuritis, retinitis, and ophthalmoplegia occur rarely.

Late (weeks to months after the outbreak)   Immune stromal or neurotrophic keratitis may occur.

Treatment

A. *Conjunctival involvement:* Cool compresses and erythromycin ointment to the eye and periorbital lesions tid.

B. *Corneal epithelial lesions:* Same as (A).

C. *Stromal keratitis with uveitis:* Topical steroid (e.g., prednisolone acetate 1% qid), cycloplegic (e.g., atropine 1% bid), and erythromycin ointment qhs.
D. *Neurotrophic keratitis:* See "Neurotrophic Keratopathy," Section 4.5.

NOTE Do *not* give aspirin to these children due to the possible risk of Reye's syndrome. Immunocompromised children with chicken pox may require IV acyclovir.

Follow-up Follow-up in 1-7 days, depending on the severity of ocular disease. Taper the topical steroids slowly. Watch for stromal or neurotrophic keratitis weeks to months after the chicken pox resolves.

14.6 Diabetes Mellitus

I. Diabetic Retinopathy

Signs

A. *Background* Dot and blot hemorrhages, microaneurysms, and hard exudates, generally most prominent in the posterior pole. Nearly always bilateral.
B. *Preproliferative* Cotton wool spots, venous beading and loops, intraretinal microvascular abnormalities (IRMA), and widespread capillary nonperfusion (seen on fluorescein angiography) plus findings in (A).
C. *Proliferative* Neovascularization within 1 disc diameter of or involving the optic disc (NVD), retina (NVE), or iris (NVI), fibrous tissue along the posterior surface of the vitreous and adherent to the retina, retinal detachment, vitreous hemorrhage. The findings in (A) and (B) are sometimes present. Usually bilateral. Almost always in the posterior pole.

NOTE Macular edema may be present in any of the above stages.

Differential Diagnosis

A. *Background and preproliferative*
  • Central retinal vein occlusion (CRVO) (Optic-disc swelling is present, veins are more tortuous, hard exudates are usually absent, hemorrhages

are more prominent, and it is generally unilateral and of more sudden onset.)
- Branch retinal vein occlusion (BRVO)   (The hemorrhages are distributed along the course of a vein, and do *not* extend across the horizontal raphé [midline].)
- Ocular ischemic syndrome   (The hemorrhages are larger and mostly in the mid-periphery, exudate is absent.)
- Hypertensive retinopathy   (The hemorrhages are more commonly flame-shaped and rarely abundant, microaneurysms occur less frequently, and the retinal arteries are narrowed.)
- Radiation retinopathy   (Microaneurysms are rarely present. Follows radiation therapy to the eye or adnexal structures such as the brain, sinus, or nasopharynx when the eye is irradiated inadvertently. May develop anytime after the radiation therapy, but most commonly within a few years. Generally 3000 rads are necessary, but it has been noted to occur with 1500 rads.)

B. *Proliferative*
- Neovascular complications of BRVO, CRVO, or central retinal artery occlusion   (History of one of these events. See above.)
- Sickle-cell retinopathy   (Retinal neovascularization occurs peripherally, generally not in the macula. "Sea-fans" of retinal neovascularization are present.)
- Embolization from IV drug abuse (e.g., talc retinopathy)   (History of IV drug abuse, peripheral retinal neovascularization, may see particles of talc in macular vessels.)
- Sarcoidosis   (May have uveitis, exudates around veins ["candle wax drippings"], or systemic findings.)
- Ocular ischemic syndrome   (Generally accompanied by pain, mild anterior-chamber reaction, corneal edema, episcleral vascular congestion, a mid-dilated, poorly reactive pupil, and pulsations of the central retinal artery.)

Work-up

1. Examine the iris carefully for neovascularization. (Check the angle with gonioscopy, especially if the intraocular pressure is elevated.)
2. Dilated fundus examination using a 90 or 60 diopter lens (or a fundus contact lens) with a slit lamp to obtain a stereoscopic view of the posterior pole. Rule out neovascularization and macular edema. Use indirect ophthalmoscopy to examine the retinal periphery.
3. Fasting blood sugar and, if necessary, a glucose tolerance test if the diagnosis is not established.
4. Check the blood pressure.

5. Obtain fluorescein angiography if uncertain about the presence of macular edema or neovascularization.
6. Consider blood tests for hyperlipidemia if extensive exudate is present.

Treatment

INDICATIONS

A. *Focal laser treatment should be considered when any of the following forms of macular edema is present.*
   1. Retinal thickening within 500 microns (⅓ disc diameter) of the center of the macula.
   2. Hard exudates within 500 microns of the center of the macula if associated with thickening of the adjacent retina.
   3. Retinal thickening greater than 1 disc area in size, part of which is within 1 disc diameter of the center of the macula.
B. *Panretinal photocoagulation (laser) is indicated for any one of the following conditions.*
   1. NVD greater than ¼-⅓ of the disc area in size.
   2. Any degree of NVD when associated with preretinal or vitreous hemorrhage.
   3. NVE greater than ½ disc area in size when associated with a preretinal or vitreous hemorrhage.
   4. NVI.

NOTE   Some physicians treat NVE or any degree of NVD without preretinal or vitreous hemorrhage.

(If the ocular media is too hazy for an adequate fundus view, yet one of the above conditions is met, peripheral retinal cryotherapy may be indicated if there is no vitreous traction.)

C. *Vitrectomy may be indicated for any one of the following conditions.*
   1. Dense vitreous hemorrhage causing decreased vision (especially when present for several months).
   2. Traction retinal detachment involving the macula.
   3. Macular epiretinal membranes or recent onset displacement of the macula.
   4. Severe retinal neovascularization and fibrous proliferation, unresponsive to laser photocoagulation.

NOTE   B-scan ultrasonography and/or a visual evoked potential may be required to rule out tractional detachment of the macula in eyes with dense vitreous hemorrhage obscuring a fundus view.

Follow-up

>*Diabetes without retinopathy* Dilated fundus examination yearly.
>*Background diabetic retinopathy* Dilated fundus examination every 6 months.
>*Preproliferative retinopathy* Dilated fundus examination every 2-4 months.
>*Proliferative retinopathy not meeting treatment criteria* Dilated fundus examination every 1-3 months.

(See Section 14.8, for pregnancy-related follow-up in diabetics.)

II. Neuro-ophthalmic Problems

Cranial-nerve Abnormalities

An isolated third-, fourth-, or sixth-cranial-nerve palsy, often associated with pain in or around the eye may result from diabetic microvascular disease. Only very rarely are two nerves involved simultaneously. Typically, third-nerve involvement spares the pupil (i.e., it does not become dilated). A diabetic cranial-nerve paralysis usually resolves within three months. No treatment is indicated.

Acute Disc Edema

Benign disc edema may occur in one or both eyes of a diabetic, most commonly with mild visual loss. It generally resolves after several weeks. There is no correlation with the severity of diabetic retinopathy. Telangiectasia of disc vessels may accompany the disc edema, simulating neovascularization. No treatment is indicated.

III. Glaucoma

Primary Open-Angle Glaucoma

Diabetics are at an increased risk for this form of glaucoma. When treating with a topical beta-blocker, additional care must be exercised in monitoring for side effects. A diabetic being treated with a beta-blocker may not experience the warning symptoms of hypoglycemia (e.g., sweating, shaking, nightmares, and restlessness), and may, therefore, remain hypoglycemic for a dangerously long period of time without correcting the situation.

Neovascular Glaucoma

As discussed above, neovascularization of the iris (and glaucoma) is a complication of diabetes, and panretinal photocoagulation is indicated as soon as possible.

IV. Miscellaneous

Refractive Changes

Acute hyperglycemia may produce a sudden hyperopic or myopic shift, causing bilateral blurred vision. Glasses should not be prescribed until the patient's blood sugar has been stable for several months.

Cataract

Diabetics are at an increased risk of cataract, especially posterior subcapsular cataracts.

Mucormycosis

A rare but life-threatening orbital infection by mucormycosis can occur in diabetics, particularly those with ketoacidosis. Any diabetic or compromised host with the appearance of orbital cellulitis (eyelid edema, proptosis, external ophthalmoplegia, and fever) should be further examined for necrosis of the skin, nasal mucosa, or palate. An emergency CT scan of the sinuses, orbit, and brain should be performed to aid in diagnosis. A biopsy should be obtained from any necrotic tissue as well as the nasopharynx and paranasal sinuses if this condition is suspected. Treatment is with amphotericin B. See "Cavernous Sinus/Superior Orbital Fissure Syndrome," Section 11.8.

REFERENCES

THE DIABETIC RETINOPATHY VITRECTOMY STUDY RESEARCH GROUP. Early vitrectomy for proliferative diabetic retinopathy in eyes with useful vision: Results of a randomized trial—Diabetic retinopathy vitrectomy study report 3. *Ophthalmology* 95:1307, 1988.
THE DIABETIC RETINOPATHY STUDY RESEARCH GROUP. Photocoagulation treatment of proliferative diabetic retinopathy: The second report of diabetic retinopathy study findings. *Ophthalmology* 85:82, 1978.

THE EARLY TREATMENT DIABETIC RETINOPATHY RESEARCH STUDY GROUP; Photocoagulation for diabetic macular edema. ETDRS Report #1. *Arch Ophthalmol* 103. 1796, 1985.

14.7 Albinism

Symptoms   Decreased vision and photophobia.

Signs   Nystagmus, iris transillumination defects, visible choroidal vasculature, absent foveal pit, absence of macular hyperpigmentation, failure of the retinal vessels to wreathe the fovea, and a pink reflex through an undilated pupil.

Types

  I. Oculocutaneous: Hair, skin, and eye affected.
     A. Tyrosinase positive: Some pigment as adults.
     B. Tyrosinase negative: No pigment, ever.
  II. Ocular: Decreased ocular pigment only. Skin may be lighter than siblings, but appears normal.

NOTE   The only reliable ocular finding (which is always present) is foveal hypoplasia.

Associated Disorders

  • Hermansky-Pudlak syndrome   (A bleeding disorder secondary to platelet dysfunction. There is a high incidence in patients of Puerto Rican descent.)
  • Chediak-Higashi syndrome   (An autosomal recessive disorder affecting white blood cell function, causing a high susceptibility to infection and a predisposition for a lymphoma-like condition.)

Work-up

  1. History: Easy bruisability? Frequent nosebleeds? Prolonged bleeding after dental work? Frequent infections?
  2. Family history.
  3. External examination (check hair and skin color).
  4. Complete ocular examination including a slit-lamp evaluation (nystagmus, iris color, and iris transillumination) and a dilated fundus examination.
  5. Obtain a bleeding time if the patient is planning to undergo surgery. Some physicians feel a bleeding time should be obtained in all albinos. If the

Hermansky-Pudlak syndrome is suspected, a bleeding time, platelet aggregation studies, and platelet electron microscopy are indicated.
6. If the Chediak-Higashi syndrome is suspected, polymorphonuclear leukocyte function should be evaluated by a hematologist.

Treatment There is currently no effective treatment of albinism, but the following may be helpful:

1. Tinted eyeglasses may reduce photophobia.
2. Low-vision aides may be helpful in adults.
3. Genetic counseling.

NOTES

1. Albinos with strabismus rarely achieve binocularity after strabismus surgery, possibly due to a lack of the necessary neuronal connections.
2. Albinos do poorly after retinal detachment repair due to nystagmus and inherently weak retinal pigment epithelium–retinal adhesions.
3. Patients with the Hermansky-Pudlak syndrome may require platelet transfusion prior to surgery.

14.8 Pregnancy

Many ocular problems can arise as a result of pregnancy. Below are listed some of the complaints that induce pregnant women to seek eye care and some of the disorders that should be considered in pregnancy.

Blurred or Decreased Vision

CHANGE IN REFRACTIVE ERROR

(Visual acuity decreased with current glasses, but can be improved to normal status with a new refraction or a pin hole. No other findings on examination.)

The patient's change in refraction is probably due to a shift in fluid and/or hormonal status and will most likely revert back to normal after delivery. Unless the patient has a strong desire (e.g., occupational need) to change her glasses prescription, it is best to wait several weeks postpartum before giving a new prescription.

PREECLAMPTIC/ECLAMPTIC HYPERTENSIVE RETINOPATHY

(Occurs after 20 weeks' gestation. Same clinical findings as hypertensive retinopathy of other etiologies: Focal or generalized narrowing of the arterioles, flame-shaped hemorrhages, cotton wool spots, $+/-$ disc swelling. An exudative retinal detachment can occur. Bilateral occipital lobe infarction and cortical blindness can rarely occur.)

The severity of retinal changes correlates with the risk of fetal mortality and possibly with the risk of damage to the mother's kidneys. If severe retinopathy is present and progressing, strong consideration should be made with regard to terminating the pregnancy. Sometimes the clinical findings (e.g., exudative retinal detachment) resolve with blood pressure control.

CENTRAL SEROUS CHORIODOPATHY

(Localized detachment of the sensory retina from the underlying pigment epithelium by clear serous fluid in the macular area. The margins of the detachment are sloping and merge gradually into attached retina. No blood is present.)

With rare exception, observation is the treatment of choice with most cases resolving postpartum. A more hyperopic correction may be provided as a temporary visual aid. Focal laser therapy is rarely needed.

RETINAL DETACHMENT

Usually exudative, resolving a few weeks after delivery. The visual prognosis is generally good and no treatment is indicated. The pregnancy does not have to be terminated if preeclampsia/eclampsia can be ruled out.

DIABETIC RETINOPATHY

Visual loss from diabetes may occur in patients who had diabetes prior to gestation. Following are our recommendations for management.

A. Gestational diabetes: Not at risk for retinopathy. No treatment or retinal follow-up is required.
B. No retinopathy or only minimal background retinopathy prior to pregnancy: Baseline examination in the first trimester and a repeat examination in the third trimester. No treatment is needed.
C. Background retinopathy (microaneurysms, dot and blot hemorrhages, hard exudates): Examination every trimester. No treatment is needed.
D. Preproliferative retinopathy (cotton wool spots, venous beading and loops, intraretinal microvascular abnormalities): Examine every month. No treatment is indicated.
E. Proliferative retinopathy (during any stage of pregnancy; neovascularization of the disc, retina, or iris): Laser panretinal photocoagulation as usual. Earlier, more aggressive institution of therapy is important in pregnant women due to a tendency of proliferative diabetes to progress rapidly. This is not an indication to terminate pregnancy.

NOTE   Active proliferative retinopathy at the time of labor may indicate a need for Caesarean section since Valsalva at the time of delivery may cause vitreous hemorrhage.

Headache

PITUITARY ADENOMA

Pituitary adenomas may enlarge during pregnancy, producing a visual field disturbance (classically a bitemporal hemianopsia) or headache. As subclinical pituitary adenomas may produce amenorrhea, women who underwent treatment to induce ovulation should be examined with a high index of suspicion.

A possible cause of pituitary adenoma enlargement during pregnancy is pituitary apoplexy, a potentially life-threatening event. Therefore, any woman with a diagnosis of a pituitary adenoma who presents with a headache or a new visual field defect should receive an MRI +/− a lumbar puncture (LP) to rule out subarachnoid hemorrhage from the tumor. Women with growing pituitary adenomas (especially with evidence of subarachnoid blood on imaging) should be delivered by Caesarean section to avoid the risk of apoplexy during the delivery. Postpartum hemorrhage or shock can cause an infarction of the pituitary gland leading to hypopituitarism (Sheehan's syndrome).

PSEUDOTUMOR CEREBRI

There may be an increased incidence of this entity in pregnant women. Headache, papilledema, a normal CT scan of the head, and a high opening pressure on LP with a normal spinal fluid composition confirm the diagnosis. Treatment may be difficult since many of the medications generally used to treat this entity are contraindicated in pregnant women. This entity typically worsens with pregnancy.

PREECLAMPTIC/ECLAMPTIC HYPERTENSIVE DISEASE

As discussed above. Refer to the obstetrician for blood pressure control.

MIGRAINE HEADACHE

Usually worse during pregnancy and immediately postpartum.

MENINGIOMA OF PREGNANCY

Very aggressive growth pattern. Difficult to treat.

OTHERS

For example cortical vein thrombosis.

NOTE   All pregnant women complaining of a headache should have their blood pressure, visual fields, and fundus checked (particularly looking for papilledema). A CT scan of the head without contrast, shielding the abdomen, may need to be performed. As mentioned above, MRI +/− LP is often required if a hemorrhage is suspected.

Difficulty Wearing Contact Lenses

CORNEAL CHANGES

Physiological changes in the cornea may hinder contact lens wear. As corneal sensitivity is also known to decrease during pregnancy (possibly increasing the risk of infection), discontinuation of contact lenses is often advisable.

14.9   Stevens-Johnson Syndrome

(Erythema Multiforme Major)

Symptoms   Acute onset of fever, rash, red eye, often with generalized malaise and arthralgias.

Critical Signs   "Target" lesions on the skin (red centered vesicles surrounded by a pale ring which is surrounded by a red ring), hemorrhagic crusting of the lips, bilateral conjunctivitis.

Other Signs   Skin vesicles, bullae, and maculopapular lesions concentrated on the hands and feet, ruptured bullae of the mouth, and ulcerative stomatitis. Corneal neovascularization, scarring of the conjunctiva and/or cornea, dry eyes, symblepharon, eyelid deformities, corneal ulcers, corneal perforation, and/or endophthalmitis may develop. Patients may appear toxic. The mortality rate is 10-33%.

Etiology   May be precipitated by many agents, including any of the following:

- Drugs (e.g., sulfonamides, barbiturates, chlorpropamide, thiazide diuretics, phenytoin, salicylates, tetracycline, codeine, and penicillins)
- Infectious agents (e.g., various bacteria, viruses, and fungi, especially herpes and mycoplasma)

Differential Diagnosis

- Ocular pemphigoid   (Slowly progressive scarring of the conjunctiva with symblepharon formation, forniceal shortening, and dry eye. Mucous membrane vesicles or ruptured or formed bullae are evident.)

Work-up

1. History: Attempt to determine the precipitating factor.
2. Slit-lamp examination: Be certain to evert the eyelids and examine the fornices.
3. Conjunctival and corneal scrapings for stains and cultures if infection is suspected, see "Infectious Corneal Infiltrate/Ulcer," Section 4.12.
4. Electrolyte profile, CBC.

Treatment

1. Hospitalize.
2. Treat the precipitating factor (e.g., remove the antibiotic, treat the infection, etc.).
3. Topical steroid (e.g., prednisolone acetate 1% 4-8 × /day, depending on the severity of the anterior-segment inflammation).
4. Systemic steroids (e.g., prednisone 80-100 mg po q day) (controversial) + an H_2 blocker (e.g., ranitidine 150 mg po bid.) See Appendix 5 for a systemic steroid work-up.
5. Topical antibiotic (e.g., erythromycin or bacitracin ointment 2-3 × /day).
6. Artificial tears (e.g., Refresh drops q 1-2 hours) prn.
7. Cycloplegic (e.g., atropine 1% tid).
8. Break symblepharon with a glass rod bid after instilling a topical anesthetic (e.g., proparacaine).
9. Supportive systemic care prn (i.e., hydration, local mouth and skin care, systemic antibiotics, etc.).

Follow-up

- Follow daily in the hospital watching for the development of an infectious ulcer or elevated intraocular pressure. When the acute phase has resolved, weekly outpatient follow-ups are initiated, watching for long-term ocular complications.
- Steroid and antibiotic treatment are maintained for 48 hours after the eye is healed and then tapered.
- Artificial tears and lubricating ointment may need to be maintained indefinitely if the conjunctiva has been severely scarred.
- If trichiasis develops, cryotherapy or surgical repair may be indicated.
- Consider a keratoprosthesis in a scarred endstage eye with visual potential.

14.10 Vitamin A Deficiency

Symptoms Dry eye, foreign-body sensation, ocular pain, night blindness, or severe loss of vision. Gradual onset in most cases.

Critical Signs Patients often appear malnourished or are victims of a process causing defective vitamin A absorption or utilization. Bilateral conjunctival and corneal dryness with lack of the normal luster, Bitot's spot (paralimbal, silvery-white dots in a triangular patch), and a decreased tear film break-up time are typical.

Other Signs Sterile corneal ulceration with a sharp delineation between normal and abnormal stroma; corneal perforation or secondary bacterial infection may occur. There may be loss of pigment in the retinal periphery.

Etiology

  Primary Dietary lack of vitamin A (usually from malnutrition or an extreme dietary habit—relatively uncommon in developed countries).
  Secondary Vitamin A deficiency in the presence of an adequate dietary intake, often from cystic fibrosis in children and young adults, chronic pancreatitis, postgastrectomy surgery, inflammatory bowel disease, post–intestinal bypass surgery for obesity, chronic liver disease, abetalipoproteinemia (Bassen-Kornzweig syndrome), others.

Differential Diagnosis See "Dry Eye Syndrome," Section 4.2.

Work-up

  1. History: Malnutrition? Poor or extreme diet? GI or liver disease? Previous surgery?
  2. Complete ophthalmic examination: Be certain to test eyelid closure, inspect the eyelid margins, and pull down the lower eyelids to examine the inferior fornices.
  3. Serum vitamin A level before treatment is initiated (typically <20-80 ug/dl).
  4. Impression cytology of the conjunctiva if available.
  5. Dark adaptation electroretinogram (may be more sensitive than the serum vitamin A level which may not fall until the body's reserves are depleted).
  6. If a corneal ulcer exists and appears infected, scrapings for stains and cultures are obtained. See "Infectious Corneal Infiltrate/Ulcer," Section 4.12.

Treatment

1. Vitamin A replacement therapy: Vitamin A palmitate in oil 200,000 i.u. (60,000 μg) po daily for 2 days (an additional dose is occasionally given 2 weeks later).

   • ½ dose for children under 1 year of age and for pregnant women.
   • If unable to utilize the oral route (e.g., due to gastroenteritis) the equivalent dose is given intramuscularly in the water-dispersible form.

2. Intensive ocular lubrication with artificial tears (e.g., Refresh drops) q 15-60 minutes and artificial tear ointment (e.g., Refresh PM) qhs.
3. Topical vitamin A ointment 2-4×/day may be of some benefit.
4. Treatment of malnutrition if present.
5. Consider supplementing the patient's diet with zinc.
6. Consider a penetrating keratoplasty or keratoprosthesis for corneal scars in eyes with potentially good vision.

Follow-up Determined by the clinical presentation and response to treatment. Some patients need to be admitted to the hospital, while others can be followed every several days to weeks.

14.11 Neurofibromatosis

(von Recklinghausen's Syndrome)

Ocular Signs Lisch nodules (multiple light-brown iris nodules), plexiform neurofibroma of the eyelid (''S''-shaped configuration of the upper eyelid with a ''bag of worms'' feeling on palpation), glaucoma, optic-nerve glioma, pulsating proptosis (from the absence of the greater wing of the sphenoid bone with herniation of an encephalocele), astrocytic hamartoma of the retina, conjunctival plexiform neurofibroma, enlarged corneal nerves, diffuse uveal thickening, uveal nevi (and rarely melanoma), myelinated nerve fibers, optic-nerve meningioma, orbital neurofibromas and schwannomas.

Critical Systemic Signs Café-au-lait spots (6 or more lesions larger than 1.5 cm in diameter is diagnostic), axillary freckling, cutaneous neurofibromas.

Other Systemic Signs Intracranial astrocytomas (gliomas), pituitary tumors, bilateral acoustic neuromas, mental deficiencies (mental retardation, hyperactivity, learning disabilities), malignant degeneration of peripheral nerve sheath tumors, pheochromocytoma, gastrointestinal and genitourinary malignancies, including Wilms' tumor, and a variety of other malignancies.

Inheritance Autosomal dominant with incomplete penetrance.

Work-up

1. Family history: Examination of family members is also very important.
2. Complete general and ophthalmic examinations.
3. CBC, electrolytes.
4. CT scan (axial and coronal views) or MRI of the orbit and brain.
5. IQ and psychological testing.
6. Electroencephalogram.
7. Audiography.
8. Urine for levels of epinephrine and norepinephrine.

Treatment

1. Dependent upon findings.
2. Genetic counseling.
3. Psychological support and counseling.

Follow-up Every 6-12 months in the absence of a disorder requiring therapy.

14.12 Tuberous Sclerosis

(Bourneville's Syndrome)

Ocular Sign Astrocytic hamartoma of the retina or optic disc (a white, semi-transparent or "mulberry-appearing" tumor in the superficial retina that may undergo calcification with age; there are no prominent feeder vessels and no associated retinal detachment.)

Critical Systemic Signs Adenoma sebaceum (yellow-red papules in a "butterfly" distribution on the upper cheeks, apparent in the prepubertal years), astrocytic hamartomas of the brain with seizures and/or subnormal intelligence or mental retardation.

Other Systemic Signs Subungal angiofibromas (yellow-red papules around and beneath the nails of the fingers or toes), shagreen patches, ash leaf sign (depigmented macules on the skin), café-au-lait spots, renal angiomyolipoma, cardiac rhabdomyoma, pleural cysts causing spontaneous pneumothorax, cystic bone lesions, and hamartomas of the liver, thyroid, pancreas, or testes.

Inheritance   Autosomal dominant with incomplete penetrance.

Differential Diagnosis

- Retinoblastoma   (Flat or elevated white retinal tumor which has prominent feeder vessels, may be bilateral and/or multifocal. Vitreous seeding, retinal detachment, pseudohypopyon, iris neovascularization, or vitreous hemorrhage may be present. No systemic signs initially.)

Work-up

1. Family history: Examination of the family members is also important.
2. Complete general physical and ophthalmic examinations.
3. CBC, electrolytes.
4. CT scan (axial and coronal views) or MRI of the brain.
5. Electroencephalogram.
6. Echocardiogram.
7. Chest x-ray.
8. Abdominal CT scan.

Treatment

1. Retinal astrocytomas generally require no treatment.
2. Genetic counseling.

Follow-up   Yearly in the absence of a disorder requiring therapy.

14.13   Sturge-Weber Syndrome

(Encephalofacial Cavernous Hemangiomatosis)

Ocular Signs   Diffuse choroidal hemangioma ("tomato catsup" fundus—the lesion obscures all detail of the choroidal vasculature and produces a uniform red fundus background; best appreciated when compared to the other eye), unilateral glaucoma (facial hemangioma of the upper eyelid increases the risk of glaucoma), iris heterochromia, blood in Schlemm's canal (seen on gonioscopy), secondary serous retinal detachment, secondary retinal pigment epithelial alterations (retinitis pigmentosa-like picture).

Critical Systemic Sign Port wine stain—"nevus flammeus" (facial hemangioma along the first and second divisions of the trigeminal nerve).

Other Signs Subnormal intelligence or mental retardation, Jacksonian-type seizures, peripheral arteriovenous communications, facial hemihypertrophy ipsilateral to "nevus flammeus," leptomeningeal angiomatosis, cerebral calcifications.

Inheritance Sporadic.

Work-up

1. Complete general and ophthalmic examinations.
2. CT scan (axial and coronal views) or MRI of the brain.
3. Electroencephalogram.

Treatment

1. Treat glaucoma if present: First-line drugs are aqueous suppressants, e.g., timolol or levobunolol and/or methazolamide; pilocarpine and epinephrine compounds are less effective due to high episcleral venous pressure. See "Primary Open-Angle Glaucoma," Section 10.1.
2. Consider treating serous retinal detachments which are large or are threatening or involving the macula (laser photocoagulation is often used, but the success rate is low).
3. Anticonvulsants for epilepsy.

Follow-up Every 6 months, watching carefully for glaucoma or a serous retinal detachment.

- If glaucoma is present, closer follow-up may be required.
- If skin involvement is only in the mandibular area, the risk of glaucoma is much lower and the interval for follow-up may be extended to one year.

14.14 von Hippel-Lindau Syndrome

(Retinocerebellar Capillary Hemangiomatosis)

Critical Ocular Signs Retinal capillary hemangioma (small yellow-red tumor with a tortuous dilated feeder artery and a draining vein), sometimes associated with subretinal exudations and/or a retinal detachment.

Other Signs   Cerebellar hemangioblastoma, hypernephroma, pheochromocytoma, renal cysts, pancreatic cysts, epididymal cysts, syringomyelia.

Inheritance   Autosomal dominant with incomplete penetrance.

Differential Diagnosis

- Racemose hemangiomatosis   (No definable tumor present, large dilated tortuous vessels forming arteriovenous communications.)
- Coats' disease   (Characteristic aneurysmal dilatation of blood vessels is found with prominent subretinal exudate. No identifiable tumor is present.)

Work-up   (Indicated when multiple or bilateral retinal capillary hemangiomas are discovered, or when a unilateral retinal capillary hemangioma is found along with characteristic systemic findings or a positive family history.)

NOTE   Some physicians work-up all retinal capillary hemangiomas.)

1. Family history and examination of family members.
2. Complete general physical and ophthalmic examinations.
3. CBC, electrolytes.
4. MRI of the brain (visualizes the posterior fossa better than CT scan).
5. Urine for levels of epinephrine and norepinephrine.
6. Abdominal CT scan.
7. Fluorescein angiogram if treatment of the retinal capillary hemangioma is planned.

Treatment

1. Photocoagulation or cryotherapy of a retinal hemangioma is often indicated if it is affecting or threatening vision.
2. Genetic counseling.
3. Systemic therapy dependent upon findings.

Follow-up   Every 3-6 months, depending on the retinal condition.

14.15   Wyburn-Mason Syndrome

(Racemose Hemangiomatosis)

Ocular Signs   Enormously dilated, tortuous retinal vessels with arteriovenous communications. No distinct mass or subretinal exudate is present. Rarely, proptosis from a racemose hemangioma of the orbit is present.

Systemic Signs   Midbrain racemose hemangiomas, seizures, hemiparesis, mental changes, and ipsilateral pterygoid fossa, mandible, and maxillary hemangiomas. Intracranial hemorrhage from a midbrain hemangioma can occur.

Inheritance   Sporadic.

Differential Diagnosis

- Retinal capillary hemangioma   (A distinct mass is present, sometimes with subretinal exudate.)

Work-up

1. Complete general and ophthalmic examinations.
2. MRI of the brain.
3. Electroencephalogram.

Treatment

1. No treatment is required for the retinal lesions. The condition is congenital and does not progress.
2. Warn the patient of the risk of massive hemorrhage with ipsilateral dental and facial surgery.

Follow-up   Yearly.

14.16   Ataxia Telangiectasia

(Louis-Bar Syndrome)

Ocular Signs   Dilated conjunctival vessels, strabismus, impaired convergence, nystagmus, oculomotor apraxia.

Critical Systemic Signs   Cerebellar ataxia that becomes apparent after the child learns to walk, cutaneous telangiectasias in a butterfly distribution on the face, antecubital and popliteal fossa, behind the ears or at the base of neck during the first decade. Recurrent sinopulmonary infections due to IgA deficiency and impaired T-cell function can occur.

Other Systemic Signs   Leukemia or lymphoma (often leading to death in childhood or early adulthood), mental retardation, seborrheic dermatitis, pigmentary changes of the skin, testicular or ovarian atrophy, a hypoplastic or atrophic thymus.

Inheritance   Autosomal recessive.

Work-up

1. Family history   (Examination of the family members often aides in the diagnosis.)
2. Complete general and ophthalmic examinations.
3. CBC.
4. Chest x-ray.
5. MRI of the brain.

Treatment

1. Systemic treatment dependent upon findings.
2. Genetic counseling.

Follow-up   Patients need close medical follow-up. Routine eye examinations should be performed every 1-2 years.

15

General Ophthalmic Problems

15.1 Acquired Cataract

Symptoms Slowly progressive visual loss or blurring, usually over months to years, affecting one or both eyes. Glare, particularly from oncoming headlights while driving at night and reduced color perception may occur. The particular symptoms are based on the location and density of the opacity.

Critical Sign Opacification of the normally clear lens (see types below).

Other Signs The retina often appears indistinct on funduscopic examination and the dilated red reflex may be dim on retinoscopy. The patient may be found to be more myopic than previously. A cataract alone does not cause a relative afferent pupillary defect.

Types of Cataracts

A. Nuclear   (Yellow or brown discoloration of the central part of the lens on slit-lamp examination. Typically blurs distance vision more than near vision.)
B. Posterior subcapsular   (Opacities appear near the posterior aspect of the lens, often forming a plaque. They are best seen in retroillumination against a red fundus reflex. Glare and difficulty reading are common

complaints. May be associated with ocular inflammation, prolonged steroid use, diabetes, trauma, or radiation. Classically in patients under 50 years of age.)

C. Cortical (Radial or spokelike opacities in the lens periphery expand to involve the anterior and posterior lens. Often asymptomatic until the changes develop centrally.)

NOTE A mature cataract is defined as anterior cortical changes sufficiently dense to totally obscure the view of the posterior lens and posterior segment of the eye.

Etiology

- Age-related.
- Trauma (Ocular or head contusion, others.)
- Toxic (Steroids, anticholinesterases, antipsychotics [e.g., phenothiazines], others.)
- Intraocular inflammation (e.g., uveitis).
- Radiation.
- Intraocular tumor (A ciliary body malignant melanoma may produce a sector cortical cataract.)
- Degenerative ocular disease (e.g., retinitis pigmentosa).
- Systemic disease:

A. Diabetes (The juvenile form is characterized by white "snow flake" opacities in the anterior and posterior subcapsular locations. It often progresses rapidly. Adults develop "age-related" cataracts as above, but at an earlier age.)

B. Hypocalcemia (Small white iridescent cortical changes, usually seen in the presence of tetany.)

C. Wilson's disease (Red-brown pigment colored deposition in the cortex beneath the anterior capsule, a "sunflower" cataract. Seen with a corneal Kayser-Fleischer ring.)

D. Myotonic dystrophy (Multicolored opacities behind the anterior capsule.)

E. Others (e.g., Down's syndrome, atopic dermatitis).

Work-up Determine the etiology, whether the cataract is responsible for the decreased vision, and whether surgical removal would improve vision.

1. History: Medications? Systemic diseases? Trauma? Ocular disease or poor vision in youth or young adulthood (before the cataract)?

2. Complete ocular examination, including distance and near vision, pupillary examination, and refraction. A dilated slit-lamp examination using both direct and retroillumination techniques is usually required to properly view the cataract. Fundus examination, concentrating on the macula, is essential in ruling out other causes of decreased vision.
3. B-scan ultrasound when the fundus is obscured by a dense cataract to rule out posterior segment pathology.
4. The potential acuity meter or laser interferometry can be used to estimate the visual potential when cataract extraction is being considered in an eye with age-related macular degeneration changes.

   NOTE Laser interferometry and the potential acuity meter often overestimate an eye's visual potential in the presence of macular holes or macular pigment epithelial detachments. Interferometry also makes an overprediction in cases of amblyopia. Near vision is often the most accurate manner of evaluating macular function if the cataract is not too dense.

5. When surgery is planned, keratometry readings and an A-scan ultrasound measurement of axial length are required for determining the power of the desired intraocular lens. An evaluation of the corneal endothelium, usually done at the slit lamp, but occasionally requiring an endothelial cell count, is also needed.

Treatment

1. Cataract surgery may be performed:
   a. To improve visual function in patients with symptomatic visual disability.
   b. As surgical therapy of ocular disease (e.g., lens-related glaucoma or uveitis).
   c. To facilitate management of ocular disease (e.g., to monitor or treat diabetic retinopathy or glaucoma).
2. Correct any refractive error if the patient declines cataract surgery.
3. A trial of mydriasis (e.g., scopolamine ¼% q day) may be used successfully in some patients if the patient opts not to have the cataract removed.

Follow-up Unless there is a secondary complication from the cataract (e.g., glaucoma) (quite rare), a cataract itself does not require urgent action. Patients who decline surgical removal are reexamined yearly, sooner if there is a symptomatic decrease in visual acuity.

If congenital, see "Congenital Cataract," Section 9.6.

15.2 Subluxed or Dislocated Lens

Subluxation = Partial disruption of the zonular fibers; the lens is decentered, but remains partially in the pupillary aperture.
Dislocation = Complete disruption of the zonular fibers; the lens is displaced out of the pupillary aperture.

Symptoms Decreased vision, double vision which persists when covering one eye (monocular diplopia).

Critical Signs Decentered or displaced lens, iridodonesis (quivering of the iris), phakodonesis (quivering of the lens).

Other Signs Marked astigmatism, cataract, angle-closure glaucoma due to pupillary block, acquired high myopia, vitreous in the anterior chamber, asymmetry of the anterior chamber.

Etiology

- Trauma (Most common cause. Results in subluxation if greater than 25% of the zonular fibers are ruptured. Need to rule out a predisposing condition [see other etiologies]. Often associated with syphilis.)
- Marfan's syndrome (Cardiomyopathy, aortic aneurysm, tall stature with long extremities and kyphoscoliosis. Typically bilateral lens subluxation, superiorly and temporally. Patients are at increased risk for a retinal detachment. Often autosomal dominant.)
- Homocystinuria (Frequent mental retardation, skeletal deformities, resembles Marfan's syndrome in stature, high incidence of thromboembolic events [particularly with general anesthesia]. Typically bilateral lens subluxation, inferiorly and nasally. Increased risk of retinal detachment. Autosomal recessive.)
- Weill Marchesani syndrome (Short fingers and short stature, seizures, microspherophakia [small round lens], myopia, no mental retardation. Often autosomal recessive.)
- Others (Acquired syphilis, congenital ectopia lentis, aniridia, Ehlers-Danlos syndrome, Crouzon's disease, hyperlysinemia, sulfite-oxidase deficiency, high myopia, chronic inflammations, hypermature cataract, and others.)

Work-up

1. History: Family history of the disorders listed above? Trauma? Systemic illness (e.g., syphilis, seizures)?

2. Complete ocular examination: At the slit lamp note if the condition is unilateral or bilateral and the direction of the displaced lens.
3. Systemic examination: Evaluate stature, extremities, hands, and fingers; often in conjunction with an internist.
4. RPR and FTA-ABS, even if there is a history of trauma.
5. Sodium nitroprusside test of the urine (rule out homocystinuria).
6. Echocardiogram (rule out Marfan's syndrome).

Treatment

I. Lens dislocated into the anterior chamber
 A. Dilate the pupil, place the patient on his back, and replace the lens into the posterior chamber by head manipulation. It may be necessary to indent the cornea after topical anesthesia (e.g., proparacaine) with a Zeiss gonioprism or a cotton swab to reposition the lens. After the lens is repositioned in the posterior chamber, constrict the pupil with chronic pilocarpine ½-1% qid, and perform a peripheral laser iridectomy.
 or
 B. Surgically remove the lens (usually performed if the lens is a cataract, if "A" fails, if the patient develops recurrent dislocations, or if the patient cannot be trusted to take the pilocarpine.)
II. Lens dislocated into the vitreous
 A. Lens capsule intact, patient asymptomatic, no signs of inflammation: Observe.
 B. Lens capsule broken, patient symptomatic, eye inflamed: Surgical removal of the lens.
III. Subluxation
 A. Asymptomatic: Observe.
 B. High uncorrectable astigmatism or monocular diplopia: Surgical removal of the lens.
 C. Symptomatic cataract: Options include surgical removal of the lens, mydriasis (e.g., scopolamine ¼% q day) and aphakic correction, pupillary constriction (e.g., pilocarpine 4% gel qhs) and phakic correction, or a large optical iridectomy (away from the lens).
IV. Pupillary block: Treatment is identical to aphakic pupillary block, see "Postoperative Glaucoma," Section 10.15.

• If Marfan's syndrome is present: Refer the patient to a cardiologist for an annual echocardiogram and management of any cardiac-related abnormalities. Prophylactic systemic antibiotics are required if undergoing surgery (or a dental procedure) to prevent endocarditis.
• If homocystinuria is present:
 1. Pyridoxine 50-1000 mg po q day.
 2. Reduce dietary methionine.

3. Avoid surgery if possible due to the risk of thromboembolic complications. If surgical intervention is necessary, anticoagulant therapy is indicated.

Follow-up   Depends on the etiology, degree of subluxation/dislocation, and symptoms.

15.3   Headache

Most headaches are not dangerous nor ominous symptoms, however, they can be symptoms of a life- or vision-threatening problem. Below are listed accompanying signs and symptoms pointing toward a life- or vision-threatening headache and some of the specific signs and symptoms of various headaches.

A. *Warning symptoms and signs of a serious disorder*
   - Scalp tenderness, weight loss, pain with chewing, muscle pains, or malaise in patients at least 55 years of age (giant-cell arteritis)
   - Optic-nerve swelling
   - Fever
   - Altered mentation or behavior
   - Stiff neck
   - Neurologic signs
   - Decreased vision
   - Subhyaloid (preretinal) hemorrhages on fundus examination
B. *Less alarming, but suspicious, symptoms and signs*
   - Onset in a previously headache-free individual
   - A different, more severe headache than the usual headache
   - One which is *always* in the same location
   - One that awakens the person from sleep
   - One that does not respond to pain medications that previously relieved it
   - Nausea and vomiting, particularly "projectile" vomiting

Etiology

LIFE- OR VISION-THREATENING

- Giant-cell arteritis (GCA)   (Age ≥55 years, weight loss, fever, malaise, anorexia, muscle aches, scalp tenderness, pain on chewing, palpable tender nodule or cordlike pulseless area along the temporal artery, or decreased vision. May have a high ESR.)

- Acute angle-closure glaucoma   (Decreased vision, red and painful eye, cloudy cornea, fixed mid-dilated pupil, high intraocular pressure [IOP].)
- Ocular ischemic syndrome   (Periorbital eye pain, mid-peripheral retinal hemorrhages, dilated retinal veins, neovascularization of the iris, disc, or retina.)
- Malignant hypertension   (Marked elevation of blood pressure often accompanied by retinal cotton wool spots, hemorrhages, and when severe, optic-nerve swelling. Headaches typically are occipital in location.)
- Increased intracranial pressure   (May have papilledema, loss of venous pulsations[1] in the disc vessels, or a sixth-cranial-nerve palsy.)
- Infectious central nervous system disorder (meningitis/brain abscess)   (Fever, stiff neck, mental status changes, photophobia, neurological signs.)
- Structural abnormality of the brain (tumor/aneurysm/arteriovenous malformation)   (Mental status change, signs of increased intracranial pressure, or neurologic signs during, and often after, the headache episode.)
- Subarachnoid hemorrhage   (Extremely severe headache, mental status change, rarely seen subhyaloid hemorrhages on fundus examination, usually from a ruptured aneurysm.)
- Epidural or subdural hematoma   (Follows head trauma, altered level of consciousness, may produce anisocoria.)

OTHERS

- Migraine   (See Section 15.4.)
- Cluster   (See Section 15.5.)
- Tension
- Herpes zoster virus   (Headache/pain may precede the herpetic vesicles. See Section 4.16.)
- Sinus disease   (NOTE   A sinus headache can be a serious headache in diabetics and immunocompromised hosts since Mucormycosis may be responsible.)
- Tolosa Hunt syndrome   (See "Cavernous Sinus Superior Orbital Fissure Syndrome," Section 11.8.)
- Cervical spine disease
- Temporomandibular joint syndrome
- Dental disease
- Tic douloureux
- Anterior uveitis   (See Section 13.1.)
- Post spinal tap
- Paget's disease

---

[1]While the presence of spontaneous venous pulsations indicates normal intracranial pressure at that moment, the absence of pulsations has little significance. A significant number of normal individuals do not have spontaneous venous pulsations.

- Depression/psychogenic
- Convergence insufficiency (See Section 15.6.)
- Accommodative spasm (See Section 15.7.)

Work-up

1. History: Ask about the location, intensity, frequency, possible precipitating factors, and time of day of the headaches. Determine the age of onset, what relieves the headaches, and whether there are any associated signs or symptoms. Specifically ask about the serious or suspicious symptoms/signs listed above, trauma, medications and birth control pills, a family history of migraine, and whether the patient experienced motion sickness or cyclic vomiting as a child.

2. Complete ocular examination, including pupillary, motility, and visual field evaluation; IOP measurement, optic-disc and venous pulsation assessment, and a dilated retinal examination. Manifest and cycloplegic refractions may be helpful.

3. Neurologic examination (check neck flexibility and other meningeal signs).

4. Palpate the temporal arteries in potential GCA cases (are they swollen, hard, and tender?).

5. Temperature and blood pressure.

6. Immediate ESR $+/-$ temporal artery biopsy when giant-cell arteritis is suspected (see Section 11.15).

7. CT scan (axial and coronal views) or MRI of the brain when an intracranial abnormality is suspected.

8. Carotid noninvasive flow studies when the ocular ischemic syndrome is suspected.

9. Lumbar puncture (in the hospital) is obtained in suspected cases of meningitis or subarachnoid hemorrhage.

10. Referral to a neurologist; ear, nose and throat specialist; internist; or family doctor as indicated.

Treatment/Follow-up   See individual sections.

15.4 Migraine

Symptoms   Typically unilateral (although it may occur behind both eyes or across the entire front of the head) throbbing or boring head pain accompanied by nausea, vomiting, mood changes, fatigue, or photophobia. Visual disturbances, including flashing (zigzagging) lights, blurred vision, or a visual field defect lasting 15-50 minutes, may precede the headache. The headache is often preceded by an "aura," a sensation of an impending migraine. Neurological deficits may occur. A positive family history is common as is a history of car sickness or cyclic vomiting as a child. Migraine in children may present as recurrent abdominal pain and malaise.

NOTE   The majority of unilateral migraine headaches at some point change sides of the head. Patients who *always* have a headache on the same side of the head may have a more serious headache disorder.

Signs   Usually none. Complicated migraines may have a permanent neurological or ocular deficit (see below).

Classification   Definitions and classifications vary.

I. *Common migraine*   (80%) Nausea, vomiting, fatigue, and mood changes are associated with this variant.
II. *Classical migraine*   (10%) The headache is *preceded* by a 15 to 50-minute visual disturbance or transient focal neurological change. See "complicated migraine" below for specific types of visual and neurological defects.
III. *Visual migraine without headache*   The patient experiences the visual aura of a classical migraine without the subsequent headache. Some of these patients have and some have not had migraine headaches in the past.
IV. *Complicated migraine*   A subset of migraine in which neurological deficits outlast the headache. Rarely, a deficit may be permanent.
   A. Cerebral: A neurological deficit involving the motor, sensory, or visual systems. Onset can be at the height of a migraine headache, but more commonly it follows the headache. Examples include focal motor deficits, speech disorders, and paresthesias of the extremities, face, tongue, or lips. "Hemiplegic migraine" consists of total paralysis or weakness on one side of the body.
   B. Ophthalmoplegic: Ipsilateral paralysis of one or more extraocular muscles, usually occurring during a migraine attack in childhood. The ophthalmoplegia usually occurs as the headache is resolving.
   C. Retinal: Sudden monocular visual loss in a migraine patient. Light flashes and headache do not usually occur.
   D. Basilar artery migraine: Mimics vertebrobasilar artery insufficiency with bilateral blurring or blindness, vertigo, gait disturbances, formed hallucinations, and dysarthria in a patient with migraines.

Associations or Precipitating Factors   Birth control or other hormonal pills, puberty, pregnancy, menopause, foods containing tyramine or phenylalanine (e.g., aged cheeses, wines, chocolate), alcohol, fatigue, emotional stress, refractive errors, or bright lights.

Differential Diagnosis   See "Headache," Section 15.3.

Work-up   See Section 15.3 for a general headache work-up.

1. History: May establish the diagnosis.
2. Ocular and neurologic examinations, including refraction.
3. CT scan or MRI of the head is indicated for:
    a. Atypical migraines (e.g., migraines that are always on the same side of the head, those which begin in middle age in a person with no family history nor a history of car sickness or cyclic vomiting as a child, or those with an unusual sequence—e.g., visual disturbances persisting into or occurring after the headache phase).
    b. Complicated migraines.

Treatment

1. Avoid agents which precipitate the headaches (e.g., stop using birth control pills; avoid alcohol and any foods that may precipitate attacks; reduce stress).
2. Correct any significant refractive error.
3. Medication to be used at the onset of the headache (the earlier the better) in patients with infrequent headaches:
    a. Initial therapy: Aspirin or acetaminophen 650 mg po q 4-6 hours as needed.
    b. More potent therapy (when initial therapy fails):

    Aspirin 325 mg/caffeine 40 mg/butalbital 50 mg (e.g., Fiorinal)[2] 1-2 tablets q 4 hours, not to exceed 6 tablets per day.
    Acetaminophen 325 mg/caffeine 40 mg/butalbital 50 mg (e.g., Fioricet)[2] 1-2 tablets q 4 hours, not to exceed 6 tablets per day.
    Ergotamine derivative (e.g., ergotamine tartrate 1 mg/caffeine 100 mg, [e.g., Cafergot][3] 2 tablets po initially, then 1 tablet q 30 minutes, not to exceed 6 tablets in 24 hours or 10 tablets in 1 week).

    NOTE   Cafergot is available in suppository form, the maximum

---

[2]Contraindicated in patients with porphyria. Patients are warned about drowsiness and cautioned about driving. They are told that alcohol and other CNS depressants can potentiate the drowsiness. Drug dependency can develop with prolonged use.

[3]Contraindicated in patients with cardiovascular disease, renal or hepatic disease, and pregnancy. Muscle weakness and pain or even cardiac ischemic pain can occur.

dosage being 2 suppositories in 24 hours and not more than 5 suppositories in 1 week.

4. Prophylactic medication to be used in patients with frequent or severe headache attacks or those with neurological changes:

Propranolol (e.g., Inderal)[4] 10-80 mg po q day in divided doses initially; slowly increase the dose by 10-20 mg every 2-3 days until the desired effect is obtained (can go up to 160-240 mg/day).

Amitriptyline (e.g., Elavil)[5] 25-200 mg po qhs (start at a low dose and increase the dose by 25 mg every 1-2 weeks if needed).

Calcium channel blockers (e.g., verapamil 240 mg po q day); we rarely use these.

5. Antinausea medication as needed for an acute episode (e.g., prochlorperazine 25 mg rectally bid).

Follow-up   Patients are generally reevaluated in 4-6 weeks to assess the efficacy of the therapy.

15.5   Cluster Headache

Symptoms   Typically unilateral, very painful, periorbital, frontal, or temporal headache associated with ipsilateral tearing, rhinorrhea, sweating, nasal stuffiness, and/or a droopy eyelid. Usually lasts minutes to hours. Typically recurs once or twice daily for several weeks, followed by a headache-free interval of months to years. The cycle can then repeat itself.

Signs   Ipsilateral conjunctival injection, facial flush, or a Horner's syndrome (third-order neuron etiology) may be present.

Precipitating Factors   Alcohol, nitroglycerin.

Differential Diagnosis

• Migraine headache   (Positive family history of migraines or a history of car sickness or cyclic vomiting in many cases. The associated symptoms listed above are typically absent.)

---

[4]Do not give to patients with asthma, congestive heart failure, bradycardia, or hypotension. Do *not* stop this drug suddenly; it must be tapered slowly.

[5]Do not give to patients taking a monoamine oxidase inhibitor or patients with narrow anterior-chamber angles or benign prostatic hypertrophy.

• Others   (See "Headache," Section 15.3.)

Work-up

1. History and complete ocular examination.
2. Neurologic examination, particularly a cranial-nerve evaluation.
3. Consider an hydroxyamphetamine (e.g., Paredrine) test if a Horner's syndrome accompanies a suspected cluster headache to confirm a third-order neuron etiology (see Section 11.2).
4. Obtain a CT scan (axial and coronal views) or MRI of the brain when the history is atypical or a neurologic abnormality other than a third-order neuron Horner's syndrome is found.

Treatment

1. No treatment is necessary if the headache is mild.
2. Aspirin or acetaminophen should be tried initially.
3. No alcoholic beverages or cigarette smoking during a cluster cycle.
4. When headaches are moderate to severe and unrelieved with nonprescription medication, one of the following drugs may be an effective prophylactic agent during cluster periods:

   • Methysergide 2 mg po tid with meals. Do not use for longer than 3-4 months due to the significant risk of retroperitoneal fibrosis. Methysergide is not recommended in patients with coronary artery or peripheral vascular disease, thrombophlebitis, hypertension, pregnancy, or hepatic or renal disease.
   • Oral steroids (e.g., prednisone 40-80 mg po for one week, tapering rapidly over an additional week if possible) plus an antiulcer agent (e.g., ranitidine 150 mg po bid). See Appendix 5 if considering systemic steroids.
   • Lithium 600-900 mg po q day is administered in conjunction with the patient's medical doctor. Baseline renal (BUN, creatinine, urine electrolytes) and thyroid function tests (T3, T4, TSH) are obtained. Lithium intoxication may occur in patients using indomethacin, tetracycline, or methyldopa.

   Some physicians administer an ergotamine inhaler (9 mg/ml, containing 0.36 mg per inhalation) 1 inhalation q 5 minutes × 3 (maximum every 12-24 hours) or ergotamine 2 mg sublingual q 30 minutes × 3 (maximum in 24 hours) to be started at the onset of an attack. Ergotamine pills may be used in prophylaxis. Ergotamine has the same contraindications as methysergide. We do not use ergotamine as a first-line agent.

   If necessary, an acute severe attack can be treated with IV diazepam.

Follow-up Patients started on systemic steroids are seen within a few days and then every several weeks to evaluate the effects of treatment and monitor intraocular pressure. Patients on methysergide or lithium are reevaluated in 7-10 days. Plasma lithium levels are monitored in patients on this agent.

15.6 Convergence Insufficiency

Symptoms Eye discomfort, headache, sleepiness, or blurred vision from reading or doing near work. It is most common in teenagers and young adults, but may be seen in presbyopes.

Critical Sign An inability to maintain fusion at near due to a reduced amplitude of fusional convergence power (see Work-up below).

Other Signs A distant near point of convergence, an exophoria greater at near than at distance, and a reduced amplitude of accommodation.

Etiology Fatigue or illness, drugs, uveitis, Adie's tonic pupil, or glasses inducing a base-out prism effect. Often idiopathic.

Differential Diagnosis (Other causes of eyestrain with reading.)
- Uncorrected refractive error (especially hyperopia and astigmatism)
- Accommodative insufficiency (AI) (Symptoms develop after 20-40 minutes of reading, same age group as convergence insufficiency (CI), but these patients have normal fusional capacities. When a 4 diopter base-in prism is placed in front of an eye while reading, the print is noted to blur in AI, but become clearer in CI. Patients with AI usually benefit from reading glasses; those with CI do not.)

Work-up

1. Manifest (without cycloplegia) refraction.
2. Determine the near point of convergence: Ask the patient to focus on an accommodative target (e.g., the eraser of a pencil) and to inform you when double vision develops as you bring the target in towards him; a normal near point of convergence is <6-8 cm.
3. Check for exo- (or eso-) deviations at distance and near using the cover tests (Appendix 2) or the Maddox rod test.
4. Measure the patient's fusional ability at near: Have the patient focus on an accommodative target at his reading distance. With a prism bar, slowly increase the amount of base-out prism in front of one eye until the patient notes double vision (the break point). Now slowly reduce the amount of

base-out prism until a single image is again noted (the recovery point). A low break point (i.e., 10-15 prism diopters) and/or a low recovery point is consistent with convergence insufficiency.
5. Place a 4 diopter base-in prism in front of one eye while the patient is reading and determine whether the print becomes clearer or more blurred (rule out accommodative insufficiency).
6. Cycloplegic refraction (performed after the above tests and measurements).

NOTE   The above tests are performed with the patient's spectacle correction in place (if glasses are worn for near work).

Treatment

1. Correct any refractive error (hyperopia should be slightly undercorrected, while myopia should be fully corrected).
2. Near-point exercises (e.g., pencil push-ups): The patient is taught to focus on the eraser of a pencil while slowly moving it in from arm's length toward the face. The patient must concentrate on maintaining one image of the eraser. When double vision results, the maneuver is repeated. An attempt is made to draw the pencil in closer each time while maintaining single vision. The exercise is repeated 15 times, 5 times per day.
3. Near-point exercises with base-out prisms (for patients whose near point of convergence is satisfactory or for those who have mastered pencil push-ups without a prism): Pencil push-ups as described above are performed while the patient additionally holds a six diopter base-out prism in front of one eye.
4. Encourage use of good lighting and time for relaxation between periods of concentrated close work.
5. For older patients or those whose condition shows no improvement despite near-point exercises, reading glasses with base-in prism can be useful.

Follow-up   This is not an urgent condition. Patients are reseen in 1 month.

15.7   Accommodative Spasm

Symptoms   Bilateral blurred distance vision or fluctuating vision, headache, and eyestrain while reading. Typically patients are teenagers who are under stress.

Critical Signs   Cycloplegic refraction reveals substantially less myopia (or more hyperopia) than was originally found when the refraction was performed without cycloplegia (the manifest refraction). Manifest myopia may be as high as 10 diopters.

Other Signs Abnormally close near point of focus, miosis, a normal amplitude of accommodation that may appear low.

Etiology Inability to relax the ciliary muscles. Accommodative spasm is involuntary and is associated with stressful situations or functional neuroses. Fatigue and prolonged reading may also precipitate episodes.

Differential Diagnosis

- Uncorrected hyperopia (Patients accept plus lenses during the manifest refraction.)
- Other causes of pseudomyopia (Hyperglycemia, medication induced [e.g., sulfa drugs], forward displacement of the lens.)

Work-up

1. Complete ophthalmic examination, including an initial manifest refraction. The manifest refraction may be highly variable, but it is important to determine the least amount of minus power or the most amount of plus power that provides clear distance vision.
2. Cycloplegic refraction.

Treatment

1. True refractive errors should be corrected. If a significant amount of esophoria at near is present, additional plus power (e.g., $+2.50$ diopters) in reading glasses or bifocal form may be helpful for close work.
2. Gentle counseling of the patient and parents to provide a more relaxed atmosphere, avoiding stressful situations is important.
3. Cycloplegics, including atropine, have been used to break the spasm, but are rarely needed except in the most resistant cases.

Follow-up Reevaluate in several weeks. The physician should also be available for additional consultative support.

15.8 Hypotony

Symptoms May be asymptomatic or complain of mild-to-severe pain. Vision may be reduced.

Critical Signs   Low intraocular pressure (IOP), usually less than 6 mm Hg.

Other Signs   Corneal folds, aqueous cell and flare, shallow anterior chamber, retinal edema, chorioretinal folds, choroidal detachment, or the appearance of optic-disc swelling.

Etiology

- Postsurgical   (e.g., wound leak, cyclodialysis cleft [disinsertion of the ciliary body from the sclera at the scleral spur], perforation of the sclera from a superior rectus bridle suture or retrobulbar injection, iridocyclitis, retinal or choroidal detachment, others).
- Post-traumatic   (Same causes as postsurgical.)
- Pharmacological   (Usually from a carbonic anhydrase inhibitor or topical beta-blocker.)
- Systemic (Bilateral hypotony)   (Conditions which cause blood hypertonicity [e.g., dehydration, uremia, exacerbation of diabetes], myotonic dystrophy, others.)

Work-up

1. History: Recent ocular surgery or trauma? Other systemic symptoms (nausea, vomiting, twitching, drowsiness, polyuria)? History of renal disease, diabetes, or myotonic dystrophy? Medications?
2. Complete ocular examination, including a slit-lamp evaluation of surgical or traumatic ocular wounds (check for poor wound apposition), IOP check, gonioscopy of the anterior-chamber angle (rule out a cyclodialysis cleft), and indirect ophthalmoscopy (rule out a retinal and/or choroidal detachment and look for signs of a scleral perforation).
3. Seidel test to rule out a wound leak (see Appendix 4).

   NOTE   A wound leak may drain under the conjunctiva, producing a filtering bleb. The Seidel test will then be negative.

4. B-scan ultrasound when the fundus cannot be seen clinically.
5. Blood tests in bilateral cases: Glucose, BUN, and creatinine.

Treatment   Repair the underlying disorder.

WOUND LEAK

- Large wound leaks: Suture the wound closed.
- Small wound leaks: Can be sutured closed or can be patched with a pressure dressing and an antibiotic ointment (e.g., erythromycin) for one night to allow the wound to close spontaneously. A carbonic anhydrase inhibitor and

a nonselective topical beta-blocker (e.g., acetazolamide 500 mg sequel po and a drop of levobunolol ½% or timolol ½%) are usually given if patching is to be employed. (NOTE Occasionally cyanoacrylate glue is applied to small wound leaks and covered with a bandage contact lens.)

- Wound leaks under a conjunctival flap (only repaired if the hypotony is affecting vision or producing a secondary ocular complication such as a flat anterior chamber or endophthalmitis): Consider cryotherapy or argon laser after painting the conjunctiva with methylene blue or rose bengal.

CYCLODIALYSIS CLEFT

Reattach the ciliary body to the sclera via suturing, cryotherapy, or diathermy. Other techniques have been used.

SCLERAL PERFORATION

The site may be closed by suturing or cryotherapy.

IRIDOCYCLITIS

Topical steroid (e.g., prednisolone acetate 1% q 1-6 hours) and a topical cycloplegic (e.g., scopolamine ¼% tid).

RETINAL DETACHMENT

Surgical repair.

CHOROIDAL DETACHMENT

Treated as iridocyclitis. Surgical drainage of the choroidal effusion along with reformation of the eye and anterior chamber is indicated for any of the following:

1. Retinal apposition ("kissing choroidal detachments").
2. Lens-corneal touch.
3. A flat or persistently shallow anterior chamber accompanied by a failing filtering bleb or an inflamed eye.

PHARMACOLOGICAL

Reduce or discontinue the IOP-lowering medication.

SYSTEMIC DISORDER

Refer to an internist.

NOTE In myotonic dystrophy, the hypotony is rarely severe enough to produce deleterious effects, and treatment from an ocular standpoint is unnecessary.

Follow-up If vision is good, the anterior chamber is well formed, and there is no wound leak, retinal detachment, nor "kissing choroidal detachments," then the low IOP poses no immediate problem, and treatment and follow-up are not urgent. Fixed retinal folds in the macula may develop from long-standing hypotony.

15.9 Blind, Painful Eye

A patient with a nonseeing eye and unsalvageable vision may develop mild-to-severe pain in it for a variety of reasons. The etiology, work-up, and treatment are discussed below.

Causes of Pain (Most common.)

- Corneal decompensation (Fluorescein staining defect on slit-lamp examination.)
- Uveitis (Anterior-chamber or vitreal white blood cells. If the cornea is opaque, the cells may not be seen.)
- Extremely high intraocular pressure (IOP) (May result from neovascular glaucoma and angle closure, uveitis, or intraocular tumor-related glaucoma. IOP may be difficult to measure if the corneal surface is irregular.)

Work-up

1. History: Determine the etiology and duration of the blindness.
2. Ocular examination: Stain the cornea with fluorescein to detect an epithelial defect and measure the IOP. If the cornea is not opaque, look for neo-vascularization of the iris and angle (with gonioscopy), and inspect the anterior chamber for cells and flare. Attempt a dilated retinal examination to rule out an intraocular tumor.
3. B-scan ultrasound of the posterior segment is required to rule out an intraocular tumor when the fundus cannot be adequately visualized.

Treatment

A. *Sterile corneal decompensation* (If it appears infected see "Infectious Corneal Infiltrate/Ulcer," Section 4.12.)
   1. Antibiotic ointment (e.g., erythromycin), cycloplegic (e.g., atropine 1%) and a pressure patch × 24-48 hours.
   2. Lubricating ointment (e.g., Refresh PM) qhs (after the patch is removed) for weeks to months (or even permanently).
   3. Consider teaching the patient to patch his own eye nightly.
   4. Consider a tarsorrhaphy in refractile cases.

B. *Uveitis*
1. Cycloplegic (e.g., atropine 1% tid).
2. Topical steroid (e.g., prednisolone acetate 1% q 1-6 hours).

C. *Markedly elevated IOP*
1. Treat uveitis if it is present or if the cornea is opaque and its presence cannot be ruled out.
2. Topical beta-blocker (e.g., levobunolol ½% bid or timolol ½% bid) +/− an epinephrine compound (e.g., dipivefrin 0.1% bid) (carbonic anhydrase inhibitors are effective, but their potential systemic side effects may not warrant their use for pain relief; miotics may increase ocular irritation).
3. If the IOP remains markedly elevated and is thought to be responsible for the pain, a cyclodestructive procedure (e.g., YAG laser cyclophotocoagulation or cyclocryotherapy) may be attempted.
4. If pain persists despite the above treatment a retrobulbar alcohol block may be given. *Technique*: 2-3 cc of lidocaine is administered in the retrobulbar region. The needle is then held in place while the syringe of lidocaine is replaced with a 1-cc syringe containing 95%-100% alcohol (some physicians use 50% alcohol). The contents of the alcohol syringe are then injected into the retrobulbar space through the needle being held in place. The syringes are again switched, so a small amount of lidocaine can rinse out the remaining alcohol. The retrobulbar needle is then withdrawn. Patients are warned that transient eyelid droop or swelling, limitation of eye movement, or anesthesia may result.

D. *Cause of pain unknown*
1. Cycloplegic (e.g., atropine 1% tid).
2. Topical steroid (e.g., prednisolone acetate 1% q 1-6 hours).

- When the above treatment fails to relieve the pain, enucleation is offered to the patient.
- The patient should wear protective glasses (e.g., polycarbonate lens) at all times to prevent injury to the fellow eye.

Follow-up Depends on the degree of pain and the clinical abnormalities present. Once the pain resolves, patients are rechecked every 6-12 months.

Appendix 1

Dilating Drops

(MYDRIATIC AND CYCLOPLEGIC AGENTS)

Drops	Approximate Maximum Effect	Approximate Duration of Action
MYDRIATIC:		
Phenylephrine 2.5, 10%	20 minutes	3 hours
CYCLOPLEGIC/MYDRIATIC:		
Tropicamide 0.5, 1%	20-30 minutes	3-6 hours
Cyclopentolate 0.5, 1, 2%	20-45 minutes	24 hours
Homatropine 2, 5%	20-90 minutes	2-3 days
Scopolamine 0.25%	20-45 minutes	4-7 days
Atropine 0.5, 1, 2%	30-40 minutes	1-2 weeks

The usual regimen for a dilated examination is:

Adults Phenylephrine 2.5% and tropicamide 1%. Repeat these drops in 15-30 minutes if the eye is not dilated.

Children Phenylephrine 2.5%, tropicamide 1%, and cyclopentolate 1-2%. Repeat these drops in 25-35 minutes if the eye is not dilated.

Infants Phenylephrine 2.5% and tropicamide 0.5%. Homatropine 2% or cyclopentolate 0.5% (generally reserved for infants more than 1-2 months of age) may also be used. The drops can be repeated in 35-45 minutes if the eye is not dilated.

NOTES

1. Dilating drops are contraindicated in most types of angle closure glaucoma and in eyes with severely narrow anterior-chamber angles.
2. Dilating drops tend to be less effective at the same concentration in darkly pigmented eyes.

419

Appendix 2

Cover/Uncover and Alternate Cover Tests

A. Cover/Uncover Test

Differentiates a phoria (the eyes are straight when fixating on a target, but misaligned when tired or not focusing) from a tropia (the eyes are misaligned at all times).

Requirements Full range of ocular motility, vision adequate enough to see the target of fixation, foveal fixation in each eye, attention, and patient cooperation. This test should be performed before the alternate cover test.

1. The patient is asked to fixate on an accommodative target at distance (e.g., a letter on the vision chart).
2. Cover one of the patient's eyes while observing the uncovered eye. A refixation movement of the uncovered eye suggests the presence of a tropia.
3. Remove the cover. A phoria is identified by refixation of the eye now being uncovered while the fellow eye maintains its position and fixation.
4. Repeat the procedure covering the opposite eye.

NOTE   A tropia may be unilateral, the same eye is always turned in or out, or it may alternate between eyes. In an alternating tropia, the contralateral eye is sometimes deviated after the cover/uncover test.

5. The patient is next asked to fixate on an accommodative target at near. Both eyes are tested at near in the manner described above.

NOTES   An esodeviation is detected by a refixation movement temporally (the eye being observed turns away from the nose). An exodeviation is detected by a refixation

420

movement nasally (the eye being observed turns toward the nose). A hyperdeviation is detected by a refixation movement inferiorly.

B. Alternate Cover Test (Prism and Cover Test)

Measures the total deviation, phoria combined with tropia.

Requirements   Same as for the cover/uncover test.

1. The patient is asked to fixate on an accommodative target at distance.
2. An occluder is held over one eye for a few seconds, and then quickly switched to the other eye. As the occluder alternately covers each eye for a few seconds, the eye being uncovered may be noted to swing into position to refixate on the target. Such eye movement indicates the presence of a deviation.
3. To measure the deviation, prisms are placed in front of one eye until eye movement ceases as the cover is alternated from eye to eye. The base of the prism is placed in the direction of eye movement. The strength of the weakest prism which eliminates eye movement during the alternate cover test is the amount of the deviation.
4. Measurements may be done for any direction of gaze by turning the patient's head away from the target while asking him to maintain fixation on it (i.e., right gaze is measured by turning the patient's head toward his or her left shoulder and asking the patient to look at the target).
5. In general, measurements are taken in the straight-ahead position (both at distance and near), in right gaze, left gaze, down-gaze (the chin is tilted up while the patient focuses on the target), up-gaze (the chin is tilted down while the patient focuses on the target), and with the patient's head tilted toward his or her left shoulder and then toward his or her right shoulder. Measurements are taken both with and without glasses in the straight-ahead position.

Appendix 3

Amsler Grid

Used to test macular function or to detect a central/paracentral scotoma.

1. Have the patient wear his or her glasses and occlude the left eye while you hold an Amsler grid approximately 12 inches in front of the right eye (Fig. A-1).
2. The patient is asked what is in the center of the page. Failure to see the central dot may indicate a central scotoma.
3. Have the patient fixate on the central dot (or the center of the page if he or she cannot see the dot) and ask if all four corners of the diagram are visible. Are any of the boxes missing?
4. Again, while staring at the central dot, the patient is asked if all of the lines are straight and continuous or if some are distorted and broken.
5. The patient is asked to outline any missing or distorted areas on the grid with a pencil.
6. Repeat the procedure, covering the right eye and testing the left.

NOTES

1. It is very important to monitor the patient's eye for movement away from the central dot.
2. A red-colored Amsler grid may pick up more subtle defects.

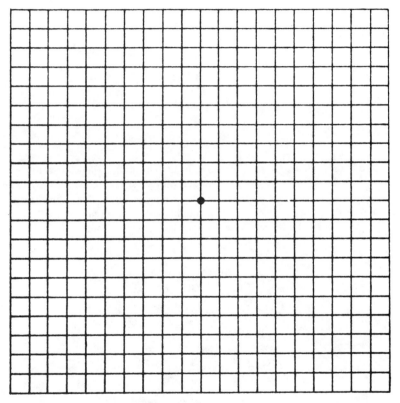

Figure A-1. Amsler grid. See text.

Appendix 4

Seidel Test to Detect a Wound Leak

Concentrated fluorescein dye (from a moistened fluorescein strip) is applied directly over the potential site of perforation while observing the site with the slit lamp (using the white light) (Fig. A-2). If a perforation and leak exist, the fluorescein dye will be diluted by the aqueous and will appear as a green (dilute) stream within the dark-orange (concentrated) dye. The stream of aqueous may also be seen with the blue light of the slit lamp.

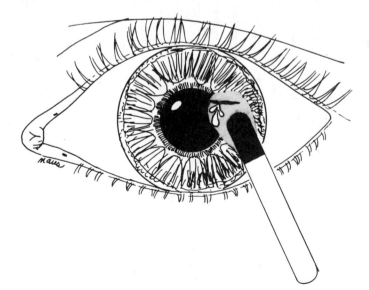

Figure A-2. Seidel test.   See text.

Appendix 5

Systemic Steroid Work-up

Contraindications to systemic steroids: Peptic ulcer disease, tuberculosis, active infection, psychosis, or pregnancy. Note that diabetics started on systemic steroids often have difficulty controlling their blood sugar.

Work-up   (often performed by an internist)

1. Blood tests: Fasting blood sugar and/or glucose tolerance test, CBC with a differential, pregnancy test as needed.
2. PPD with an anergy panel.
3. Chest x-ray.
4. Stool guaiac test.
5. Blood pressure.

NOTE   Systemic steroid therapy should be accompanied by an anti-ulcer regimen, such as antacids or an H_2 blocker (e.g., ranitidine 150 mg po bid).

Appendix 6

Forced Duction Test and Active Force Generation Test

A. Forced Duction Test

This test distinguishes restrictive causes of decreased ocular motility from other motility disorders. One technique is the following:

1. Place a drop of topical anesthetic (e.g., proparacaine) into the eye.
2. Place a cotton-tipped applicator soaked with cocaine 10% on the muscle to be grasped (i.e., the muscle away from the "paretic" field) for about 1 minute.
3. The anesthetized muscle is grasped firmly with toothed forceps (e.g., Graefe fixation forceps) and the eye is rotated in the "paretic" direction (Fig. A-3). If there is resistance to passive rotation of the eye, a restrictive disorder is diagnosed.

B. Active Force Generation Test

The patient is asked to look in the "paretic" direction while a sterile cotton swab is held just beneath the limbus on that same side. The amount of force generated by the "paretic" muscle is compared with that generated in the normal contralateral eye.

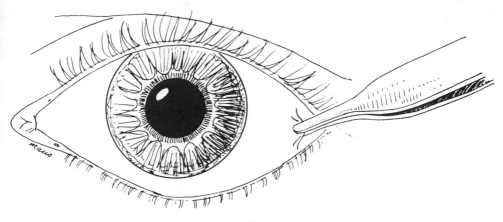

(a)

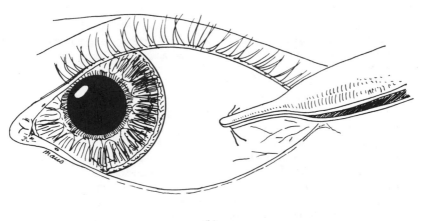

(b)

Figure A-3. Forced ductions.   In the case illustrated, the left eye could not look inward. (a) The lateral rectus muscle is grasped with forceps. (b) The eye can be moved in the paretic direction (inward in this case) without resistance, ruling out a restrictive muscle condition.

Appendix 7

Technique for Diagnostic Probing and Irrigation of the Lacrimal System

1. Anesthetize the eye with a drop of topical anesthetic (e.g., proparacaine) and hold a cotton-tipped applicator soaked in the topical anesthetic on the involved punctum for several minutes.
2. Dilate the punctum with a punctum dilator.
3. Gently insert a small Bowman probe into the punctum 2 mm vertically, and then 8 mm horizontally—toward the nose (Fig. A-4). Pull the involved eyelid laterally while slowly moving the probe horizontally to facilitate the procedure and to avoid creating a false passageway.
4. In the presence of an eyelid laceration, a torn canaliculus may be diagnosed by the appearance of the probe in the site of the eyelid laceration.
5. Irrigation of the lacrimal system is performed after removing the probe and inserting an irrigation canula in the same manner in which the probe was inserted. 5-10 cc of saline is gently pushed into the system. Leakage through a torn eyelid also diagnoses a severed canaliculus. Resistance to injection of the saline, ballooning of the lacrimal sac, or leakage of the saline out of either punctum may be due to a lacrimal-system obstruction. A patent lacrimal system usually drains into the throat quite readily and the arrival of saline may be noted by the patient.

NOTE   If solely evaluating the patency of the lacrimal system, and not ruling out a laceration, the system can be irrigated as above, right after punctum dilatation.

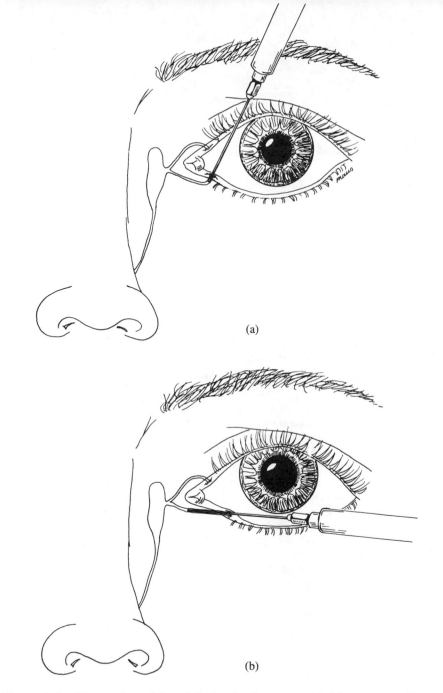

Figure A-4. Diagnostic probing of the lacrimal system. (a) After punctum dilatation, the probe or irrigation needle is directed inferiorly for 2 mm. (b) The instrument is rotated horizontally and, with the eyelid stretched laterally, is inserted toward the nose.

Appendix 8

Technique for Subtenons and Subconjunctival Injections

A. Technique for Subtenons Injection

1. Topical anesthesia is applied to the area to be injected (e.g., topical proparacaine and/or a cotton-tipped applicator soaked in proparacaine held on the area for 1-2 minutes). If subtenons steroids are to be injected, then 0.1 cc of lidocaine may be injected in the same manner as next described, several minutes before the steroids. The inferotemporal quadrant is usually the easiest location.
2. With the aperture of a 25-gauge-⅝ inch needle facing the sclera, the bulbar conjunctiva is penetrated 2-3 mm from the fornix, avoiding the conjunctival blood vessels (Fig. A-5).
3. As the needle is pushed in, lateral motions of the needle are made to ensure that the needle has not penetrated the sclera (at which point lateral motions would be inhibited).
4. The curvature of the eyeball is followed, attempting to place the aperture of the needle near the posterior sclera.
5. When the needle has been pushed in up to the hilt, the stopper of the syringe is pulled back to ensure against intravascular penetration.
6. The contents of the syringe are injected, and the needle is removed.

B. Technique for Subconjunctival Injection

1. Topical anesthesia is applied as above.
2. Forceps are used to tent up the conjunctiva, allowing the tip of a 25-gauge-⅜ inch needle to penetrate the subconjunctival space. The needle is placed several millimeters below the limbus at the 4 or 8 o'clock position with the aperture facing the sclera and the needle pointed inferiorly toward the fornix (Fig. A-6).

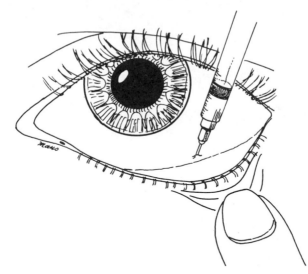

Figure A-5. **Subtenons injection.** The needle is placed 2-3 mm from the fornix, through conjunctiva and tenon's capsule. If possible, angle the injection so the syringe does not lie over the cornea.

3. When the entire tip of the needle is beneath the conjunctiva, the stopper of the syringe is withdrawn to ensure against intravascular penetration, the contents of the syringe are then injected, and the needle is removed.

NOTE   An eyelid speculum may be helpful in keeping the eyelids open during these two procedures.

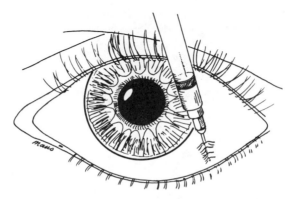

Figure A-6. **Subconjunctival injection.** The tip of the needle is placed into the subconjunctival space.

Appendix 9

Vitreous Examination
for Cells

1. Best performed in a completely darkened room with the patient's pupil widely dilated.
2. *Anterior vitreous*   Use the high-power magnification of the slit lamp, reduce the beam height to less than the pupil diameter, and narrow the beam width to focus through the pupil. Set the illumination to the brightest setting. Move the slit lamp forward with the joy stick, angling the beam of light until the anterior vitreous can be seen posterior to the lens. By moving the joy stick, several optical sections can be sampled. Patients are sometimes asked to move their eyes from left to right, facilitating the recognition of vitreous cells as they float by.
3. *Mid and posterior vitreous*   Using a Hruby (first choice), fundus contact, or 60 diopter lens, the slit beam is initially focused on the disc. The joy stick is then used to slowly pull the slit lamp away from the eye, refocusing the light on the posterior vitreous. Again, patients may be asked to look toward their left, right, and then primary position to produce movement of cells and to facilitate their recognition.

Appendix 10

Making Fortified Topical Antibiotics

Fortified Tobramycin (or Gentamicin)

With a syringe, inject 2 ml tobramycin 40 mg/ml directly into a 5 ml bottle of tobramycin 0.3% ophthalmic solution (e.g., Tobrex). This gives a 7 ml solution of fortified tobramycin (approximately 15 mg/ml). These drops need to be kept in the refrigerator. They expire in 7 days.

Fortified Cefazolin

Add enough sterile water (without preservative) to 500 mg of cefazolin dry powder to form 10 ml of solution. This provides a strength of 50 mg/ml. Refrigerate. Expires after 4 days.

Fortified Bacitracin

Add enough sterile water (without preservative) to 50,000 units bacitracin dry powder to produce a 5 ml solution. This yields a 10,000 unit/ml solution. Refrigerate. Expires after 7 days.

Appendix 11

Tetanus Prophylaxis

History of Tetanus Immunization (doses)	Clean Minor Wounds		All Other Wounds	
	Tetanus Toxoid	Immune Globulin	Tetanus Toxoid	Immune Globulin
Uncertain	Yes	No	Yes	Yes
0-1	Yes	No	Yes	Yes
2	Yes	No	Yes	No*
3 or more	No†	No	No‡	No

Dose of tetanus toxoid is 0.5 cc im.

*Unless wound is more than 24 hours old
†Unless more than 10 years since last dose
‡Unless more than 5 years since last dose

Source: From U.S. Public Health Service, Advisory Committee on Immunization Practices. Morbidity and Mortality Weekly Report, Supplement. vol. 21, no. 25, June 24, 1972. Atlanta, Centers for Disease Control.

Drug Glossary
Contraindications and Side Effects

Listed below are drugs commonly used in ophthalmology along with some contraindications and side effects which assume clinical importance. Most of these drugs should not be used in pregnant or breast-feeding women, infants, in those with significant renal or hepatic disease, or when an allergy to the drug is suspected or known (therefore these contraindications are not listed separately for each drug, and should be investigated further if therapy is desired under one of these circumstances).

Acetazolamide (e.g., Diamox) Contraindicated with sulfa allergy, metabolic acidosis, adrenal insufficiency, and a history of kidney stones (a relative contraindication). Be careful in patients using another diuretic, a systemic steroid, or digoxin since the potassium level may be lowered to a dangerous level. Side effects: Blood dyscrasias, kidney stones, others.

Aminocaproic acid (e.g., Amicar) Contraindicated with an intravascular clotting disorder. Side effects: Hypotension (particularly postural), nausea, vomiting, others.

Atropine (topical) Contraindicated in most angle-closure situations, infants, albinos, and Down's syndrome patients. Use cautiously in pediatric patients as the margin for toxicity is low. Side effects: Urinary retention, tachycardia, delirium, others. *Treatment of anticholinergic (e.g., atropine) overdose* Physostigmine 1-4 mg iv, repeating 0.5-1.0 mg iv q 15 minutes until the symptoms improve.

Carbachol (topical) See **Pilocarpine**.

Carbogen (95% O_2, 5% CO_2) Contraindicated in patients with pulmonary disease or an electrolyte disorder.

Clindamycin Side effects: Pseudomembranous colitis, others.

Cocaine (topical) Contraindicated with compromised cardiovascular or cerebrovascular status.

Cyclopentolate (topical)   See **Atropine**.
Dipivefrin (e.g., Propine) (topical)   See **Epinephrine**.
Echothiophate iodide (e.g., Phospholine iodide) (topical)   See **Pilocarpine**. Patients (or parents) are told that succinylcholine should never be given for general anesthesia (the combination of the two drugs can be lethal).
   Treatment of anticholinesterase overdose   Atropine 2 mg iv q 5 minutes until relief of symptoms or pralidoxime 25 mg/kg iv in 500 ml of 5% D5W over 2 hours (do *not* use in overdose of neostigmine and physostigmine).
Epinephrine (topical)   Contraindicated with severe cardiovascular disease. Side effects: Macular edema in aphakic patients, conjunctival reaction, precipitation of narrow-angle glaucoma, others. Allergic conjunctivitis is common.
Fluorometholone (topical)   See **Prednisolone acetate**.
Gentamicin   Side effects: Nephrotoxicity, ototoxicity, neuromuscular blockade (myasthenialike syndrome), others.
Homatropine (topical)   See **Atropine**.
Isosorbide   See **Mannitol**.
Ketoconazole   Side effects: Hepatotoxicity (patients are told to return immediately if anorexia, nausea and vomiting, dark urine, pale stools, or jaundice is noted), others.
Levobunolol (e.g., Betagan) (topical)   See **Timolol**.
Mannitol   Contraindicated with hypotension, cardiovascular compromise, or concomitant administration of another osmotic agent. Side effects: Congestive heart failure, subarachnoid or subdural hemorrhage, mental confusion, others.
Methazolamide (e.g., Neptazane)   See **Acetazolamide**.
Neomycin (topical)   Side effects: Superficial punctate keratitis and allergic conjunctivitis are common.
Phenylephrine (e.g., Neosynephrine) (topical)   Contraindicated with significant cardiac disease, sympathetic denervation (i.e., those on MAO inhibitors and diabetics with neuropathy), most angle-closure glaucomas, and in the presence of occludable anterior-chamber angles.
Pilocarpine (topical)   Side effects: Exacerbates iritis, can precipitate or exacerbate angle-closure glaucoma when used in high concentrations (usually 4-6% or greater), retinal detachment (especially high concentrations or other strong miotic agents such as echothiophate), brow ache, others.
Prednisolone acetate (topical)   Often contraindicated with herpes simplex or fungal keratitis. Side effects: Increased intraocular pressure, cataract, increased susceptibility to infectious organisms, others.
Prednisone   See Appendix 5 for contraindications and a work-up to be implemented to establish the safety of systemic treatment. Side effects: Hyperglycemia, hypokalemia, hypertension, peptic ulcer, increased intraocular pressure, cataract, pseudotumor cerebri, mental status changes, aseptic necrosis of bone, osteoporosis, decreased wound healing, growth suppression in children, fluid retention, others.
Proparacaine (topical)   Side effects: Corneal epithelial erosions with repeated and prolonged use.
Scopolamine (topical)   See **Atropine**.
Sulfacetamide (topical)   Side effects: Stevens-Johnson syndrome, bone marrow suppression, others.
Sulfadiazine   See **Sulfacetamide**.

Tetracycline   Contraindicated in children less than 8 years of age (tooth discoloration). Side effects: Gastrointestinal upset, pseudotumor cerebri, hepatotoxicity, skin sensitivity to sunlight (patients are told upon starting the drug to avoid sunlight if possible), others.

Timolol (e.g., Timoptic) (topical)   Contraindicated with asthma or other breathing problems, bradycardia (the patient's pulse is checked before administering a beta-blocker), arrhythmias, congestive heart failure, hypotension, others.

Tobramycin   See **Gentamicin**.

Tropicamide (topical)   See **Atropine**.

Vancomycin   Side effects: Nephrotoxicity, ototoxicity, others.

General Glossary

Accommodation   an increase in the refractive power of the natural lens of the eye; it is generally employed while doing near work, e.g., reading

Amaurosis fugax   monocular blurring of vision developing completely by 30 seconds and lasting from 10 minutes to 2 hours. It may be associated with visible emboli in the retinal vessels.

Amblyopia   a unilateral or bilateral reduction of best-corrected central visual acuity in the absence of a visible organic lesion corresponding to the degree of visual loss

Anisocoria   a difference in size between the two pupils

Anisometropia   a difference in refractive error between the two eyes (e.g., one eye may be farsighted and one nearsighted, one eye may be relatively normal and the other very nearsighted, etc.)

Anterior chamber   the space in the eye bordered anteriorly by the cornea and posteriorly by the iris and the pupil

Applanation tonometer   an instrument which measures intraocular pressure

Astigmatism   the refracting power of the eye is not the same in all meridians (e.g., more hyperopic vertically than horizontally)

Bulbar conjunctiva   a freely movable tissue which forms the most superficial covering of the globe from the limbus to the fornices

Buphthalmos   distention of the globe in response to elevated intraocular pressure; seen in congenital glaucoma

Chemosis   edema of the conjunctiva

Coloboma   congenital absence of any eye structure

Conjunctivitis   inflammation of the conjunctiva

Cotton wool spot   a superficial retinal infarction appearing as a fluffy white lesion, sometimes obscuring retinal vessels

Crowding phenomenon   individual letters can be read better than a whole line; most commonly seen in amblyopic patients

439

Cycloplegic   anything which causes paralysis of the ciliary muscle and therefore paralysis of accommodation

Descemet's membrane   an inner (posterior) corneal layer

Diplopia   double vision

Ectopia lentis   dislocated lens

Ectropion iridis (ectropion uveae)   eversion of the iris at the pupillary rim such that the pigmented posterior aspect of the iris is visualized

Enophthalmos   a measurable depression of the globe within the bony orbit

Enucleation   removal of the eye

Episcleritis   inflammation of the external surface of the sclera (beneath the bulbar conjunctiva)

Esophoria   the eyes are aligned during binocular vision, but have a latent tendency to cross (e.g., while not focusing)

Esotropia   ocular misalignment in which the nonfixating eye is turned inward ("cross-eyed")

Exenteration   removal of the eye and orbital contents

Exophoria   the eyes are aligned during binocular vision, but have a latent tendency to turn out away from one another

Exophthalmos   a measurable protrusion of the globe from the bony orbit

Exotropia   ocular misalignment in which the nonfixating eye is turned outward ("wall-eyed")

Flare   increased protein in the anterior-chamber fluid, permitting visualization of the slit-lamp beam

Floaters   visual perception of dots or spots which may seem to "swim" or shift location when the position of gaze is shifted

Fluorescein angiography   a diagnostic test utilizing intravenously injected fluorescein to highlight vascular abnormalities in the eye, most commonly in the fundus

Fovea   an area of the retina corresponding to central vision, approximately 1.5 mm in diameter, located temporal and slightly inferior to the center of the optic disc

Foveola   the center of the fovea, 0.5 mm in diameter

Ghost vessels   corneal stromal blood vessels containing no blood

Gonioscopy   examination of the anterior-chamber angle structures of the eye, including the trabecular meshwork

Guttata (corneal)   dropletlike excresences on the posterior surface of Decemet's membrane

Hard exudates   deep retinal lipid, often glistening-yellow in appearance

Heterochromia   a difference in coloration, especially between the two irides in a given patient

Hyperopia (farsightedness)   a condition in which the eye is too short or the refractive power too weak to bring objects at distance or near into clear focus (without the use of accommodation)

Hyphema   blood in the anterior chamber; when layering or clotting of the blood is present, the term *hyphema* is used; when only suspended red blood cells are present, the term *microhyphema* is employed

Hypopyon   layering of white blood cells inferiorly in the anterior chamber

Hypotony   abnormally low intraocular pressure, usually below 6 mm Hg

Indirect ophthalmoscopy   the use of a relatively large lens located between the patient and the observer, in combination with a light source, to view the fundus

Intraretinal microvascular abnormalities (IRMA)   dilated, often telangiectatic, retinal capillaries that act as shunts between arterioles and venules

Iritis (anterior uveitis, iridocyclitis, cyclitis)   inflammation of the iris or ciliary body or both

Keratic precipitates   cellular aggregates that form on the corneal endothelium, often inferiorly in a base-down triangular pattern

Krukenberg spindle   a narrow, vertically oriented band of pigment, located along the central corneal endothelium

Leukocoria   a grossly visible white pupil

Macula   an area 3-4 disc diameters in size centered at the posterior part of the retina

Meibomianitis   inflamed, inspissated oil glands along the eyelid margins, reflecting . inflammation of the meibomian glands

Microphthalmia   a congenitally small, disorganized eye

Miosis   constriction of the pupil

Mydriasis   dilatation of the pupil

Myopia (nearsightedness)   a condition in which the eye is too long or the refractive power too great to bring objects at a distance clearly into focus

Nanophthalmos   a congenitally small but otherwise normal eye

Neovascularization   growth of abnormal new blood vessels

Nystagmus   rhythmic oscillations or tremors of the eyes that occur independently of normal movements

Ophthalmoplegia   paralysis of the extraocular muscles

Optic neuritis   inflammation of the optic nerve

Ora serrata   the most peripheral portion of the retina

Oscillopsia   the perception that the environment is moving back and forth

Palpebral conjunctiva   the most superficial covering of the underside of the eyelids from the fornices to the eyelid margins

Papilledema   optic-disc swelling produced by increased intracranial pressure

Peripapillary   surrounding the optic disc

Peripheral anterior synechiae   adhesions between the peripheral iris and anterior-chamber angle or peripheral cornea

Peripheral iridectomy   removal of a portion of the peripheral iris

Phoria   the eyes remain well aligned under conditions of normal binocular vision but have a latent tendency to become misaligned (e.g., when not focusing)

Photophobia   ocular pain on exposure to light

Photopsia   a sensation of instantaneous flashes of light; most commonly indicative of retinal traction

Polycoria   presence of many openings in the iris

Posterior synechiae   adhesions between the iris and the anterior lens capsule, most commonly at the pupillary border

Proptosis   protrusion of the globe from the bony orbit

Pseudohypopon   a layered collection of noninflammatory cells in the anterior chamber, usually associated with neoplastic conditions

Ptosis (blepharoptosis)   drooping of the upper eyelid

Punctum   the opening of the tear drainage system in the eyelid margin

Pupillary block   when aqueous humor is prevented from flowing from the posterior chamber into the anterior chamber between the iris and lens

Radial keratotomy   a surgical technique in which radial incisions are made into the superficial cornea in an effort to change the corneal topography and therefore the patient's refractive error

Relative afferent pupillary defect (RAPD)   a decreased pupillary constriction to light in one eye as compared to the other eye using the swinging flashlight test

Retinitis   inflammation of the retina

Retinoscopy   a technique by which the reflex from a streak of light shined on the retina is used to estimate the refractive error of the eye

Rhegmatogenous retinal detachment   detachment of the retina due to a retinal break (hole)

Scleral depression   a technique by which indentation of the peripheral retina is combined with indirect ophthalmoscopy in order to view the peripheral retina

Scleritis   inflammation of the sclera

Scotoma   an area of loss of sensitivity in the visual field

Staphyloma   an outpouching of the sclera which involves the uvea

Strabismus   ocular misalignment

Tarsorrhaphy   a surgical technique by which the margins of the upper and lower eyelids of an eye are joined together, either partially or completely

Trabeculectomy   a surgical technique used for glaucoma to improve aqueous outflow

Tropia   ocular misalignment

Vitritis   inflammation of the vitreous

Bibliography

AMERICAN ACADEMY OF OPHTHALMOLOGY. Basic and clinical science course. Volumes 1-11, 1988-1989. San Francisco: American Academy of Ophthalmology, 1988.

BENSON WE. Retinal detachment: diagnosis and management. 2nd ed. Philadelphia: JB Lippincott, 1988.

BENSON WE, BROWN GC, TASMAN W, eds. Diabetes and its ocular complications. Philadelphia: WB Saunders, 1988.

BURDE RM, SAVINO PJ, TROBE JD, eds. Clinical decisions in neuro-ophthalmology. St. Louis: CV Mosby, 1985.

COHEN E. Contact lenses and external disease. *Int Ophthalmol Clin* 26:1, 1988.

DEUTSCH TA, FELLER DB, eds. Paton and Goldberg's management of ocular injuries. 2nd ed. Philadelphia: WB Saunders, 1985.

DUANE TD, JAEGER EA, eds. Clinical Ophthalmology., Rev. ed. Philadelphia: Harper & Row, 1987.

GASS, JDM. Stereoscopic atlas of macular diseases: diagnosis and treatment. 3rd ed. St. Louis: CV Mosby, 1987.

KANSKI, JJ. Uveitis: A colour manual of diagnosis and treatment. London: Butterworths, 1987.

KAUFMAN HE, BARRON BA, McDONALD MB, WALTMAN SST, eds. The Cornea. New York: Churchill Livingstone, 1988.

ROY FH. Ocular differential diagnosis. 4th ed. Philadelphia: Lea & Febiger, 1989.

SHIELDS JA. Diagnosis and management of intraocular tumors. St. Louis: CV Mosby, 1983.

SHIELDS JA. Diagnosis and management of orbital tumors. Philadelphia: WB Saunders, 1989.

SHIELDS MB. Textbook of glaucoma. 2nd ed. Baltimore: Williams & Wilkins, 1987.

SMOLIN G, THOFT RA, eds. The Cornea: scientific foundations and clinical practice. Boston: Little, Brown, 1987.

SPOOR TC, NESI GA, eds. Management of ocular, orbital and adnexal trauma. New York: Raven Press, 1988.

WALSH TJ. Neuro-ophthalmology: clinical signs and symptoms. Philadelphia: Lea & Febiger, 1985.

Index

Figures are indicated by f after the page number; tables are indicated by t after the page number. Page numbers in bold indicate a major discussion.

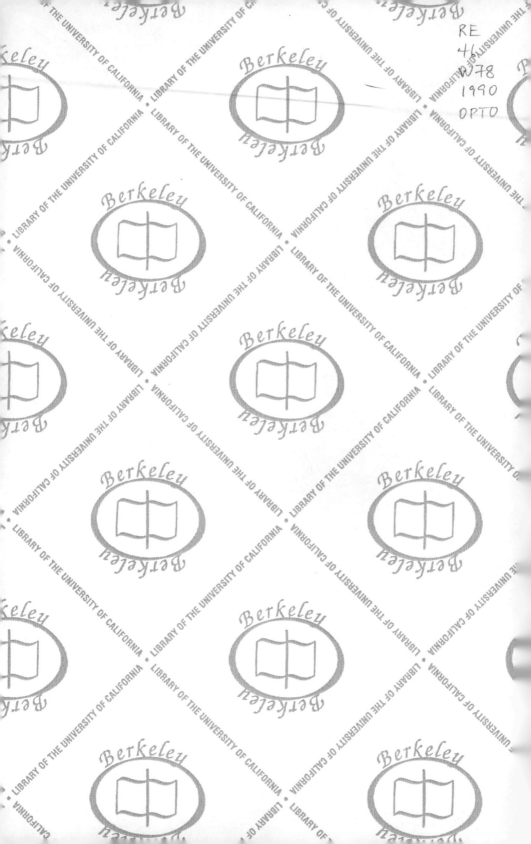